Modern
Hospital
Psychiatry

A NORTON PROFESSIONAL BOOK

Modern Hospital Psychiatry

John R. Lion, MD
Wolfe N. Adler, MD
William L. Webb, Jr, MD

Editors

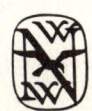

W. W. Norton & Company • New York • London

Copyright © 1988 by John R. Lion, Wolfe N. Adler, William L. Webb, Jr.

All rights reserved.

Published simultaneously in Canada by Penguin Books Canada Ltd., 2801 John Street, Markham, Ontario L3R 1B4.

Printed in the United States of America.

First Edition

Library of Contress Cataloging-in-Publication Data

Modern hospital psychiatry.

"A Norton professional book."
1. Psychiatric hospital care. I. Lion, John R.,
1938-   . II. Adler, Wolfe N. III. Webb,
William L., 1930-   . [DNLM: 1. Hospitals,
Psychiatric. 2. Mental Disorders—therapy.
WM 400 M691]
RC439.M73   1988   362.2′1   87-23979

ISBN 0-393-70048-8

W. W. Norton & Company, Inc., 500 Fifth Avenue, New York, N.Y. 10110

W. W. Norton & Company Ltd., 37 Great Russell Street, London WC1B 3NU

1 2 3 4 5 6 7 8 9 0

Preface

This volume stems from our desire to clarify the experience of psychiatric hospitalization. For the average patient and family—and the outside clinician as well—the inpatient experience appears mysterious and indeterminate. A psychiatric milieu is foreign in comparison with the traditional medical ward, and psychosocial interventions within the hospital itself often seem without clear rationale. It is our attempt to describe the various aspects of inpatient care, from admission to discharge, and to comment upon various types of hospitals and the role of staff within these institutions.

We have emphasized readability to our authors, and asked them to make their chapters clinically relevant. This volume is for the mental health worker, but we also envisioned it for nonpsychiatrist professional, whether clinician or administrator. Case examples are utilized as a means of conveying to the reader the diagnostic and therapeutic complexities involved with inpatient work.

Our volume also reaffirms our belief in the psychiatric facility at a time when society reevaluates the problems of deinstitutionalization. We trust the chapters within this text draw attention to the care that goes on within a hospital.

John R. Lion, M.D.
Wolfe N. Adler, M.D.
William L. Webb, Jr., M.D.

Baltimore and Hartford, 1987

Contents

Preface v
Contributors xi

SECTION I: The Institution *1*

1. The Private Psychiatric Hospital 3
    William L. Webb, Jr.

2. The Public Mental Hospital 22
    *James T. Barter and
    Patricia A. Marshall*

3. The Psychiatric Unit in the General Hospital 39
    Manoel W. Penna

4. The Forensic Hospital 48
    *Stuart B. Silver and
    Jose A. Gelpi*

SECTION II: The Admissions Process *71*

5. The Psychiatric Emergency Room 73
    *Andrew Edmund Slaby and
    Mary Eileen McNamara*

6. The Admissions Process 88
    Barry Rudnick

SECTION III: Hospitalization — 97

7. The Diagnostic Process — 99
   *Bruce Leopold and
   John R. Lion*

8. Milieu Therapy — 109
   Wolfe N. Adler

9. Inpatient Psychotherapy — 129
   *Melvin Prosen and
   Donald Ross*

10. Inpatient Cognitive Behavior Therapy — 136
    James McGee

11. The Use of Medication in a Hospital Setting — 169
    *John R. Lion and
    Joe P. Tupin*

12. Activity Therapy in Hospital Psychiatry — 179
    Diane Gibson

13. The Role of the Psychiatric Nurse — 208
    Ann Marie T. Brooks

14. Inpatient Psychiatric Research Units — 228
    John J. Boronow

15. Regulation, Insurance, and the Medical Record — 251
    *Robert W. Gibson and
    Lynn Flanigan*

16. Forensic Issues — 271
    Jonas R. Rappeport

17. Violence and Suicide within the Hospital — 291
    John R. Lion

18. Treatment Considerations for Children and Adolescents — 300
    *Donald H. Saidel and
    Richard M. Sarles*

19. Inpatient Treatment Considerations of the Elderly — 322
    *Barry W. Rovner and
    Marshal F. Folstein*

20. The Medically Ill Patient — 334
    *Michael Edelstein and
    Peter Hartmann*

21. The Inpatient Care of the Chronic Mentally Ill 352
    John A. Talbott and
    Ira D. Glick

SECTION IV: Discharge *371*

22. Discharge Planning 373
    Charles P. Peters and
    Faith B. Dickerson

23. Following Hospitalization: Residential Aftercare 384
    Richard D. Budson

Index 403

Contributors

Wolfe N. Adler, M.D.
Director, Division of General Adult Inpatient Programs,
Sheppard and Enoch Pratt Hospital,
Towson, Maryland

James T. Barter, M.D.
Professor of Psychiatry,
Abraham Lincoln School of Medicine,
University of Illinois at Chicago;
Director,
Illinois State Psychiatric Institute

John J. Boronow, M.D.
Chief of Service, Chronic Schizophrenia Rehabilitation Unit,
Sheppard and Enoch Pratt Hospital,
Towson, Maryland

Ann Marie Brooks, R.N., D.N. Sc., M.B.A.
Director, Department of Nursing,
Sheppard and Enoch Pratt Hospital,
Towson, Maryland

Richard D. Budson, M.D.
Service Chief and Director,
Community Residential and Treatment Services,
McLean Hospital,
Belmont, Massachusetts;
Associate Professor of Psychiatry,
Department of Psychiatry,
Harvard Medical School

Faith Dickerson, Ph.D.
Assistant Chief of Service, Chronic Schizophrenia Rehabilitation Unit,
Sheppard and Enoch Pratt Hospital,
Towson, Maryland

Michael Edelstein, M.D.
Staff Psychiatrist,
Sheppard and Enoch Pratt Hospital;
Clinical Assistant Professor of Family Medicine,
University of Maryland School of Medicine,
Baltimore, Maryland

Lynn Flanigan, R.N., M.S.W.
Quality Assurance Administrator,
Sheppard and Enoch Pratt Hospital,
Towson, Maryland

Marshal Folstein, M.D.
Professor of Psychiatry,
Department of Psychiatry and
 Behavioral Sciences,
Johns Hopkins Hospital
 School of Medicine,
Baltimore, Maryland

Jose A. Gelpi, M.D.
Clinical Director,
Clifton T. Perkins Hospital Center,
Jessup, Maryland;
Assistant Clinical Professor,
University of Maryland School of
 Medicine,
Baltimore, Maryland

Diane Gibson, M.S., O.T.R.
Director, Activity Therapy Department,
Sheppard and Enoch Pratt Hospital,
Towson, Maryland

Robert W. Gibson, M.D.
President and Chief Executive
 Officer,
Sheppard and Enoch Pratt Hospital,
Towson, Maryland;
Training and Supervisory Analyst,
Washington Psychoanalytic Institute

Ira D. Glick, M.D.
Professor of Psychiatry,
Cornell University Medical College,
The Payne Whitney Psychiatric
 Clinic,
The New York Hospital

Peter Hartmann, M.D.
Medical School Associate Professor
 of Family Medicine,
Assistant Professor of Psychiatry,
University of Maryland School of
 Medicine,
Baltimore, Maryland

Bruce C. Leopold, M.D.
Chief of Service, Short-Term
 Evaluation Unit,
Sheppard and Enoch Pratt Hospital,
Towson, Maryland

John R. Lion, M.D.
Clinical Professor of Psychiatry,
University of Maryland School of
 Medicine,
Baltimore, Maryland;
Consultant Psychiatrist,
Sheppard and Enoch Pratt Hospital

James McGee, Ph.D.
Director, Department of Psychology,
Sheppard and Enoch Pratt Hospital,
Towson, Maryland

Mary Eileen McNamara, M.D.
Assistant Professor of Psychiatry
 and Human Behavior,
Brown University,
Providence, Rhode Island

Patricia A. Marshall, Ph.D.
Director, Child Life Program and
 Family Education
Wyler Children's Hospital,
University of Chicago,
Chicago, Illinois

Manoel W. Penna, M.D.
Clinical Associate Professor of
 Psychiatry,
University of Maryland School of
 Medicine,
Baltimore, Maryland

Contributors

Charles Peters, M.D.
Chief of Service, Personality Disorder Program,
Sheppard and Enoch Pratt Hospital,
Towson, Maryland

Melvin Prosen, M.D.
Chief of Service, Intermediate Treatment Service,
Sheppard and Enoch Pratt Hospital,
Towson, Maryland;
Instructor in Psychiatry,
Johns Hopkins University School of Medicine

Jonas Rappeport, M.D.
Chief Medical Officer,
Circuit Court of Baltimore,
Baltimore, Maryland;
Clinical Professor of Psychiatry,
University of Maryland School of Medicine

Donald Ross, M.D.
Director, Residency Training,
Sheppard and Enoch Pratt Hospital,
Towson, Maryland;
Clinical Assistant Professor of Psychiatry,
University of Maryland School of Medicine

Barry Rovner, M.D.
Assistant Professor of Psychiatry,
Department of Psychiatry and Behavioral Sciences,
Johns Hopkins University School of Medicine,
Baltimore, Maryland

Barry Rudnick, M.D.
Admissions Officer,
Sheppard and Enoch Pratt Hospital,
Towson, Maryland

Donald Saidel, Ph.D.
Manager, Child and Adolescent Inpatient Programs,
Sheppard and Enoch Pratt Hospital,
Towson, Maryland;
Clinical Assistant Professor of Psychiatry,
University of Maryland School of Medicine

Richard Sarles, M.D.
Director, Child and Adolescent Psychiatric Services,
Sheppard and Enoch Pratt Hospital,
Towson, Maryland;
Clinical Professor of Psychiatry and Pediatrics,
University of Maryland School of Medicine

Stuart B. Silver, M.D.
Superintendent,
Clifton T. Perkins Hospital Center
Jessup, Maryland;
Assistant Clinical Professor of Psychiatry,
University of Maryland School of Medicine

Andrew Edmund Slaby, M.D., Ph.D., M.P.H.
Medical Director,
Fair Oaks Hospital,
Summit, New Jersey;
Adjunct Professor of Psychiatry and Human Behavior,
Brown University,
Providence, Rhode Island

John Talbott, M.D.
Professor and Chairman,
Department of Psychiatry,
University of Maryland School of
    Medicine,
Baltimore, Maryland

Joe P. Tupin, M.D.
Professor of Psychiatry,
University of California — Davis
    Medical Center,
Sacramento, California

William L. Webb, Jr., M.D.
Psychiatrist-In-Chief,
The Institute of Living,
Hartford, Connecticut;
Clinical Professor of Psychiatry,
University of Connecticut School of
    Medicine,
Farmington, Connecticut

The Institution

I

The Private Psychiatric Hospital

William L. Webb, Jr.

A HISTORICAL PERSPECTIVE

The traditions of the modern private psychiatric hospital began in the early part of the 19th century with the introduction of the concept of moral treatment. Prior to that time the mentally ill were regarded as beasts and, therefore, insensitive to their surroundings. They were subject to a variety of abusive treatments designed to drive out the toxic influences thought to be responsible for the animal-like behavior. Emanating from the influence of Pinel in France, and the Tuke family in England, moral treatment took an entirely different approach.

Operating from a humanistic and religious position, the treatment emphasized kindness and the conception that the mentally ill continued to have internal resources that, if encouraged, would restore them to mental health. The attendants were encouraged to treat the patients with patience and dignity. The institutions were generally small and under the careful direction of a physician with the title of superintendent. The superintendent and his family most often lived on the grounds and interacted daily with the patients. Every effort was made to involve the patients in the normal process of daily living appropriate to that time. Patients were invited to tea with the superintendent and they frequently shared meals. The hospitals were carefully designed to provide a healthy and esthetically pleasing environment. Great care was taken in landscaping the grounds to provide a sense of refuge and asylum. Patients were encouraged to engage in some kind of work, usually on a farm, and restraints for violence discouraged.[1]

Throughout the 19th century, seven private hospitals exerted significant influence on the course and development of the practice of hospital psychiatry. These include the Pennsylvania Hospital, the first hospital to set aside psychiatric beds, established in 1752 in Philadelphia, and the McLean Hospital in Belmont, Massachusetts. Established expressly in the moral treatment tradition were the Hartford Retreat in Hartford, Connecticut, the Bloomingdale Asylum (New York Hospital) in White Plains, New York, Friends Hospital in Philadelphia, and the Butler Hospital in Providence, Rhode Island.

Initially some of these hospitals provided care for the indigent patient, as well as for those able to pay. However, the care of the indigent increasingly shifted to the state supported hospitals that were rapidly developing toward the end of the 19th century. The private hospitals to the present are almost exclusively reserved for those patients who are able to pay. Grob points out that despite considerable popularity in their local region, they were generally too small to become "the forerunners of a large geographically dispersed system of institutions capable of caring for a considerable proportion of the nation's mentally ill."[2]

Despite this rather narrow focus, the superintendents of these private hospitals exerted enormous influence on the professional development of psychiatry as a specialty. The American Psychiatric Association was initially organized by the 13 superintendents of prominent psychiatric hospitals, most of which were private. Thomas Kirkbride, the superintendent of the Pennsylvania Hospital, published a book on the organization and construction of "hospitals for the insane" in 1854 that exerted influence throughout most of the 19th century. Isaac Ray, superintendent of Butler Hospital, wrote the first classical treatise on forensic psychiatry. Amariah Brigham, superintendent of the Hartford Retreat, started the *American Journal of Insanity*, later to become the *American Journal of Psychiatry*.

During the first half of the 20th century, the major sites of treatment for the severely mentally ill were the private psychiatric hospitals and the state hospital systems. The private system consisted of many small hospitals, usually owned and directed by a single physician with one or two attending staff. The Sheppard and Enoch Pratt Hospital admitted its first patient in 1891 and assumed its position along with the northeastern hospitals as a national referral source for the smaller hospitals and small number of practicing psychiatrists.[3] A notable development was the expansion of a small proprietary hospital in Topeka, Kansas, into the Menninger Foundation. Founded in 1921 by the two brothers, Karl and William, Menninger established an international reputation by developing the first comprehensive treatment program based on psychoanalytic principles.

Chestnut Lodge in Rockville, Maryland, became a center for an intensive psychoanalytic psychotherapeutic treatment approach to the treatment of schizophrenia. Frieda Fromm-Reichmann at Chestnut Lodge and Harry Stack Sullivan at Sheppard Pratt utilized the full resources of the hospital environment to treat schizophrenia psychotherapeutically. Sullivan established one of the first specialized treatment programs in a private psychiatric hospital. His program for the treatment of the young schizophrenic adult required a special unit and trained staff and offered a continuous therapeutic environment.

Most of the large psychiatric hospitals enjoyed an international clientele. Patients came and remained for long periods of time. Characteristic of many of these hospital campuses were private dwellings where wealthy patients and their private attendants resided for life.

The Hartford Retreat provides a good example of the innovative way in which a private hospital coped with the attitudes toward mental illness and fashioned a treatment program responsive to the cultural and emotional needs of the American public during the 1930s and 1940s, following the Great Depression. The Retreat, until that time, had continued in its tradition of moral treatment, offering, as they came available, whatever treatments were available. The Depression had worked a significant hardship on the institution. In 1931, Dr. C. Charles Burlingame became psychiatrist-in-chief. Dr. Burlingame was by nature energetic and innovative. He changed the name of the Retreat to The Institute of Living. He referred to the patients as guests and publicized The Institute as "a combination of hospital, university and country club."[4] He improved the appearance of the campus to look like an English Tudor village and completed it with a five-hole golf course. Guests were encouraged to attend a number of self-improvement courses, including cooking, sewing, woodworking, leather craft and metal craft. Guests were also treated to Sunday afternoon rides in a fleet of black limousines.

At the same time, Burlingame significantly improved the quality of the medical staff and placed a premium on whatever new therapeutic modality that was available for the treatment of the mentally ill. He encouraged research and, at one time, the Institute supported a neurochemistry laboratory and a primate colony. The result was instant success. The Institute developed a national and international reputation as a private psychiatric hospital for the famous and affluent. Extraordinary means were taken to protect the identity and confidentiality of the guests.

Following the second World War, a strong interest developed in the therapeutic effects of group process in a structured setting. Main and Jones described their experience with the "therapeutic community."[5,6] Faced with the treatment of veterans who displayed serious characterological and adjustment problems in the post war era, they devised a system of care that maximized patient participation in their treatment through group process (community meetings and self-help groups) and deemphasized the traditional authoritative hierarchy of staff and patient relationships. Everyone dressed in civilian dress and addressed each other by first name. Decisions were made by democratic process and ostensibly everyone had more or less equal vote. Although this mode of intervention has not proven effective with more seriously disturbed patient populations, its influence was pervasive and traveled under the name of milieu therapy. Nearly all private hospital settings employ some form of community meeting, organized groups and directed activities programs. Emphasis on the milieu has been a valuable addition because it focuses the staff's attention on the importance of daily ward interactions in the therapeutic process, allows patients a mode of expression and encourages the participation of the entire staff in decision-making. However, carried to an extreme it can diffuse the implementation of a treatment plan and produce unnecessary interstaff rivalry and dissension.

During the last 20 years enormous changes have taken place in the character and quality of private psychiatric hospitals. The community mental health movement, beginning in the 1960s, and the appearance of psychiatric units in general hospitals were major influences. Both of these developments placed a premium on a shortened length of hospital stay. This was accompanied by significant advances in psychopharmacology. Neuroleptics were effective in bringing the acute symptomatology of the major psychoses under fairly rapid control and many chronically mentally ill heretofore confined to hospitals were able to be discharged and followed in the community.

There developed among many community psychiatry advocates a deep antihospital bias. The community mental health movement, through the process of deinstitutionalization, reduced the resident patient populations in state hospitals by 75% or approximately 420,000 occupied beds by 1980. Those elderly psychotics not able to be discharged were transferred to nursing homes. Whether the disposition was the community or nursing home, the treatment resources were woefully inadequate. Community services were either totally unavailable or so fragmented as to constitute a nonsystem.

In recent years a new, young, chronic patient population has emerged. Usually diagnosed schizophrenic or character disorder with substance abuse, these patients are heavy utilizers of psychiatric services. Many are recidivists and revolve in and out of private and public inpatient facilities.

Insurance coverage has become available to a wider segment of the population in the last 20 years. Although there have been increasing limitations on all types of coverage, of the 141,209 admissions to private psychiatric facilities in 1980, 96.9% were covered by some form of third-party carrier. This has produced a broader patient mix in private hospitals. Once available only to the very wealthy, private hospitals offer services to patients from a variety of social and economic backgrounds.

The 1960s witnessed the entrance of the for-profit, investor-owned hospital chains into the private psychiatric hospital business. They have steadily grown and, according to the membership records of the National Association of Private Psychiatric Hospitals, there are 240 nongovernmental (private), free-standing hospitals operating in the country in 1986. Forty-eight percent are affiliated with for-profit (investor-owned) hospital chains and 32% are independently owned for-profit, and 25% are voluntary (not-for-profit). The chains have enjoyed a number of economic advantages (economy of scale, equity financing, and corporate-wide management services and policy) which have offered them a competitive advantage.

The for-profits have stirred some controversy. Levenson points out, "Some persons believe it is morally wrong for a hospital to be operated as a for-profit enterprise; others believe that for-profit ownership is proper and socially advantageous."[7] Issues of quality and efficiency of management have also been debated. The not-for-profit sector has raised the question of quality of care in for-profit hospitals. Currently no good research has demonstrated that the quality of care provided by the for-profits is inferior to the voluntary hospitals. The for-profits in turn have argued that they are more efficiently managed. A recent study suggests that their profitability has been derived more from aggressive pricing strategies than from more efficient management.[8]

During the last five years, we have witnessed a revolution in the economics of medical delivery. Fueled by skyrocketing health care costs (10.9% of the Gross National Product in 1986), the federal government, the corporate section, and the insurance industry have set in motion a series of initiatives that will exert a major impact on the financial foundation of private psychiatric hospitals. Examples include the prepayment (diagnostic related groupings), discounts (preferred provider organizations), case management (independent physician associations), and capitation (health maintenance organizations).

Although private psychiatric hospitals are exempt from DRGs, they feel increasing pressure to reduce the length of stay, operate in a cost-effective manner, and above all, provide sufficient documentation to support the need for the patient to be in the hospital. Most hospitals experience extended delays in obtaining reimbursement from third-party carriers. At times this can constitute a serious cash flow problem. These cost-savings initiatives often spell additional administrative costs for the hospital to comply. The biggest burden is borne by those hospitals dedicated to the care of the more severely and chronically mentally ill. The weak link in all these systems is chronic illness. Patients with chronic illnesses can easily be squeezed out of all the cost-saving systems. Unfortunately, mental illness is predominantly a chronic illness.

THE DISTINGUISHING FEATURES OF THE PRIVATE PSYCHIATRIC HOSPITAL

What are the distinguishing features of the private psychiatric hospital? This is a difficult question to answer primarily because there is such a wide variation among different private hospitals. As Gralnick points out, "No two hospitals are the same."[9] They run the gamut from a for-profit community psychiatric hospital dedicated to short-term care to a much larger voluntary hospital dedicated to psychoanalytically oriented long-term care. Perhaps the best way to approach their commonality and distinction is to outline some of the issues with which all must cope.

A major philosophical issue common to all private, free-standing, psychiatric hospitals is the dual responsibility to two conflicting ethics — a humanistic concern for patients and the economic pressures of the free market. By their tradition they are dedicated to the humanistic concern for the individual patient, but they must be equally responsive to economic forces. This is not a new dilemma. It has been with the private hospitals since their beginnings. It is significant that one of the major sources of interstaff conflict cited in the classic study of Chestnut Lodge by Stanton and Schwartz was derived from the budget.[10] Financial issues exercise a very significant influence in a private facility because economic resources are the lifeblood of an institution. The private hospital, voluntary or for-profit, is buffeted by free market forces. Whereas the chronic underfunding of state facilities produces a state of apathy and low morale, the constant uncertainty of revenues in a private institution can be a serious source of anxiety and frustration for the staff and administration. Frequently there is a major split in communication between the clinical and administrative staff around the issue of expenses and revenue.

Secondly, most private psychiatric hospitals must have an explicit or implicit marketing strategy. As economic competition has picked up in recent years this has become much more blatant, but it has always been true. Private facilities place a great premium on reputation. This is commonly fostered by special courtesies to referring doctors and various participations in community education activities.

The need to remain competitive has concentrated a high level of therapeutic expertise in the private hospital sector. The large hospitals are becoming regional referral centers for those cases unresponsive to short-term interventions. Nearly all have developed specialized services that offer special treatments or are designed for a given patient population. These include adolescent services, geriatric services, young adult services, alcohol and substance abuse services, programs for personality disorders, phobia clinics, and comprehensive programs for eating disorders. Many of these programs are continuous and offer the widest variety of interventions available.

Thirdly, in order to survive, private hospitals usually must strive for an acceptable level of therapeutic competence. If they are open staff facilities, they must attempt to attract the best local psychiatrists to the staff. If they are closed with regard to staff, efforts should be made to maintain and sustain the development of staff. Various regulatory bodies act as watchdogs on quality. Accreditation by the Joint Commission on Accreditation of Hospitals is not only a feather in the cap, but also essential for the economic survival of the institution. Responsiveness to regulatory functions is often a double-edged sword. Private psychiatric hospitals are commonly subject to many regulatory agencies. Many of these are designed to insure a standard of quality, but in recent years a new set of regulators have appeared that are primarily concerned with cost containment. These include case management review for third-party payers, State Cost Review Commissions for Hospitals, and Medicare regulations. With these conflicting regulatory agencies, private hospitals frequently are caught in the middle.

The major responsibility for the treatment of the severely mentally ill falls to the state programs and the private psychiatric hospitals. What are some of the major differences between these two treatment resources? Are the differences strictly cosmetic, as some say? There are a number of significant differences. The state hospitals operate in highly charged political environment, often competing unsuccessfully for necessary resources. The private hospitals, through their board of trustee structure, more often have greater community support and a greater opportunity to combat the stigma of mental illness through public education programs. Generally, the private hospitals are more esthetically constructed and located. In the tradition of moral treatment, many are located in bucolic settings that are tastefully landscaped. The somewhat longer length of stay provides an opportunity for convalescence. This is a neglected concept in many systems that stress ultra-short hospital stays and quick returns to the community. Finally, the governance structure of private hospitals and the competitive environment in which they exist stimulate more creative approaches to treatment.

Traditionally, the private hospitals have been the seat of education; in some, major research has taken place. Pottash, Sweeney, Gold and Extein have expressed the opinion, "the system we believe is most likely to ensure both high quality patient care and professional satisfaction is the closed staff system in a private psychiatric hospital." They go on to point out that considerable "clinical research is being done in the private psychiatric system"[11] and that the overhead costs for research in this system are considerably less than in most academic centers. Many private hospitals either participate in affiliated education in a variety of professional disciplines or have their own training programs.

The "free-standing" aspect of the private psychiatric hospitals deserves special mention. It places a special burden of responsibility on the medical and nursing staff to be sensitive to the medical aspects of treatment. Hall, et al., demonstrated that in 100 randomly selected psychiatric patients there was a prevalence of 28% undiagnosed medical illnesses that either contributed to or were the sole cause of the abnormal behavior.[12] Most important are medical emergencies that occur at inopportune times. Many hospitals employ full- or part-time medical consultants, but nothing takes the place of a medical and nursing staff that can manage medical emergencies and a good working relationship with a general hospital emergency service, hopefully not too far away.

The positive side of the private psychiatric hospital's free-standing status is its removal from the hustle and bustle of the general hospital. Psychiatric units in general hospitals are generally space-limited. In other situations psychiatric patients are scattered among medical and surgical patients. For very short stays this is feasible, but for longer stays patients need more living room and an organized activities program to enhance their recovery. For those patients who need a longer stay, the greater privacy and the more tranquil environs of the private psychiatric hospital are important for recovery.

Private psychiatric hospitals continue to be small. Most are under 150 beds. The largest, The Institute of Living in Hartford, has 401 beds. Even the larger hospitals are divided into smaller units, which may have considerable autonomy. The individual patient units usually number between 20 and 30 beds. Staff/patient ratios are usually pretty good. Maxmen et al. provide the following staff/patient ratios rating. By staff they mean "the total number of full-time professional staff, including nurses, social workers, psychiatrists, aides, etc. who work on the unit in a 24-hour period." "Arbitrarily" they consider a staff patient ratio of 1 : 1 very high, 1 : 1 1/2 high, 1 : 1 1/2–3 medium, 1 : 3–10 low medium, and less than 1 : 10 as low. A relatively high staff/patient ratio means that patients have a better chance of having individual attention and an individualized treatment program in a private hospital.

Characteristically private hospitals have a somewhat longer length of stay than general hospital units, but currently the length of stay in most private hospitals seldom exceeds 60 days. A selected few are dedicated to long-term care (length of stay longer than six months), but even these hospitals treat many more short-term patients than in the past. The added length of stay in private hospitals also provides an opportunity for more extensive staff/patient contact, implementation of an individualized treatment plan, and more extensive discharge planning. Most private hospitals have pleasant surroundings, activities programs and recreational opportunities.

THE ORGANIZATIONAL STRUCTURE OF THE PRIVATE HOSPITAL

A number of authors have emphasized the importance of the formal and informal organizational structure in psychiatric hospitals. This is of importance in any human organization, but it seems critically important in a psychiatric hospital because of its impact on the hospital's major goal of creating a total therapeutic environment for the patient. All aspects of the clinical and administrative organization should be dedicated to this mission, and there is ample evidence that organizational problems present a serious obstacle to achieving that goal. The best analogy is a symphony orchestra in which all the component parts are acting synergistically to produce a work of art. Essential in the organizational structure is clearly defined leadership, open communication, clear-cut objectives, job and role definition, and lines of responsibility and accountability. A critical ingredient in a psychiatric hospital is a humanistic, supportive and fair attitude among all staff. The best environment is democratic and participatory but with clear-cut direction and leadership.

The ultimate authority and responsibility in a voluntary hospital are vested in a board of trustees. Trustees vary in their commitment to this responsibility but legally they are accountable for the quality of care rendered in the hospital. In a for-profit hospital this responsibility is assumed by corporate headquarters. Boards and corporations vary somewhat in the degree to which they dictate management decisions, but both often serve the function of approving the decisions of the chief executive and his senior management staff. The relationship with the chief executive is crucial; in major decisions, he cannot act without the support of the board or corporate management.

Through the chief executive officer, the board exerts enormous influence on the planning, priorities and quality of patient care. Although boards generally look for guidance from the senior administrative staff of the hospital, they vary significantly in the scope of their vision and the priorities they are willing to support. The board also exerts an important source of communication and linkage with the community. A strong board with a balanced vision of the future is a major determinant of the success of a private nonprofit hospital.

The key leadership position in the hospital is the chief executive officer.

In most of the older private hospitals, this position is held by a physician, but the majority of the newer hospitals, particularly the for-profits, have an administrator as chief executive. With the increasing financial and managerial complexity of directing a modern health care facility, the chief executive officer certainly needs administrative experience and education. Whatever his background, the chief executive officer exerts a tremendous personal influence on the atmosphere of the hospital and the morale of the staff.

The administrative functions of the hospital usually include finance, human resources (personnel), general services (plant maintenance, laundry, housekeeping, grounds keeper, motor pool), information services, planning, development and marketing. The size and complexity of these departments are determined by the magnitude of the hospital. Whether they represent a few people or several departments, they commonly report to the chief executive officer. Since these functions influence all aspects of daily living in the hospital, it is important that they be integrated with the clinical care of patients. The administrative personnel must have the cooperation of the clinical departments and the medical staff to complete many overlapping responsibilities (preparation of budgets, billing, documentation, hiring and firing). They need to feel supported and appreciated by the clinical staff. In turn, the clinical staff should perceive the administration as sharing their concern with providing quality patient care. In times of diminishing resources, the administration is often accused by the clinical staff of being insensitive to patient needs. Further, the administration comes into direct contact with patients and families at admission, around billing issues, and around patient environment issues. The quality of that interaction bears heavily on the image projected by the institution. The negotiation of the administrative-clinical relationship lies with the chief executive officer and the medical director. The quality of that relationship often is reflected in the morale of the staff.

The clinical administrative leadership resides with the medical director. His influence may be weak or strong, broad or circumscribed, but the quality of clinical care is ultimately a reflection of him (or her). His major arena of negotiation is with the medical staff but he has an equal obligation to guard the interests of the other mental health professionals who report to him. Ideally nursing, social work, psychology and occupational therapy report to him. Any variation whereby a clinical discipline has direct access to the chief executive officer seriously weakens the authority of the medical director. His authority must be protected because he orchestrates the direction and quality of the clinical programs. In a small, open staffed hospital he negotiates this directly with the medical staff and other disciplines, organized as departments, by personal influence and the enunciation of policy. In larger hospitals he might administer through a clinical matrix, whereby several disciplines organize around a program, unit or clinical division and the clinical departmental authority is more circumscribed. Whatever the structure, he must heal the interprofessional and interdepartmental rivalries that are a part of any human enterprise. Further, he must act as an interpreter for the clinical staff to create a bridge of understanding between the clinicians and administrators.

The morale of the medical staff and the working relationship with the medical director are critical elements in the success of a private hospital. The medical staff is both a source of strength and a counterbalance to the authority of the medical director. The medical staff performs a number of important quality assurance functions. Through its committee structure, the medical staff credentials and monitors new additions to the medical staff, oversees the medical record, quality assurance, pharmacy and therapeutics, and most important, sets the standard of clinical practice in the hospital. This is true whether the staff is closed (full-time) or open (partially in private practice). These functions are set forth in the bylaws of the medical staff. Problems occur when there is an imbalance in the power relationship between the staff and director. A director who is too authoritarian may demoralize or lose the support of his staff. One who is too passive may not garner the support he needs to set an appropriate standard of care.

Areas of potential conflict with the medical staff are the medical record and the quality assurance program. Appropriate and timely documentation in the medical record not only is essential in good psychiatric practice but also serves as an indicator of the quality of patient care in the hospital. Adequate documentation has increasingly become important to regulators and peer reviewers in the matters of accreditation and reimbursement. Some staff members are compulsively late with discharge summaries or inadequate in their documentation. Interaction around these matters produces premature greying in medical directors.

The process of quality assurance has taken on increasing importance as a management tool and method of quality control. Required by the Joint Commission on Accreditation of Hospitals, the system taps a number of data sources to assess the quality of clinical care and administrative function throughout the hospital.[14] These are reviewed and ranked by a quality assurance committee. Remedial action is recommended, implemented and documented. Since the quality assurance program cuts across all administrative and clinical activities in the hospital, different groups in the hospital, with their conflicting priorities and special interests, may face different recommendations. Medical staff may bristle at this and other forms of peer review. The medical director's diplomatic skills may be sorely tested in the process of engaging the cooperation and support of all parties for the quality assurance program.

DIAGNOSTIC AND TREATMENT PROCESS IN THE PRIVATE PSYCHIATRIC HOSPITAL

The diagnostic and treatment process begins with the patient's admission to the hospital. Admission data to private psychiatric hospitals reveal that patients are predominantly white (87%), well educated (median education 12th grade), and in their mid-thirties (median age 34); slightly over half are female. The majority has experienced some kind of prior mental health care. Many have received only inpatient care (44.9%), while 21.7% have received both inpatient and outpatient treatment. Most receive the diagnosis of affective disorder and most enter on a voluntary basis. Private practicing psychiatrists are the major referral source and patients stay in the hospital two or three weeks and receive more than one kind of treatment.[15]

These statistics indicate that private psychiatric hospitals by and large treat patients with a relatively good prognosis. Statistics for some of the larger tertiary facilities would be quite different. In 1985 most of the admissions to The Institute of Living had been hospitalized elsewhere, usually in short-term facilities, four or five times previously. Good prognosis or bad, admission to a psychiatric hospital is a double crisis, external and internal. It is a major crisis for the patient, family and referring doctor. Mezzich et al., in a study of 792 patients admitted to hospitals, identified four patient factors in the decision to hospitalize: delusional psychosis, hyperactivity, antisocial behavior, and dangerousness.[16] Such behaviors produce a sense of urgency for all concerned. Admissions create an internal crisis for similar reasons. A new disruptive patient places a burden on the patients and staff in the hospital.

Despite these obvious tensions around admission, the process in a private hospital is generally less adversarial than in a public hospital or general hospital psychiatric unit. Most of the admissions are voluntary; commonly, they are transfers from a short-term facility. The leisurely pace of admissions to private hospitals, associated with waiting lists and extensive pre-admission interviews, is largely a thing of the past.

The diagnostic process begins the minute the patient is admitted. Some hospitals incorporate the initial comprehensive medical and psychiatric evaluation into the admission process. Others have some time limit within which the initial evaluation must be completed and on the chart. As lengths of stay have shortened, there is more pressure to complete the comprehensive evaluation, including complete history, physical, laboratory findings, ward behavior observations, and information from significant others, in a timely manner, usually within 72 hours.

Planning treatment in the modern, private psychiatric facility is a cooperative venture. This is contrasted with a general hospital unit, which usually is organized on a medical model. A therapeutic team is formed in which several disciplines cooperate in the diagnostic process that identifies significant dynamic issues, target behaviors usually symptomatic of the disorder, social skills and vocational deficits, and environmental conflicts with significant others. Treatment objectives should be practical, obtainable and observable. The plan should not dehumanize the patient to a list of treatment objectives but create a flexible, responsive environment sensitive to individual needs and problems. The capacity to maintain a balance between structured direction and flexible human responsiveness is, in the final analysis, what distinguishes a therapeutic environment from a sterile procedural exercise. The somewhat slower pace of the private hospital acts to support this humanistic balance.

The clinical program is usually centered on a 20-to-30-bed unit. Maxmen, Tucker and LeBow[13] noted that the characteristics of the treatment program are significantly influenced by two factors, the length of stay and the primary treatment modality. Those programs with a longer length of stay and a psychotherapeutic orientation place a greater emphasis on the dynamic understanding of the patient and the influence of the ward milieu. Most of these programs have a strong psychoanalytic orientation. The major therapy is individual psychoanalytically oriented therapy provided by a member of the psychiatric or psychological staff. The group therapies and milieu activities are organized to support the patient's increased self-understanding and maturation. Chestnut Lodge is a good example of such a facility. With only 90 beds, the hospital employs a full-time medical staff of 30. Levine and Wilson[17] suggest that the primary function of such a psychiatric holding environment is the delivery of the normative services which the nuclear family customarily provides.

Hospitals with a shorter length of stay have a more generic ward environment and place a greater emphasis on careful medical and psychiatric evaluation, pharmacotherapy and crisis intervention. Whether long-term or short-term, the program and organization of the unit should encourage staff involvement with patients. Too often staff find ways to hide behind paperwork or glass partitions.

All modern psychiatric programs should be orchestrated to provide the psychotherapeutic and medical interventions necessary to move the patient toward a return to the community or the least restrictive environment. Discharge planning should begin shortly after the patient's admission. O'Sullivan and Brody write that the essential determinants in the discharge planning process include living arrangements, physical health (medication and diet), psychiatric status, economic status, vocational training/education, social abilities (leisure activities), family and other supports, self-care abilities, and access to transportation. They conclude, "success is measured by suitable placement that brings about a period of stability and independence consistent with the patient's psychiatric condition."[18]

Despite the best laid plans, most hospitalized patients progress through a series of crises that must be resolved. These can include conflicts with the staff or other patients, failure to respond to treatment, encounters with family members, or regression to a lower level of functioning. The resolution of these problems without major confrontations such as signing out against medical advice or acting-out is one measure of success for a psychiatric hospital. Invariably the biggest crisis of all is discharge. With the emphasis on decreased length of stay, most patients present a dilemma to staff around issues of placement or readiness for discharge.

SPECIAL ISSUES IN THE PRIVATE HOSPITAL

In western culture, family members seem to present problems to hospitals. In general hospitals they hang around the corridors or outside the intensive care units. Psychiatric hospitals are ambivalent about families. Most modern psychiatric programs involve the family in the patient's care, but frequently there are communication problems on both sides. The rapid growth and popularity of the National Alliance for the Mentally Ill, an organization spawned by discontented families, attest to that fact. Each hospital develops a strategy for relating to families. This may be in the person of the social worker who does a family intake and therapy with a selected few or a more elaborate program that includes family education, family night, and family/ patient group sessions. Meaningful collaboration with the family in the treatment of the patient is missing from many of these activities. While the patient's rights of confidentiality must be preserved, each institution needs a comprehensive outreach program to maximize family participation and collaboration. As an example, the short-term treatment unit at the Menninger Foundation makes it a requirement that some family member become a part of the therapeutic program for each patient admitted. As the length of stay in the hospital is shortened, relations with the family support system become even more critical.

Most private psychiatric hospitals in recent years have experienced increased geriatric admissions. This is paradoxical in that private psychiatric hospitals were initially excluded from Medicare reimbursement. Geriatric patients require special medical and rehabilitation support services that are best handled on a medical/psychiatric unit that is integrated with a day hospital and aftercare services. Stein notes that the community mental health centers and public sector have progressively turned away from the care of the elderly. He suggests that this may progressively become the province of the private psychiatric hospital.[19]

Adolescent admissions have also shown a quantum leap in the past several years. For example, the percentage of patients at The Institute of Living under the age of 20 went from 25% to 35% between the years of 1983 and 1986. The majority of these patients are between the ages of 15 and 18, but there has been increasing demand for admission of patients down to age 12. The majority of these admissions are for severe character pathology and drug abuse. Recently there has been considerable controversy over whether a psychiatric hospital is an appropriate facility for the treatment of these teenagers. The length of stay for adolescents in the National Association of Private Psychiatric Hospital's survey averages 87 days. Clearly these are intermediate care admissions, and provision of a well-thought-out program, integrated with adequate recreational and educational opportunities, is more important than whether the site is a hospital or a residential treatment center. The big question is cost. The latter is significantly less expensive. The important questions of whether the patient mix is more severe in the hospital or whether the hospital offers better treatment advantages have not been answered.

The housing of adolescent patients in a hospital generally places a major resource burden on the facility.[20] They require a well organized program, more staffing, and accessible educational facilities. Wear and tear on facilities can be a big problem. Most hospitals organize their adolescent programs separately. Bond and Auger[21] suggest housing the teenagers on wards mixed with about one-third adults. According to the authors, this reduces acting-out and destructiveness. Some of the adult patients develop positive and therapeutically beneficial relationships with teenagers. In my experience, the mixing of adult and adolescent patients is just that—a mixture but not necessarily a recipe for successful treatment.

Recent court decisions concerning patient rights that have originated in the public sector have significantly influenced the private hospital. Issues like the right to treatment and, more importantly, the right to refuse treatment have sensitized the public and private sector to the importance of the patient as an equal partner in the treatment process. Although the majority of private hospitals limit themselves to voluntary admissions, a significant minority do take involuntary committed patients. Whether the patient is voluntary or committed, the power disparity between patients and staff is significant. Most hospitals have some mechanism for patient-staff dialogue around issues of rights and privileges. This may take the form of a patient ombudsman, patient council, or a community meeting. Voluntary patients who refuse treatment are not treated without appropriate legal consultation, with reference to statutory requirements and outside medical consultation. Initially, many professionals viewed the patient advocacy movement with resentment and resistance. Recently this has evolved, particularly in the private sector, to a new patient-staff relationship that is much more in keeping with the standards of moral treatment on which the private hospitals were founded.

Under a great deal more pressure in recent years is the issue of confidentiality, particularly regarding the medical record. In a psychiatric hospital the guarantee of a patient's confidentiality is the cornerstone of the treatment process. Recent years have witnessed a steady incursion of third-party payers, cost management reviewers, and the courts into the confidentiality of psychiatric records. Many patients do not understand the magnitude of these incursions, and when they do, it may have a negative effect on their treatment. In turn, hospitals and professionals are under increasing ethical constraint as to the amount of information they can give third parties. This is an area that should be carefully scrutinized, both to study the therapeutic consequences of breaching confidentiality and to avoid unethical invasions of privacy.

OUTCOME STUDIES AND THE FUTURE OF THE PRIVATE PSYCHIATRIC HOSPITAL

Writings concerning outcome of psychiatric hospitalization have pursued two themes—the emphasis on a shorter length of stay and the narrowing of criteria for long-term stay. This has been backed up by a number of studies that purport to show that short-term hospitalizations followed by continuity of care produce better results than long-term hospitalization. Herz, Endicott, and Spitzer, working in a public sector environment with a minority population of chronically mentally ill, demonstrated that short-term hospitalization combined with day hospital produced a better outcome than prolonged hospitalization (defined as 90 to 120 days).[22] Glick et al. produced similar findings with patients arbitrarily assigned to short-term (less than 30 days) and long-term (greater than 90 days) on a research ward at Langley Porter.[23] Neither of these studies replicates the treatment experience in a long-term private psychiatric hospital; therefore, they do not adequately evaluate the efficacy of that mode of long-term intervention.

Much more relevant is the work of McGlashan, who followed up 446 (72%) of the patients discharged from Chestnut Lodge between the years of 1950 and 1975.[24,25,26] Chestnut Lodge is a small private hospital which has enjoyed a reputation for the long-term treatment of seriously disturbed patients. He found that 37% of the schizophrenics were residing in sheltered environments, compared to 26% of patients with bipolar, and 5% with unipolar, depression. Forty-one percent of the schizophrenics were continuously disabled for 15 years of follow-up. On the other hand, patients with borderline personality disorders were "comparable with unipolar patients and scored significantly better than schizophrenic patients on most indexes of outcome."

Mosher, in his reports from the Soteria House experiment, makes a strong case for a longer-term psychotherapeutic treatment program for the chronically psychotic.[27] Mosher contends that there will always be a significant population of mental patients who need longer-term psychiatric intervention in a structured, protected setting. The question for the future is whether the criteria defining this population will be so stringent as to restrict care largely to custodial maintenance in a public facility. Is there a continued role for the private psychiatric hospital in their care? There is clearly a role for the psychotherapeutically oriented private hospital in the treatment of chronic character disorders, chronically psychotic, and severely disturbed adolescents. Yet the private psychiatric hospital can no longer be unidimensional in its therapeutic offerings.

What are the implications of these findings for the future of private psychiatric hospitals? Some of the changes are already apparent. Most private psychiatric hospitals are rapidly moving toward short-term (less than 30 days) or intermediate (60 to 90 days) care. Those committed to long-term care anticipate a significant drop in the number of patients who can afford this treatment. Many are exploring the expansion of services into a comprehensive system of care that includes day hospitals, residential treatment facilities, halfway houses and supervised apartments. Whether operating as a stand-alone facility or as part of a comprehensive system, the hospital of the future will be even more sensitive to its place in a network of psychiatric care. The hospital must expand its role beyond its current perimeter of responsibility to become a facilitator in the process that returns the psychiatric patient to an adjustment in the community. A forward-looking perspective is demanded that places discharge planning on the agenda the day the patient arrives.

Careful efforts to nurture relationships with referring sources and community resources become ever more important. The for-profit private hospitals are already linked into a national system of care. Progressively, the voluntary hospitals will also link up with national systems and expand locally to include linkages with other general and specialty hospitals and alternative delivery systems (health maintenance organizations, preferred provider organizations and residential treatment centers). Access to these systems is necessary to obtain capital for facility improvements, as well as, and more importantly, patient referrals. Increasingly, the corporate sector will negotiate directly with systems of care for comprehensive mental and health benefits. Voluntary Hospitals of America (VHA) is an example of a national system of not-for-profit hospitals. The structure and function of VHA are indistinguishable from a for-profit chain, except that the individual provider hospitals maintain somewhat more autonomy.

With all of these efforts, some patients will simply demand more time and treatment effort than are allowed in the current reimbursement schemes. The needs of this sicker population must be addressed by creative working relationships between public and private resources or the development of some new source of private reimbursement (catastrophic insurance). Whatever the solution, it will carry the private psychiatric hospital further into the economic/political arena. The freestanding, private hospital is probably fast becoming a thing of the past; rather, the hospital of the future will be a critical link in a system of services carrying severely ill patients from a structured safe environment to one of least restriction.

REFERENCES

1. Grob GN: Mental Illness and American Society, 1875-1940. Princeton, NJ, Princeton Press, 1983
2. Grob GN: Mental Institutions in America. New York, Free Press, 1973
3. Forbush B: The History of the Sheppard and Enoch Pratt Hospital. Philadelphia, 1971
4. Burlingame C: Patient Handbook for The Institute of Living. Hartford, 1942
5. Main TF: The hospital as a therapeutic environment. Bull Menninger Clin 1946; 10:66-70
6. Jones M: The Therapeutic Community. New York, Basic Books, 1953
7. Levenson A: Issues surrounding the ownership of private psychiatric hospitals by investor owned chains. Hosp Community Psychiatry 1983; 34:1127-1131
8. Watt JM, Derzon A, Renn SC, Schramm CJ, Hahn JS, Pillar GD: The comparative economic performance of investor owned and not for profit hospitals. N Eng J Med 1986; 314:89-96
9. Gralnick A: The nature of the psychiatric hospital: an exploration into the development of one such. Psychiatric Hospital 1983; 14:29-33
10. Stanton AH, Schwartz MS: The Mental Hospital. New York, Basic Books, 1954
11. Pottash AC, Sweeney D, Gold MS, Extein I: Models for care and research: closed-staff private hospitals. Hosp Community Psychiatry 1983: 34:1058-1061
12. Hall RCW, Popkin MK, DeVaul R, Faillace LA, Stickney SK: Physical illness presenting as psychiatric disease. Arch Gen Psychiatry 1978; 35:1315-1320
13. Maxmen JS, Tucker GJ, LeBow, MD: Rational Hospital Psychiatry. New York, Brunner Mazel, 1974
14. Lieberman PB, Astrachan BM: The JCAH and psychiatry: current issues and implications for practice. Hosp Community Psychiatry 1984; 35:1205-1214
15. Mental Health Statistical Note No. 174, Characteristics of Admissions to Private Psychiatric Hospital Inpatient Services, United States, 1980, US Dept of Health and Human Services, NIMH, 1985
16. Mezzich JE, Evanczuk KJ, Mathias RJ, Coffman MS: Symptoms and hospitalization decisions. Am J Psychiatry 1984; 141:764-769
17. Levine I, Wilson A: Dynamic interpersonal process and the inpatient holding environment. Psychiatry 1985; 48(4):341-57
18. O'Sullivan AO, Brody M: Discharge Planning for the Mentally Disabled, QRB; 1986
19. Stein EM: Treating the aged: how the public system affects the private system. Psychiatric Hospital 1983; 14:82-86

20. Johansen K: The impact of patients with chronic character pathology on a hospital inpatient unit. Hosp Community Psychiatry 1983; 34:842-846
21. Bond TC, Auger N: Benefits of the geriatric milieu, in Adolescent Hospital Treatment, Adolescent Psychiatry. Edited by Feinstein SC, Looney J, Schwartzberg AL, Sorasky AD, Chicago, University of Chicago Press, 1986
22. Herz MI, Endicott J, Spitzer RL: Brief hospitalization: a two year follow-up. Am J Psychiatry 1977; 134:502-507
23. Glick ID, Hargreaves WA, Drues J, et al: Short vs long hospitalization: a controlled study: III. Inpatient results for nonschizophrenics. Arch Gen Psychiatry 1976; 33:78-83
24. McGlashan TH: The chestnut lodge follow up study, 1. Follow up methodology and study sample. Arch Gen Psychiatry 1984; 41:573-585
25. McGlashan TH: The chestnut lodge follow up study 2. Long term outcome of schizophrenia and the affective disorders. Arch Gen Psychiatry 1984; 41:586-601
26. McGlashan TH: The chestnut lodge follow up study 3. Long term outcome of borderline personalities. Arch Gen Psychiatry 1986; 43:20-30
27. Wendt RJ, Mosher LR, Matthews SM, Menn AZ: Comparisons of two treatment environments for schizophrenia, in Principles and Practice of Milieu Therapy. Edited by Gunderson JG, Will OA, Mosher LR et al, New York, Jason Aronson, 1983

2
The Public Mental Hospital

James T. Barter
Patricia A. Marshall

For over a hundred years the public mental hospital has been the major national resource for the treatment of the mentally ill. These hospitals were started as humane alternatives to the almshouse, the jail, or a life of homeless wandering from town to town. Their history has been characterized by cycles of reform and scandal.[1] When adequately supported by legislatures and sufficiently staffed, public hospitals were able to provide excellent levels of care and treatment. All too often, however, they suffered repeated budgetary crises, became overcrowded and understaffed, with consequent public reaction. The resultant deterioration in conditions led to exposés and public outrage.

In the early 1960s, the rationale for large public hospitals was challenged by the community mental health movement and over the subsequent two and a half decades the population of these facilities dropped almost 80%. As hospitals shrank in size and some closed, new community programs began to provide alternative treatment settings. Now a reassessment of the role of the state hospital in the care of the mentally ill has resulted because of the failure of responsible governmental agencies to provide adequate and continuing fiscal support for community programs. Unfortunately, this has taken the form of a debate about the advantages of institutional care over community care, rather than a thoughtful assessment of the kind of system of care needed for the mentally ill.[2-4] Here we will describe public hospitals, their current status and the problems they face. While we will not necessarily resolve the debate about the need for a unified system of care with a well-defined role for public hospitals, perhaps we will stimulate thinking about the issues.

The term "public mental hospital" as used in this chapter refers to state hospitals, publicly funded county and municipal hospitals, and Veterans Administration (VA) hospitals. Common characteristics of public hospitals include: deriving a major share of their funding from a governmental entity, enmeshment in a larger bureaucracy with multiple levels of oversight, and little or no control over service load or patient characteristics. Public mental hospitals differ significantly from private or proprietary hospitals. No attempt is made in this chapter to deal with all these differences. Other chapters in this volume will describe the characteristics of alternative settings. It is sufficient to keep in mind that governance is often the prime issue which defines such major differences as patient characteristics, funding sources and referral patterns. Governance of state hospitals is usually vested in the executive branch and dependent on legislative mandate. Because of its pre-eminent and durable role in the treatment of the mentally ill, the state mental hospital will be used as the prototype for the public mental hospital in this chapter.

CHARACTERISTICS OF PUBLIC MENTAL HOSPITALS

Location

In the sixties, nearly every state had at least one state hospital. By tradition public facilities such as state hospitals were often located in rural areas. With the advent of the community mental health movement in the early sixties this policy began to be questioned. Philosophically the community mental health movement proposed locating psychiatric services as close to the patient's home as possible, not only to ease the transition back to the community but also to facilitate the involvement of family and significant others in the treatment process. Rural location of state hospitals was antithetical to this tenet.

Between 1960 and 1980, the number of states having a state hospital in their first or second ranked most populous city grew from 23 to 32, an increase of 39%. Thus, new state hospitals were built in major population centers. There was also a distinct pattern of closing rural hospitals. During the decade of 1970–80, half of the 37 state hospitals closed were in sparsely populated areas. In the same time period 34 new state hospitals were opened, only one of which was built in a sparsely populated rural area. In spite of this trend, many states still favor rural hospital locations. The data seem to indicate that there are two subsets, one a "central city" set which favors location of public psychiatric hospitals in urban settings and the other a "nonurban" set which prefers nonpopulous area locations.[5]

Numbers

Although there was a decline in state and county hospitals from 310 in 1970 to 280 in 1980, this was offset by the rise in general hospital psychiatric units and expansion of the VA system.[6] Psychiatric units in general hospitals rose from 797 in 1970 to 923 in 1980.[7] This growth was consistent with the community mental health philosophy and was aided by the availability of Hill-Burton construction monies and federal reimbursement programs such as Medicaid and Medicare. In 1980 there were 136 VA medical centers with separate psychiatric treatment services. These have become a major factor in delivery of public mental health services, providing inpatient units and, in many locales, outpatient clinics. Within the VA, 32% of all beds are devoted to psychiatric care, accounting for 10% of all psychiatric beds in the U.S.[8]

Functions

Public mental hospitals have filled numerous functions during the past century. The moral treatment movement defined the role of the public hospital as humane treatment of the mentally ill enabling them to return to their families and to society and as asylums for those whose prognosis was considered hopeless. The decline of the moral treatment movement around the turn of the century coupled with the rapid rise of inmate population and penurious funding by state legislatures led to a largely custodial role for public hospitals until the late fifties and early sixties. The rise of the community mental health movement, along with the advent of effective treatments such as insulin coma therapy, electroconvulsive treatment and psychotropics, revived interest in treatment and rehabilitation. The expectation that the mentally ill could be treated outside of state hospitals raised questions among legislators and mental health professionals over the future role of the public hospital.[9-12]

Throughout this period, suggestions on adapting the hospital to social and political realities ranged from closing them entirely to maintaining them as specialized tertiary care centers.[13-15] Nevertheless, they have continued to fulfill the traditional roles and functions they have always had.[16] These include treatment and rehabilitation, detention of societal undesirables, and protection of those unable to function outside of an asylum. To a lesser extent research and training have also continued as important roles. Finally, for many communities, there is an economic benefit of having a state hospital in their locale.

Treatment and rehabilitation have always been the overt purpose for public hospitals, even though during their most custodial phases little active treatment was carried out. One of the benefits of the depopulation of state hospitals was that staff/patient ratios rose, permitting active milieu treatment for acute and chronic patients in conjunction with the use of psychotropics. Psychosocial rehabilitation techniques aimed at returning the patient to community living became a feature of many hospitals. The length of stay decreased at the same time that admissions and readmissions rose, reflecting the redefinition of priorities from long-term custodial care to more active treatment programs. Many hospitals redefined themselves as providing active treatment for acute as well as chronic patients and also started special treatment programs for alcoholics and other substance abusers.

Detention and seclusion of socially undesirable individuals and those who are unresponsive to rehabilitative attempts have been, in the past, an important role for the public hospital. The problems of deinstitutionalization, particularly the apparent rise in homeless mentally ill and concerns about "dangerous" individuals has resulted in renewed pleas for seclusion and detention.[17] However, recent court decisions and public opinion have mitigated against this. The idea of detention without treatment is abhorrent and in the Wyatt v. Stickney decision the Fifth Circuit Court of Appeals held that it was unconstitutional to involuntarily hold a mentally ill individual and not provide active treatment.[18] If this role becomes paramount, then a real danger exists that state hospitals will revert to removing undesirables from society. Similar to the population of "socially undesirables" are mentally ill persons who are unable to care for themselves because of the severity and persistence of their illness. Before the advent of the public mental hospital these individuals often roamed the countryside untended and generally despised. The state hospital as asylum became an answer for their plight. Recently several authorities have advocated a resurrection of this protective role for state hospitals.[2,19-20] The role of the asylum as a refuge is a meaningful one,[21] but whether the state hospital is the appropriate institution to fulfill this role is debatable.[22]

In addition to providing treatment and rehabilitation for the mentally ill and protective services for socially undesirables, the state hospital also has served as a research and training ground for psychiatric practitioners and academicians. However, this role has diminished significantly. State hospitals are no longer a major resource for training psychiatric residents or other mental health professionals although VA hospitals are. In the five years between 1975 and 1980 alone there was a decrease in state hospital resident positions from 1175 to 640. This is a 46% decrease and is greater than the corresponding 34% decrease in patient population during the same period of time.[23]

The reasons for this decreased importance in training are multiple. Many state hospital programs were criticized because they were not affiliated with university training programs, had poorer standards for training than university programs, and enrolled disproportionately high numbers of foreign medical graduate trainees. Veterans Administration training programs have affiliated with universities and have maintained a high quality. A few other isolated models of training utilizing public hospitals and community mental health settings exist, but they are not a dominant national influence on training.[24,25] This decline in the importance of the public sector in training has spawned a host of problems regarding the recruitment of psychiatrists into public service. The future of training programs in the public sector may well rest on the success of state-university collaborations.[26]

Earlier in this century research was a significant mission for some state hospitals; in fact, many psychiatric institutes in the U.S. arose out of public or state hospital roots. The legislation establishing these prestigious public hospitals stressed the tripartite role of (1) promoting research into the causes of mental illness and improvement of treatment and care, (2) providing training and education to mental health professionals, and (3) maintaining a standard of excellence in treatment for mentally ill persons. Thus, many public hospitals were committed to research in addition to training professionals and treating patients. Today research is not a major role for most state hospitals. Instead, research has become largely a university function and virtually all psychiatric institutes have been assimilated by universities. However, the resurgence of interest in chronic mental illness and treatment resistance, coupled with state-university collaborative efforts, may well make state hospitals more attractive as sites for research.

Finally, there is a less obvious function of the public hospital which is not directly related to the treatment or care of the mentally ill. State hospitals are of economic benefit to the host community. Particularly in rural locales the state hospital or VA hospital may be the major employer and thus a significant industry. The closure of state hospitals in California was resisted strongly by cities such as Modesto and Mendocino on economic grounds. The potential for economic disruption was compared to the closing of a cannery or other industrial enterprise. Significant pressure was put on the legislature to delay or rescind these closures, not only by the municipalities but also by the employee unions. In recent years, labor unions have become one of the more potent political forces opposing the closure or reduction of staffing for state hospitals, largely on economic grounds. (For similar reasons many rural communities are welcoming the placement of new prisons in their midst because of the benefit of a labor intensive industry in what is often an economically depressed area.)

OPERATIONS

Administration

Public hospitals are usually administered under the policymaking guidance of a governmental agency. For the VA this is the central office of the Veterans Administration and ultimately the federal government.[27] Most state hospitals are administratively responsible to a state department of mental health within the executive branch of government. Fiscal resources and broad policy issues are often determined by the legislature. The complex bureaucracy created by these overlapping and often overburdening levels of government impede the delivery of optimal care. Moreover, the year to year budget process, influenced as it is by political considerations, makes long-range planning impossible.

In addition, the rigid civil service system in most governmental hospitals discourages the hiring of high quality staff and imposes long delays in filling positions. It also makes the firing of incompetent staff so cumbersome that many supervisors are reluctant to attempt to discharge such a staff member. The added protection of collective bargaining agreements establishes further constraints in managing human resources. Staffing patterns evolve on the basis of a formula developed by budget analysts whose interest is not quality care but fiscal restraint.

Inflexibility concerning most phases of administration in the public hospital system seems to be the norm. Considering the magnitude of changes which would be necessary at several bureaucratic levels to approximate the management efficiency of private or proprietary hospitals, there is little room for optimism that this situation will change in the near future.

Leadership

Earlier in this century the position of state hospital director was prestigious, and many leaders of psychiatry were associated with state institutions. Indeed, a group of directors of state institutions founded the forerunner to the American Psychiatric Association. Increasingly, directorships are now being filled by business administrators or nonphysician, nonpsychiatrist mental health directors.[28,29] This loss of medical leadership effects the degree of attention paid to professional care issues in favor of "efficient management," by which is meant the primacy of business oriented concerns. Business and health care are not incompatible, but frequently the concerns of professionals over the standard and quality of clinical care are losing out to management efficiency. In a ten-year period in California, there was a significant decline in physician administrators in public hospitals and other public mental health programs in favor of nonmedical administrators, a trend which appears to be true for the country as a whole. Usually when the top administrator is not a physician than there is a bifurcated organizational chart with an associate director for clinical programs (a physician or in some cases a mental health professional) and an associate director for administration who is responsible for the business office, the personnel department, and facilities maintenance.

Funding

Public hospitals have the worst of fiscal worlds. Generally they are not funded on a capitation or fee-for-service basis and have difficulty qualifying for or getting third-party payments. Since they cannot control their admissions or population, their finances do not increase or decrease in proportion to their census. Their source of funding is tax dollars appropriated by a legislative body. Many public hospitals have gone after and been able to secure third-party revenue from such federal resources as Medicaid and Medicare as a survival strategy to maintain an acceptable level of service.

Usually budgets are voted by the legislature for annual periods and are subject to the pressures of competing interests. Rarely is a public mental hospital judged on its own merits as a provider of service. Instead the hospital is considered along with prisons, police, fire, welfare, and public health. Funding can vary significantly from year to year depending on the state's fiscal resources and the political skill of the administrator of the state department of mental health. Lobbying efforts by representatives of the mentally ill have been inadequate and generally have had little impact on the level of funding. This may change as the National Alliance for the Mentally Ill and other consumer groups become more widely known and politically active.

It is not uncommon in the budget process to submit multiple versions of the budget as it goes through the department of mental health, the executive branch, and then the legislature. Changes are often made during this process without consultation with the administrator of the hospital, and so the ultimate appropriation may have little relationship to what was submitted or what is necessary to run the hospital. Skillful administrators learn the tricks necessary to massage an appropriation to meet their needs. Usually the administrator of a public hospital is trying to settle last year's books, figure out how to stretch this year's dollars to cover current needs, and is beginning to prepare next year's budget submission. Fund transfers and creative reallocation are commonplace. Fortunately, many states still use budget categories that are so broad that some manipulation is feasible and generally accepted, as long as the total appropriation is not exceeded.

An analysis of expenditure patterns for mental health care shows some interesting trends. In 1969 state and county mental hospitals accounted for 55% of all expenditure for mental health, whereas in 1979 they had dropped to 41%. State and county hospitals accounted for 45% of all inpatient admission in 1969 but only 30% in 1979. It is important to remember than there was a marked decrease in the number of beds during this time, so that yearly cost per bed rose dramatically.

Cost of care in public hospitals is characterized by wide fluctuations from state to state. In 1980, the average cost per day in public hospitals was $120.

with a range from about $80. to $155. In the decade of the seventies, after adjustment for inflation, mental health facility expenditures rose from 3.3 billion to 4.3 billion. Most of this increase went to other than state and county hospitals. Yet, in many states 80% or more of the total dollar allocation for mental health is still spent in state hospitals.[30,31]

CLINICAL CARE

Referral Patterns

Public hospitals are open to everyone although there may be limitations. Veterans Administration hospitals, for example, are restricted to former members of the armed services and their dependents.[8] Some state and municipal hospitals restrict admission based on geography. State hospitals may take direct admissions, but many get their patients on referral from a community mental health service (so-called community treatment failures), a local public or private hospital (usually after third-party payments have run out), or from the courts (those not guilty by reason of insanity or individuals incompetent to stand trial).[16] Most of the patients treated in public mental hospitals are poor and chronically ill. Recently there have been stories of increased pressure on admissions to public hospitals as a result of transfers from private nonprofit and proprietary hospitals of patients whose third-party or Diagnostic Related Group benefits have elapsed. Whether this is a real trend or only anecdotal information has not been determined at this time.

Patient Characteristics

At one time public mental hospitals, particularly state hospitals, were repositories for large numbers of patients. Up until 1957 there was a constantly increasing census in state facilities resulting in overcrowding and horrendously low staff to patient ratios. Beginning in the mid fifties, as a result of several factors, the resident population in state hospitals began a precipitous decline, from a high of over 550,000 in 1957 to less than 140,000 by 1980.[32] Although there is debate about their relative importance, the following were probably seminal influences in this process called deinstitutionalization: the introduction of psychotropic medications; the introduction of new treatment methods such as group and milieu therapy; the change in social security and other federal reimbursement which permitted payment for community residential care and treatment; the rise of the community mental health movement; and societal changes which sanctioned community treatment for seriously mentally ill.[9,33]

Today state hospital and public hospital clientele are characterized by relatively short stays, frequent readmissions and a high frequency of mixed substance abuse and other mental disorder. "Of the total of 146,000 resident patients [on a hypothetical day in 1979], 29,000 (20%) were short-stay patients (less than 3 months), 29,200 (20%) were intermediate-stay patients (3 to 12 months), and 87,600 (60%) were long-stay patients (more than 12 months)."[16] By contrast, less than 7% of patients admitted to private psychiatric hospitals or general hospitals with psychiatric units stay longer than three months.

Types Of Patients

Acute: Contrary to popular perception, public hospitals admit a large proportion of acutely ill patients, often for short stays. It has been argued that the length of stay for these patients is too short and partially responsible for the high rate of readmission. It is difficult to verify this since there are no controlled studies relating length of hospital stay to therapeutic outcome or rate of readmission. The data which exist support a contrary view, that longer hospital stays promote readmission and extremely long stays lead to institutionalism.[34,35]

Chronic: Considering the high rate of readmission and recidivism reported, it seems reasonable to assume that large numbers of chronic mentally ill receive treatment and services in public mental hospitals. Of course this is a self-fulfilling prophecy since most chronic patients have meager resources and few alternatives for treatment outside of public programs. The apparent rise in homeless chronic mentally ill has been attributed to the lack of adequate numbers of treatment resources (beds) in the public sector.[36,37]

Alcohol and other substance abuse: Fifty percent of veterans seeking care at the VA have problems with alcoholism as a primary or secondary problem.[8] A recent survey at the Illinois State Psychiatric Institute revealed that over 50% of patients seeking admission had an associated substance abuse or alcohol problem. Craig and Laska,[12] in a comparison of admissions to Rockland State Hospital between 1972 and 1980, also report that "patients admitted with a primary diagnosis of alcohol or drug abuse or both showed the greatest increase."

Geriatrics: Whole wards of geriatric patients existed in most state hospitals ostensibly to provide protection and care. Unfortunately, conditions were often deplorable. One of the features of deinstitutionalism was the transfer of geriatric patients out of state hospitals to community care facilities such as skilled nursing facilities. This has been referred to as "transinstitutionalism" with good reason. This movement of the elderly into nursing

The Public Mental Hospital 31

homes was made possible by the availability of federal funding to support their care.

Between 1969 and 1973 the number of elderly mentally ill in nursing homes increased from 96,000 to 194,000. Occasional exposés of scandalous conditions in such facilities continue to raise concerns about the degree of protection the elderly are receiving. However, there is no evidence that the elderly living in state hospital facilities are treated more humanely.[38]

Staffing

It has been difficult to establish standards for staffing public facilities; wide variations exist. For a selected group of states, the ratio of full-time-equivalent (FTE) clinical staff to patients in state psychiatric hospitals ranges from a low of 0.14 (Alabama) to a high of 0.94 (South Dakota). The median appears to be around 0.70.[39] In Illinois the staff to patient ratio (including support staff) has ranged from 1.5 to 1.7 the past ten years. Such ratios as these are minimal; in fact, facilities with ratios of below 2 staff to 1 patient are significantly hampered in providing active treatment services. Facilities with staff/patient ratios at the lower end of the continuum struggle to be able to provide other than custodial services. Generally in public hospitals the direct care staff-to-patient ratio is 30% below that of comparable private institutions. For professional staff, this ratio is 58% below.[40]

Further compounding the problem of inadequate overall staffing numbers is the problem of the proportion of professional staff to other mental health direct care staff. In only seven states are there as many as four psychiatrists per 100 inpatients in state hospitals.[41] In most public psychiatric hospitals, the frontline staff is composed of psychiatric technicians, mental health aides, and licensed vocational nurses. These paraprofessionals generally get minimal training in therapeutics and lack the skills, attitudes and competence to deal with active treatment of patients. They feel most comfortable and function best in a custodial and control capacity.

Psychiatrists: During the decade of the seventies, the number of full-time equivalent (FTE) psychiatrists working within organized mental health programs increased from 10,100 to 18,200. The National Institute of Mental Health Division of Biometry statistics for 1976 reveal that 4,333 FTE psychiatrists were working in state and county hospitals and that 1471 were working in VA hospitals.[32] Obviously most of this increase was in community mental health centers, general psychiatric hospitals and other non-state hospital or VA hospital facility. In 1975, 58% of psychiatrists working in state hospitals were foreign medical graduates.

There has been a tendency in some public facilities to employ nonpsychiatrist physicians to manage medication for psychiatric patients. The rationale supporting this seems to be that a general physician plus a psychologist or other mental health worker is equivalent to a psychiatrist. There is no evidence to support this proposition.

Psychologists: Approximately 20,000 psychologists with at least master's degrees work in organized mental health settings. About a third of these work in public hospitals, and of these 60% are trained at less than the doctoral level.[38]

Social workers: It has been estimated that approximately 20,000 master's level social workers are in the mental health field, with about 5,000 to 6,000 employed in public mental health facilities. In contrast to nurses and psychiatrists, there seems to be little or no consensus expressed about shortages of social workers.[38]

Nursing: As of 1980, 45,000 FTE psychiatric nurses worked in organized mental health settings. Many public hospitals have problems with accreditation and certification reviews because of the shortage of qualified psychiatric nurses. Less than 5% of directors of nursing in 250 large state hospitals were master's level psychiatric nurses. Particularly missing are master's level nurses in positions of supervision and leadership.[32,42] Public hospitals have tried to make up for this deficiency by the use of licensed practical or vocational nurses and various mental health auxiliaries such as licensed psychiatric technicians or mental health aides. The higher the proportion of these less well-trained staff, the more likely that the hospital will have a custodial orientation and emphasis on psychopharmacology as the major modality of treatment.

Psychiatric technicians constitute the largest group of workers and the major care providers in the public mental facility. It is estimated that they are responsible for up to 80% of the direct care rendered to patients in mental hospitals. There is wide variation from state to state in the qualifications, training, and experience required for these positions. Much could be done to improve the quality of these workers through effective inservice and continuing education. Unfortunately, few public facilities have emphasized or mandated relevant training. In an effort to develop career ladders, increasingly responsible positions have been opened up to paraprofessionals, including administrative positions such as ward chief and state hospital director.[43]

PROS AND CONS OF WORKING IN PUBLIC HOSPITALS

There is an extensive literature dealing with the pros and cons of working in the public mental health sector.[44,45] Most of this commentary has emphasized the negative aspects of a public mental health career. Community mental health centers and state hospitals have had difficulty recruiting and retaining mental health professionals, particularly psychiatrists. Certainly at their worst public mental health programs and facilities do not offer much to the competent mental health professional. However, in well staffed and well run programs there are many attractions, such as flexible working conditions, job security, opportunities for innovation, and challenging and varied patients.

Public hospitals offer a stable salary, fringe benefits, and often flexible working conditions, which may be attractive to the beginning psychiatrist. Unfortunately, when the state hospital is used solely for transitional employment for psychiatrists establishing their practices, this leads to unacceptably high levels of turnover and makes continuity of treatment impossible. Fortunately, many psychiatrists take positions in state hospitals on a transitional basis and then find the work challenging and stay on. New staff members often have considerable freedom to innovate and develop new treatment approaches, as well as to assume leadership positions at an earlier stage in their career. For those who enjoy team work, the public hospital offers an opportunity to be a member of a functioning treatment team. There are also opportunities to take on outside activities, such as working on committees within the hospital, the department of mental health, or within the state and national professional organizations, without losing income because of the time away from work.

The patient population in state hospitals is varied and includes many unusual and unique examples of mental disorder. Contrary to popular perception, the public hospital patient population is not uniformly chronic and untreatable. Indeed, the variety of diagnoses and conditions may exceed that in almost any other setting. This makes public hospitals excellent sites for teaching rotations for medical students, psychiatric residents, psychology interns, and other mental health students. For the staff member, the opportunity to participate in teaching can be rewarding and in many locations can lead to a clinical academic appointment in a university.

The poor public image that state hospitals have suffered contributes to the negative attitude about them held by both the public and the professional. The contrary side of working in public hospitals has been extensively covered in the literature. Talbott[46] referred to dozens of problems which he grouped into three classes: internal (inadequate staff pay, low morale, frequent crises); departmental (insufficient fiscal resources, ill-defined goals); and external (legislative pressures, judicial decisions, patient advocate pressures).

The internal factors described by Talbott have been echoed by many other authors. Leehey and Misiaszek[44] looked at the contribution of poor job quality to the decline of public psychiatry as a popular career choice among young psychiatrists and concluded that lack of autonomy, antagonism to a biomedical view of mental illness, and noncompetitive salaries were major factors. There is no doubt that working in public hospitals is stressful and burnout of staff at all levels is common.[40] Greenblatt[47] emphasized the issues of criticism, vilification, and abuse that go with a high visibility job and contributes to low morale. The hazard of assaults on staff by patients and general concerns about security contribute to a crises atmosphere in many public hospitals.

Many of the departmental shortcomings have been discussed earlier in this chapter. Anyone who has worked in a public setting has experienced the frustration of inflexible administrative dicta and the ponderous organizational machinery, which results in delays in decision-making. Resource deficiencies ranging from outdated and potentially dangerous equipment to inadequate staff levels are common. In accreditation reviews, state hospitals are often cited for significant fire hazards, life-threatening conditions, and safety deficiencies, often resulting in withholding of certification. States have been reluctant to put capital construction funds into aged physical plants or to build new physical facilities.

The external pressures have been particularly intense in the past decade. Attention to due process in involuntary hospitalization and the rising interest in patient rights have led to significant oversight by the judiciary, as well as fears of malpractice litigation. An avalanche of rules and regulations has ensued. Public mental hospitals, because of the number of oversight committees and advocacy groups, are likely targets for litigation. Many mental health professionals prefer to avoid working in them for this reason.

Legislatures responding to these same social pressures tend to look for simplistic answers, the result being an increase in bureaucratization. The rise of the generic administrator with no clinical or medical experience reinforces the emphasis on political and economic decision-making rather than optimal clinical care. This attitude, when it filters down to the direct care staff, increases their stress and job dissatisfaction. Medical administrators are more likely to reflect the concerns of staff about maintaining quality clinical care. When they choose to argue for treatment concerns over budgetary issues, they are seen by higher level state bureaucrats as troublemakers and thus have short tenures. There is no easy answer to these pressures except for continued advocacy for a system of quality care for the mentally ill which is comprehensive, accessible and affordable.

FUTURE OF THE PUBLIC HOSPITAL

There is significant debate about the future of state hospitals, with positions ranging from closing them all to expanding the system.[48-50] Disillusionment with the limited results from community mental health have led many to propose that we should consider opening new state hospitals and increasing the number of beds available for treatment. Articles have been written about the need for asylum for the chronically mentally ill,[19-22] the need to get the homeless mentally ill off the streets,[36,37] and the neglect of the elderly in community nursing homes.[38] All of these needs are seen by their supporters as cogent and compelling reasons for continuation and expansion of the state hospital system. On the other side are the arguments about the current inadequacies of state hospitals in many spheres, such as physical plant, fire-life-safety deficiencies, inadequate and poor quality staffing, lack of active treatment programs, insufficient funding, bureaucratic strictures, and all the well-known panoply of woes detailed earlier in this chapter. This debate will not be easily settled, nor is it likely to dissipate.

Bachrach[51] has reviewed the status of state hospitals and offers four predictions about their future: that they will survive, that they will continue to vary from state to state, that they will be one of several loci for care, and that they will continue to have fiscal and identity crises. Certainly it is difficult to disagree with these predictions. She argues that public hospitals will survive because they provide services of a unique nature. It is more likely that public hospitals, especially state hospitals, have endured because they represent a significant portion of the psychiatric service system for which no adequate replacement has been forthcoming rather than because they have any quality of uniqueness. The variability of state hospitals from one state to another is more the result of the complexities of bureaucratic structure, financial support, and state commitment to providing adequate care for the mentally ill than it is a consequence of response to patient needs. Many states have been unable to shift mental health appropriation to community programs, so that the continued use of state hospitals becomes a self-fulfilling prophecy. The patients following the money rather than the money following the patients. For this reason alone state hospitals will continue to be important loci of care. Finally, Bachrach's prediction that state hospitals will plagued by continued financial and identity crises is all too true and pathetic. Unfortunately, this prediction could be made about the whole public mental health system whether community-based or state-hospital-based.

Okin[52] has been the most persistent critic of state hospitals and argues for the creation of a new system of care for the mentally ill. Basically, the issue is that "for the vast majority of patients these facilities provide not only an inferior quality of treatment but the wrong kind of treatment altogether." After detailing the problems of inferior and outdated physical plants, programmatic and geographic isolation, staffing inadequacies, fiscal deficiencies, and many other limitations, Okin asserts that it is unlikely that existing state hospitals can be transformed into first-class treatment centers. He proposes that the future for public mental health care of the mentally ill lies in a reorientation of the whole system of care, based on a substantial expansion and reorientation of the community mental health system backed up by general hospital services and small, community-based intermediate care facilities, along with the creation of intensive care and tertiary care units of excellence in major medical centers.[53] The probability of such a unified system of care may be, as Talbott has suggested, "utopia unrealized."[54]

REFERENCES

1. Morrisey JP, Goldman HH: Cycles of reform in the care of the chronically mentally ill. Hosp Community Psychiatry 1984; 35:785-793
2. Gralnik A: Build a better state hospital: deinstitutionalization has failed. Hosp Community Psychiatry 1985; 36:738-741
3. Okin RL: Expand the community care system: deinstitutionalization can work. Hosp Community Psychiatry 1985; 36:742-745
4. Sigel GS: In defense of state hospitals. Hosp Community Psychiatry 1984; 35:1234-1236
5. Checker A: Locus of state psychiatric hospitals in the United States, 1960-1980. Am J Psychiatry 1983; 140:994-997
6. Thompson JW, Bass RD, Witkin MJ: Fifty years of psychiatric services: 1940-1990. Hosp Community Psychiatry 1982; 33:711-717
7. Redick RM, Witkin MJ: State and County Mental Hospitals, United States, 1970-1981. Mental Health Statistical Note 165, Rockville, Md, NIMH, 1983
8. Strauss GD, Such DA, Lesser I: Which veterans go to VA psychiatric hospitals for care: a pilot study. Hosp Community Psychiatry 1985; 36:963-965
9. Bachrach LL: Deinstitutionalization: An Analytic Review and Sociological Perspective. Rockville, Md, NIMH, 1976
10. Goldman HH, Adams NH, Taube CA: Deinstitutionalization: the data demythologized. Hosp Community Psychiatry 1983; 34:129-134
11. Shore MF, Shapiro R: The effect of deinstitutionalization on the state hospital. Hosp Community Psychiatry 1979; 30:605-608
12. Craig TJ, Laska EM: Deinstitutionalization and the survival of the state hospital. Hosp Community Psychiatry 1983; 35:616-622
13. Talbott JA (Editor): State Mental Hospitals: Problems and Potentials. New York, Human Sciences Press, 1980
14. Okin RL: State hospitals in the 1980's. Hosp Community Psychiatry 1982; 33:717-721
15. Kimmel WA: The Future of State Mental Hospitals: Context, Issues, and Alternatives. Rockville, Md, NIMH, 1984
16. Goldman HH, Taube CA, Regier DA, Witkin M: The multiple functions of the state mental hospital. Am J Psychiatry 1983; 140:296-300
17. Lamb HR, Mills MJ: Needed changes in law and procedure for the chronically mentally ill. Hosp Community Psychiatry 1982; 37:475-480
18. Wyatt v Stickney, 325 F Suppl 781 (MD Ala 1971); 344 F Suppl 373 (MD Ala 1972)
19. Bachrach LL: Asylum and chronically ill psychiatric patients. Psychiatry 1984; 141:975-978
20. Lamb HR, Peele R: The need for continuing asylum and sanctuary. Hosp Community Psychiatry 1984; 35:798-802
21. Rosenblatt A: Concepts of the asylum in the care of the mentally ill. Hosp Community Psychiatry 1984; 35:244-250
22. Talbott JA: The need for asylum, not asylums. Hosp Community Psychiatry 1984; 35:209
23. Thompson JW, Checker A, Witkin MJ, et al: The decline of state mental hospitals as training sites for psychiatric residents. Psychiatry 1983; 140:704-707
24. Weintraub W, Harbin HT, Book J, et al: The Maryland plan for recruiting psychiatrists into public service. Am J Psychiatry 1984; 141:91-94
25. Cutler DL, Bloom JD, Shore JH: Training psychiatrists to work with community support systems for chronically mentally ill persons. Am J Psychiatry 1981; 138:98-101

26. Talbott JA, Robinowitz C (Editors): Working Together: State-University Collaboration in Mental Health. Washington, DC, American Psychiatric Press, 1986
27. Peele R, Lipkin JO: Public mental hospitals, in Psychiatric Administration: A Comprehensive Text for the Clinician-Executive. Edited by Talbott JA, Kaplan SR, New York, Grune & Stratton, 1983
28. Talbott JA: Why psychiatrists leave the public sector. Hosp Community Psychiatry 1979; 30:778-782
29. Gaver KD, Norman ML, Greenblatt M: Life at the state summit: view and experiences of 18 psychiatric leaders. Hosp Community Psychiatry 1984; 35:233-238
30. Frank RG, Kamlet MS: Direct costs and expenditures for mental health care in the United States in 1980. Hosp Community Psychiatry 1985; 36:165-168
31. Taube CA, Barett SA (Editors): Mental Health, United States, 1985. DHHS Publication No (ADM)85-1378. Washington, DC, Superintendent of Documents, US Govt Printing Office, 1985
32. Manderscheid RW, Witkin MJ, Rosenstein MJ, Bass RD: A review of trends in mental health services. Hosp Community Psychiatry 1984; 35:673-674
33. Lerman P: Deinstitutionalization: A Cross Problem Analysis. DHHS Publication No (ADM) 81-987, Washington, DC. Superintendent of Documents, US Govt Printing Office, 1981
34. Kirschner LA: Length of stay of psychiatric patients: a critical review and discussion. J Nerv Ment Dis 1982; 170:27-33
35. Caton CLM: Effect of length of stay for inpatient treatment for chronic schizophrenia. Am J Psychiatry 1982; 139:856-861
36. Bachrach LL: The homeless mentally ill and mental health services: an analytic review of the literature, in The Homeless Mentally Ill. Edited by Lamb HR, Washington, DC, American Psychiatric Association, 1984
37. Lamb HR (Editor): The Homeless Mentally Ill, Washington, DC, American Psychiatric Association, 1984
38. Toward a National Plan for the Chronically Mentally Ill: Report to the Secretary. Committee on the Chronically Mentally Ill, Department of Health and Human Services, Rockville, Md, NIMH, 1980
39. Lamirand L, Chown, B: Selected Information from State Mental Health Program Indicators – 1982. (A project of the National Association of State Mental Health Program Directors) Oklahoma City, Ok, Oklahoma Department of Mental Health (Offset) 1983
40. Daawkins J, Depp FC, Selzer N: Occupational stresses in a public mental hospital: the psychiatrist's view. Hosp Community Psychiatry 1984; 35:56-60
41. Knesper DJ: Psychiatric manpower for state mental hospitals. Arch Gen Psychiatry 1978; 35:15-24
42. Perlmutter DR: Recent trends and issues in psychiatric-mental health nursing. Hosp Community Psychiatry 1985; 36:56-62
43. Moffic HS, Patterson GK, Laval R, Adams GL: Paraprofessionals and psychiatric teams: an updated review. Hosp Community Psychiatry 1984; 35:61-67
44. Leehey K, Misiaszek J: Poor job quality and the decline of public psychiatry. Hosp Community Psychiatry 1985; 36:1180-1183
45. Mirabi M, Weinman ML, Maquette SM, Keppler KN: Professional attitudes towards the chronic mentally ill. Hosp Community Psychiatry 1985; 36:404-405
46. Talbott JA: The Death of the Asylum: A Critical Study of State Hospital Management, Services, and Care. New York, Grune & Stratton, 1978
47. Greenblatt M: Special problems facing the psychiatrist-administrator. Hosp Community Psychiatry 1979; 30:760-762
48. Lamb HR: Treating the Long Term Mentally Ill: Beyond Deinstitutionalization. San Francisco, Jossey-Bass, 1982
49. Talbott JA: The fate of the public psychiatric system. Hosp Community Psychiatry 1985; 36:46-50
50. Arnhoff FN: Social consequences of policy toward mental illness. Science 1975; 188:1277-1281

51. Bachrach LL: The future of the state mental hospital. Hosp Community Psychiatry 1986; 37:467–473
52. Okin RL: The future of state hospitals: should there be one? Am J Psychiatry 1983; 140:577–581
53. Okin RL, Dolnik J: Beyond state hospital unitization: the development of an integrated mental health management system. Hosp Community Psychiatry 1985; 36:1201–1205
54. Talbott JA (Editor): Unified Mental Health Systems: Utopia Unrealized. New Directions for Mental Health Services, no. 18, San Francisco, Jossey-Bass, 1983

3
The Psychiatric Unit in the General Hospital

Manoel W. Penna

The treatment of psychiatric patients within a general hospital is a historically recent development establishing a counterpoint to centuries of segregation of psychiatric patients. Before, the vast majority of patients were lodged in large public institutions, often removed from urban centers. In the fifties specialized psychiatric units were erected within the boundaries of general hospitals. The first movements in this direction were initiated by teaching hospitals although they had public support behind the initiative. It was not until the late sixties and early seventies that community hospitals joined the action. Once started, this trend rapidly gained momentum and psychiatric units in general hospitals became commonplace all over the United States. The magnitude of this change is reflected in the fact that by the end of the 1970s 58% of all psychiatric admissions in the country were to general hospitals.[1]

Many assumptions can be made about the shift of care for the psychiatric patient from the state mental hospital to the general hospital. For example, it is possible that such a move has contributed to an increased public awareness about the effectiveness of psychiatric intervention. Or, the shift may have contributed to decreased prejudice against mental illness. Or, the changes may have brought about an improvement in the quality of treatment of the psychiatric patient. But there has been no research effort designed to test these assumptions and the information available on the operation of psychiatric units remains largely descriptive in nature.[1]

CHARACTERISTICS OF PSYCHIATRIC UNITS
IN THE GENERAL HOSPITAL

While having in common their location within the physical plant of a general hospital, psychiatric units differ a great deal in regard to the treatment programs they offer and the target populations they serve. These variations in purpose and patient population are primary determinants of their structure and organization. Proprietary hospitals have also entered the picture; many contain psychiatric units. Questions have already been raised about the compatibility of the profit motive with the quality of the care delivered. At this early stage, however, there is no evidence to support the argument that they are necessarily incompatible.[2]

The psychiatric unit of the teaching general hospital presents a complex and sometimes taxing set of problems deserving close scrutiny. At the inception, its mission seemed simple and straightforward: to provide quality service for psychiatric patients, and in this context to educate medical students and psychiatric residents, train other professionals such as nurses, social workers and psychologists, and develop opportunities for research. In the course of time other demands began to be articulated. Communities surrounding many of the urban medical centers, especially the ones associated with a community mental health center, militantly raised their voices to establish priorities beyond the simple provision of medical services.[3] This demand was in conflict with the tertiary character of the patient care provided. In time, compromises were made. For example, at the University of Maryland Hospital an advisory board with representatives from the community was created to monitor the delivery of clinical services and make recommendations for changes attuned to the needs of the local population.

Later difficulties were brought on by changes in fiscal policy. Many teaching hospitals had been expected to provide a great amount of free service and depended on appropriations of public funds to maintain their functions. This was changed when units were directed to assume fiscal autonomy and become totally responsible for the financial support of their operations. But third-party payers decided that they were no longer going to provide financial support for education and training of students and residents. If this policy change generated problems for the other medical services, it created havoc in the psychiatric units of teaching hospitals. For the physician to be paid, services rendered required documentation. Thus the attending psychiatrist needed to place daily notes in the patient's chart. Yet the insurance companies recognized only psychotherapy as reimbursable treatment, and the attending psychiatrist often rendered many other valuable services outside of formal therapy, such as supervision of the staff, medication adjustment, and the like. The problems surrounding this controversy are as yet unresolved.[4]

Multiple forces influence the functions of the psychiatric unit in the teaching hospital. Some are external to the institution as a whole but others are internal and can be found even within the boundaries of a department of psychiatry itself. The liaison and consultation service is a frequent contender in conflicts with the psychiatric unit, as illustrated in the following example.

> A resident rotating in the liaison service saw a patient on the medical ward and found him to be depressed. He made arrangements for his transfer to the psychiatric service. When receiving the nursing report prior to the actual move of the patient, the psychiatric nursing staff learned that the patient was confined to his bed, receiving intravenous fluids and oxygen, and requiring extensive nursing care. It became clear to them that the patient's condition precluded his participation in the active treatment program of the unit. Since he was already receiving an antidepressant, it was highly unlikely that he would derive any additional therapeutic benefit from his transfer to the unit. The amount of nursing care which he required would significantly limit the time that the nurses would allocate to the other patients in the unit. The impending transfer created a conflict involving the psychiatric unit, the medical ward, and the consultation service, making it necessary for the unit director to intervene and stop the transfer while dealing with the ill feelings from the medical attending.

Conflicts over territory are quite common in general medical settings, sometimes leading to heated debates over the proper place to treat a patient who requires more nursing care than can be reasonably provided in the psychiatric unit. When such patients are maintained in the medical-surgical wards, the utilization of liaison psychiatric nurses to assist in management can be beneficial.

In addition to territorial disputes, conflicts may arise about the transfer of a patient who is receiving some "medical" procedure such as intravenous fluids or a nasogastric tube. Many psychiatric nurses have little experience with such procedures, and become alarmed at such patients. Education is the best means of dealing with these matters.

The psychiatric unit also has problems of its own. The division of labor among its multidisciplinary personnel often becomes problematic due to the conflicting needs of the different professional groups involved. Thus, the nursing staff is usually looking for professional growth, grasping at opportunities that provide new experiences and skills. Social workers in these settings are often primarily interested in teaching, supervision, and psychotherapy to the detriment of more traditional activities such as the identification and location of needed community resources. The psychiatric residents are invested in the enrichment of their clinical experience; these needs and interests often come into conflict with the need to manage patients on the ward, a task which involves interpersonal problem-solving.

Outside the boundaries of the unit, conflicts are even harder to resolve. Residents from other specialties have their own clinical interests, which may be at variance with the medical problems which arise in patients being treated in the psychiatric unit. Thus, territorial disputes may once again occur.

> An elderly man with cirrhosis of the liver and a portocaval shunt had been admitted several times to the hospital for treatment of hepatic encephalopathy. At one point he developed a major depression accompanied by delusional thinking and was transferred to a psychiatric unit. He was successfully treated with an antidepressant. As an outpatient, he was not compliant with treatment and was subsequently readmitted again because of behavioral changes characterized by marked withdrawal, mutism, and inadequate intake of food and fluids to the point of dehydration. On such occasions, the differential diagnosis between a new bout of encephalopathy and a relapse of depressive symptoms was necessary. In fact, twice in the course of his treatment within the psychiatric unit, the patient became more withdrawn and lethargic because of metabolic abnormalities which eventually required his transfer to the medical floor. On both occasions, however, several days of discussion, consultation, and negotiation between the psychiatric and the gastroenterology staff went by before an organic diagnosis was accepted and the transfer took place. The GI staff tended to view the patient's problem as a psychiatric one, while the psychiatric staff felt his difficulties to be organic.

In the above case example, it becomes clear that the medical staff were no longer interested in the patient; he was but one of many cases of hepatic encephalopathy which they had treated and offered no unique opportunity for learning.

SPECIALIZED PSYCHIATRIC UNITS IN THE GENERAL HOSPITAL

The majority of psychiatric units located in general hospitals are found in non-teaching community hospitals. By and large they can be divided into two groups. In the first are general units that accept patients over 18 years old with a wide range of diagnoses. In the second group are specialized units. A common way of achieving specialization is simply to restrict admissions to a predetermined age group. Thus, units have been designed to treat young children, only adolescents, and more recently, geriatric patients. There is no uniform agreement on a sharp delimitation of these age groups. Thus, a geriatric unit may accept patients in their late fifties while another one restricts admissions to patients in their sixties and older.

An advantage of segregating the patient population according to age is the implementation of programs that more specifically address the particular problems of that population. For example, geriatric patients are very sensitive to medications and are at greater risk for drug interactions and side effects such as orthostatic changes. These problems can be more systematically handled on a unit specializing in the care of such patients. On such wards, staff may routinely monitor patients with instruments such as brief mental status examinations designed to detect organic impairment or with procedures such as the routine taking of blood pressure in more than one position.

Similar arguments can be made to promote the cause of specialized adolescent units. Adolescents commonly feel more comfortable among their peers and often have problems with impulse control. They require limit-setting and need highly trained staff who are sensitive to these issues and can interact comfortably with this age group.

Mixed wards have their own advantages; the patient community becomes similar to society at large and to the family, where people of all ages live together. Adolescents and the elderly can derive mutual benefits from this interaction.

Psychiatric units may also become specialized through programmatic developments. This entails the systematic application of a particular approach to treatment, such as the development of a behavioral medicine program,[5] or results from the organization of a therapeutic program tailored to meet the needs of patients with a common problem, such as chronic pain, alcoholism, drug abuse, or dementia. A special program may exist within a general unit as well. Certain kinds of patients who are notoriously difficult to manage in a general psychiatric unit, like the ones suffering from anorexia-bulimia, are best handled on a specialized unit.

A more recent development in the realm of specialized units is the organization of medical-psychiatric units.[6] Patients with concomitant medical and psychiatric disorders are often managed with a great deal of difficulty on either a medical or a psychiatric setting, much as illustrated in the above examples. Medical-psychiatric units were conceptualized to treat patients with acute and multiple medical problems. These patients are usually older than the average psychiatric patient. In fact, in a report on the administrative and clinical implications of changing a psychiatric unit into a psychiatric-medical, Fogel[7] noticed the following: The average age of the patients increased from 46 to 54 years; the proportion of patients over 65 increased from 19% to 34.9%; the proportion of concurrent medical diagnosis increased from 54.7% to 69.1%; the length of stay increased from 19.3 to 23.1 days; and the average daily hospital bill increased by 24.6% compared to a hospital-wide increase of 16.3% during the same period of time. Of interest, though not easily explained, was the finding that disposition to a nursing home decreased from 10.5% to 8.9%.

THE PSYCHIATRIC UNIT IN THE COMMUNITY HOSPITAL

This is the most common type of psychiatric unit in general hospitals. Some units are operated by a closed medical staff under contract with the hospital. The hospital collects all the fees and pays the psychiatrists a salary for the performance of specific functions, which usually include diagnostic evaluations, direct treatment of a certain number of patients, and the supervision of other mental health professionals. This model sets the division of psychiatry apart from the other services, which follow a private practice model in which attending physicians treat their patients on a fee-for-service basis. To some extent, this arrangement of the division of psychiatry recapitulates problems encountered in the teaching hospitals. Staff psychiatrists, lacking other incentives, rarely stay for a long period of time. A recent survey of general hospitals in New England show that 56.9% had an open medical staff, thus enabling psychiatrists from the community to treat their patients in the hospital.[8] The mean number of beds is 21.7, with a standard deviation of 9[8]; size is determined to a large extent by characteristics of the physical plant. Unlike medical-surgical patients who spend most of their time in their own room, psychiatric patients are mobile and require a great deal of social space for large group meetings, community meals, and occupational and recreational therapy. Psychiatric units in community hospitals are usually geared towards acute, short-term treatment, with an average length of stay of around three weeks. In order to achieve the desired results within modern time constraints, they require a ratio of staff to patients which is considerably higher than in the usual public institution. The trend among the nursing staff has been heavily weighted in the direction of registered nurses. In addition, these units routinely have available the services of a psychiatric social worker and an occupational therapist.

On a typical 20-bed mixed ward, the census at any one time usually has a preponderance of depressed individuals. Recent figures available from New England[8] provide the following distribution of diagnoses in the inpatient services of general hospitals: depression—36.8%, schizophrenia—18.2%, mania and hypomania—9.4%, adjustment disorders—9.1%, and organic disorders—6%. The figure for personality disorders was 12.1%, for drug abuse and alcoholism 12.3%, and for eating disorders 3.1%. However these three categories were unevenly distributed among the places surveyed, with some hospitals specializing in the treatment of these patients and others refusing them admission.

If the psychiatric ward is openly staffed, the existence of many attendings admitting and treating patients is potentially problematic. Usually, one of the attendings takes on the role of unit director and devotes several hours a week to working with the staff in coordinating the multiple elements of inpatient treatment. Some form of therapeutic milieu is frequently maintained. Attendings typically come to the ward for only short periods of time, sufficient to see their patients. Consequently, communication is important to maintain consistency and continuity of the individualized treatment plan. The model of primary nursing is useful in this regard, as it places responsibility for coordinating patient care on the primary nurse, who then becomes the single most important element in the communication link between the attending and the ward staff.

An effective inpatient treatment program requires a great amount of organized therapeutic activity to structure the patient's day on the unit. Some form of a hall meeting or group therapy often takes place in the morning, followed by occupational therapy during the midportion of the day. Such group meetings and activities are probably the most common elements in the operation of inpatient treatment programs. The types of groups developed seems to be limited only by one's imagination, as clearly seen in a monograph by Yalom[9] on inpatient group psychotherapy.

COMMON PROBLEMS OF THE PSYCHIATRIC UNIT

The deinstitutionalization of mental patients has had an impact upon the community and teaching hospitals and their psychiatric unit. Many deinstitutionalized patients are those with chronic disorders with unremitting active symptoms or cyclic exacerbations and remissions. Some are poorly stabilized on medication or are noncompliant with drug regimens. Thus, most admissions to community hospitals are readmissions and hospital populations have acquired a large contingent of chronic patients with grave socioeconomic problems. These patients present new challenges to staff. Of necessity discharge planning has been expanded to include such items as housing for the homeless and vocational assessment and training.[10] Because of insurance limitations some patients are able to stay in the hospital only briefly, not allowing sufficient time for an extended diagnostic evaluation. The rapid turnover has taken its toll in staff burnout. Staff need to develop new ways of viewing patients as more chronic and less amenable to change, a fact mirrored in findings that research subjects in the United States are more impaired than their counterparts in Great Britain.[11]

The shorter length of stay, although originally determined by forces outside the unit, has become a factor influencing the daily work of the staff. Some patients are ill prepared for discharge by the time they run out of their insurance coverage and no one is surprised when they return to the hospital at a later date. This relationship between length of stay and readmission has been documented in studies like one from the Veterans Administration, system which found that an increase in the length of stay from 9 to 26 days was associated with a 55% reduction in the rate of rapid readmissions.[12]

The admission of involuntary patients to general hospital psychiatric units was at one time the fulcrum of heated debates,[13] but it has become much less of an emotional issue in the course of time. The original fear was that the ward milieu would be seriously disrupted by the admission of patients who were perceived as being violent and uncontrollable. Those units that elected to admit involuntary patients soon learned that they were not as a group significantly different from their other patients, and most of them actually changed their status to voluntary patients prior to their scheduled hearings.

Adolescent patients, on the other hand, are prone to create problems when admitted to units not specialized in their care.[14] Often they are rebellious and disrespectful of authority figures, act out in minor as well as serious ways, and if not firmly managed can become very disruptive of the ward milieu. To be able to treat adolescents adequately in a general psychiatric unit the staff must become well acquainted with the special needs and problems of this age group as well as with effective means of intervention and control. Also, the reasons for and the purpose of the admission need to be made even more clear than for patients in the adult age group. Nowadays, however, most adolescents are admitted to specialized units.

Patients with character disorders, specially antisocial individuals, are notoriously difficult when admitted to a general psychiatric unit. Such patients are frequently discharged quite soon after admission. Borderline personality disorders, however, are perceived to some extent as more legitimate members of the patient population and are commonly found in these settings.[15] To ensure success with these patients it is imperative that communication among the members of the treatment team be thorough and unambiguous. Consistency of approach must be maintained or the patient will manage to split the staff and disrupt their work.

Finally, it must be realized that the psychiatric unit in the general hospital is like an emergency room; acutely ill, often agitated, sometimes even aggressive patients are brought in to the hospital by family members or the police and then admitted directly to the unit. The unit thus needs to be prepared to work with rather disturbed individuals. Illustrating the fact that this is not a minor problem is the report of a six-month prospective study showing that in a general hospital psychiatric unit seclusion was used in the management of over one-third of the patients.[16] Staff needs to be well educated and adequately trained in the techniques of acute intervention, such as restraint and seclusion.

REFERENCES

1. Schulberg HC, Burns BJ: The nature and effectiveness of general hospital psychiatric services. Gen Hosp Psychiatry 1985; 7:249-257
2. Goplerud EN: Effects of proprietary management on general hospital psychiatric units. Hosp Community Psychiatry 1986; 37:832-836
3. Panzetta AF: Community Mental Health: Myth and Reality. Philadelphia, Lea & Febiger, 1971
4. McHugh PR: Reimbursement for inpatient psychiatry. The Psychiatric Times, Vol III, No. 12, December 1986
5. Moss GR, James CR: Pilot study of a behavioral medicine program in a community hospital setting. J Behav Ther Exp Psychiatry 1986; 17:3-9
6. Stoudemire A, Fogel BS: Organization and development of combined medical-psychiatric units: Part I. Psychosomatics 1986; 27:341-345
7. Fogel BS: A Psychiatric unit becomes a medical-psychiatric unit: administrative and clinical implications. Gen Hosp Psychiatry 1985; 7:26-35
8. Fogel BS, Godbout M: A snapshot of inpatient psychiatry in New England general hospitals: 1984. Hosp Community Psychiatry 1986; 37:841-843
9. Yalom ID: Inpatient Group Psychotherapy. New York, Basic, 1983
10. Cotton PG, Bene-Kociemba A, Cole R: The effect of deinstitutionalization on a general hospital's inpatient psychiatric service. Hosp Community Psychiatry 1979; 30:609-612
11. Vaughn CE, Snyder KS, Jones S, Freeman WB, Falloon IR: Family factors in schizophrenic relapse. Arch Gen Psychiatry 1984; 41:1169-1177
12. De Francisco D, Anderson D, Pantano R, Kline F: The relationship between length of stay and rapid-readmission rates. Hosp Community Psychiatry 1980; 31:196-197
13. Leeman CP et al: Should general hospitals accept involuntary psychiatric inpatients? A panel discussion. Gen Hosp Psychiatry 1981; 3:245-253
14. Molnar G, Bernardo A: Adolescents on a general hospital psychiatric unit: problems and remedies. Hosp Community Psychiatry 1981; 32:782-785
15. Adler G: The borderline patient in the general hospital. Gen Hosp Psychiatry 1981; 3:297-300
16. Schwab PJ, Lahmeyer CB: The uses of seclusion on a general hospital psychiatric unit. J Clin Psychiatry 1979; 40:228-231

4
The Forensic Hospital

Stuart B. Silver
Jose A. Gelpi

> These dens, for we can call them by no softer name, are the only remaining representatives of old Bedlam. They consist of dismal arched corridors, feebly lit at either end by a single window in double irons, and divided in the middle by gratings more like those which enclose the fiercer carnivora at the Zoological Gardens than anything we have elsewhere seen employed for the detention of afflicted humanity. (1857)[1]

The courts of our community confront vast numbers of citizens who appear mentally and behaviorally disordered. That branch of medicine which provides consultation to the courts is designated "forensic," from the Roman forum, the public square where legal and political transactions were conducted. From this noun was derived the Latin adjective *forensis* meaning public, which has become the English word forensic, relating to law court, public debate, or formal argument.[2] Forensic psychiatry addresses the interface between psychiatry and the law, where current and informed guidance is required concerning issues of mental illness or impairment.

Forensic psychiatry encompasses both civil and criminal issues. Within its domain are not only questions of trial competency and criminal responsibility, but also considerations of psychiatric impairment in connection with testamentary capacity, social security benefits, and tort claims including medical malpractice, worker's compensation, child custody, etc. Practitioners within the field familiarize themselves with applicable law, precedential court decisions at both state and federal levels, the mechanics of communicating with lawyers, and the art of testifying as expert witnesses in courts of law. A substantial volume of professional activity in this speciality is carried out in private practice, usually office-based. Many private hospitals admit patients for private forensic evaluations, especially in relation to matters of civil law.

In contrast, virtually all forensic hospitals are operated in the public sphere, usually by state government. These facilities generally limit themselves or are limited by statute to specific professional obligations required by the criminal justice system. Although usually governed by the state health or mental health authority, they are in some jurisdictions operated within the criminal justice system. The precise chain of governance is less critical to the quality of the program than is the commitment of the community and the institutional leadership.

Forensic hospitals specialize in the evaluation and treatment of patients with either a suspected or demonstrated propensity for violence or criminal behavior. Typical admissions to Clifton T. Perkins Hospital Center in Maryland during the past several months, for example, include:

K. J., a 19-year-old admitted for pretrial examination after a charge of assault with intent to murder. Formerly a psychiatric inpatient, Mr. J., while returning from an appointment at a local mental health clinic, demanded cash from a bus driver, whom he threatened with a knife. Arrested within minutes, he was transferred to the hospital from the local jail as acutely psychotic.

R. J., admitted as "not criminally responsible" after repeatedly molesting his stepdaughter. He had been on probation for a similar offense against the same child. In this case, the trial court found Mr. J. insane based upon testimony of a private psychiatrist who had diagnosed pedophilia.

Nearly every patient of a forensic facility comes referred from another community agency, most often one related to the criminal justice system. The boundaries between the forensic mental health system and the agencies to which it relates are rigidly defined in law and regulation. Formal communications occur within specified time limits between clearly defined entities concerning exact parameters of mental function in connection with identified events in accordance with explicit legal definitions. In summary, a special patient population and a highly formalized communication system set forensic facilities uniquely apart from other mental hospitals.

HISTORY

New York was the first state to provide a separate institution for insane criminals who, until 1859, had been transferred either to Utica State Hospital or to special units within the penal facilities. In that year, the State Lunatic Asylum for Insane Convicts was opened at Auburn adjoining the Auburn State Prison. Ten years later, the Auburn Asylum also began to accept insanity acquittees committed directly from the courts. Soon overcrowded, the Auburn program in 1892 was removed to Matteawan which, in turn, rapidly proved inadequate to cope with the volume of commitments. The opening of Dannemora State Hospital in 1900 relieved overcrowding, but only temporarily. Over the next half century, both physical and professional conditions at Matteawan and Dannemora deteriorated.[3,4] In 1966, the United States Supreme Court, in *Baxstrom v. Herold* ordered most of those detained at the two institutions summarily released or civilly committed to regional public mental hospitals.[5,6]

Not long after the Baxstrom decision, attorney Frederick Wiseman produced a documentary film about Bridgewater State Hospital in Massachusetts entitled "Titicut Follies." According to Slovenko,

> . . . this institution looks like a snake pit, what with its exposed pipes, naked lights, seatless toilets, peeling walls, and an atmosphere of dampness . . . people masturbating in open view on the grounds, standing on their heads, or campaigning for Fulton Sheen for President. . . . Work and recreation are almost totally nonexistent."[7]

In 1977, a Pennsylvania Grand Jury investigating Farview State Hospital found substantial evidence of records falsification, patients being beaten to death, and perjury. "In summary, we determine that the rumors concerning Farview were true. Patients were killed there and their deaths covered up."[8] Maximum security forensic hospitals had become caricatures of correctional facilities. The emphasis was on security and repression; there was little attention to either medical or psychiatric treatment.

During the past 20 years, however, there has been a concerted effort among mental health professionals and advocates to create forensic hospitals which promote health and humanity rather than violence and futility. A national linkage of state mental health forensic directors[9] has dedicated itself to this endeavor and many states have developed accredited forensic hospitals with pride rather than desolation. In 1983, the American Bar Association's Standing Committee on Association Standards for Criminal Justice issued the First Tentative Draft Criminal Justice Mental Health Standards,[10] which comprehensively addressed the need for quality and professionalism in all aspects of the cooperation of the legal and mental health systems.

Clifton T. Perkins Hospital Center, founded in 1960 in Maryland, has grown up during this new era and has struggled to move beyond accreditation towards excellence in staffing, program, and physical plant.[11,12] Many of the observations in this chapter are based upon the experiences of this facility.

MISSION

Gentlemen.
Wee herewith send you the Body of Richard Stafford, who is Distracted, & hath been very troublesome to their Ma(jes)ties Court at Kensington, By Dispersing Books & Pamphletts full of Enthusiasme and Sedition. Wee desire that you will receive him into your Hospitall of Bethlem, and to Treat Him in such manner, as is usual for Persons in his Condition, For which the Treasurer of the said Hospital shall receive the usual Allowance payable by this Board; Wee also desire that he may not be Discharged upon any Sollicitation whatsoever, untill wee be acquainted therewith. Wee remaine.

Gentlemen
Your Loving Friends
W:Forrester.
J Forbes.
Board of Greencloth
November. 4 1691[13]

Forensic mental hospitals are designed to minimize the chance of patient escape and to resist the destructive aspects of a patient's violent and assaultive behavior. Their mission, as reflected in the 17th century writ quoted above, is one of containment and treatment. Many also perform specific evaluations for the courts. A few accept responsibility for aftercare and monitoring of a patient's post-discharge condition. In some states, special statutes define particular missions, such as treating sex offenders, antisocial repeaters, or youthful offenders. While every jurisdiction provides a mechanism to accomplish most of these tasks, the specific duties assigned to the forensic facility reflect the balance of locally available outpatient and inpatient resources.

Court-ordered mental evaluation of those individuals charged with crimes forms a major component of the professional activity at many forensic hospitals. In these evaluations, any information which bears on the mental processes of the individual under examination is relevant, whether obtained from witnesses, other professionals, direct examination, or other sources. These data must be collated and scrutinized in specific relationship to the questions asked by the criminal justice system. Not only psychiatric or the exclusive product of any one discipline, the forensic evaluation draws on many professional and informational sources.

A distinguishing characteristic between forensic evaluations and traditional psychiatric evaluations is that in the latter patients seek help on their own and are interested in amelioration of problems or relief of symptoms. In forensic evaluations, patients are often participants as a result of legal strategy or involuntary commitment. Their truthfulness is variable, since malingering or lying may seem to promote their opportunities for more favorable conditions of confinement or legal outcomes. The forensic evaluator must be alert not only to efforts by the patient to appear ill, but also to efforts by psychotic patients to seem healthy in order to escape psychiatric disposition. Such efforts to "malinger health" are often more frequent and problematic than traditional forms of malingering. One of the most useful ways of detecting such manipulative attempts is comparing data obtained from multiple sources with respect to consistency. Is the story compatible with other facts of the case? Does the information obtained from witnesses correlate with the patient's version and with the clinical presentation?

> A defendant examined by one of the authors for a pretrial assessment related a clear account of his offense, life experiences, family and community relations, and previous legal entanglements. He suddenly began to talk about extremely involved auditory and visual hallucinations that grew in complexity as the examiner listened but provided no response. At the end of the hour, the defendant asked quizzically if the doctor realized that he was describing "hallucinations."

In most jurisdictions, the courts may order evaluation of either a particular defendant's *competency to stand trial* or *criminal responsibility*. These two distinct issues are sometimes called "trialability" and "legal insanity." Competency for trial consists of the defendant's current ability not only to understand the charges and their potential consequences, but also to assist in the legal defense and to cooperate with counsel.[14] An opinion about competency includes a short-term prediction through the time of the trial. The rules governing this question in Maryland are typical of the rest of the country. Competency evaluation may be sought at any time in court proceedings and may result from observations by the judge or at the request of other interested parties. A defendant's unusual behavior may prompt the judge to raise, on his own, the question of competency.

> T. M., a young adult, was ordered to the hospital after bizarre courtroom behavior. He had abruptly jumped up at the defense table, pointed his finger at the judge, and accused him of being " . . . a part

of the conspiracy." Turning to the spectators, he asserted that he was the one who would conduct the trial.

The defense attorney may question the client's ability to rationally communicate.

> A. Z., a 22-year-old male accused of shoplifting at a local discount store, was admitted for competency evaluation upon request of his lawyer. Mr. Z. had a long history of psychiatric hospitalizations in other states. A tall, very slender young man, he appeared disheveled and was withdrawn and apathetic. His communication on most occasions was incomprehensibly incoherent. Four years after his admission, the charges were stetted and he was transferred, still severely impaired, to a regional psychiatric hospital as a civil patient.

The issue of competency may also be raised for less legitimate reasons as, for example, to avoid incarceration for certain defendants to protect them from unsafe jails, to delay trial for a variety of reasons including unpreparedness of the lawyers on either side, to enact preventive detention when evidence is insufficient to convict, to document adequate representation of clients with even remote psychiatric histories, or simply to attempt to obtain treatment for those appearing ill to the court. In fact, the spurious uses of the competency evaluation probably are more frequent than the legitimate ones. Rarely is the court in genuine doubt about a defendant's competency to stand trial.

Whenever the issue is raised, the judge must determine upon testimony and evidence presented on the record, out of the presence of a jury, whether the accused is *unable to understand the nature or the object of the proceedings against him or to assist in his defense.*[15,16] Both parts of this test must be established before the accused may be brought to trial.[17] Generally, testimony is sought from a psychiatrist or other mental health professional according to the local court precedents, but the judge may make a determination without expert testimony if he chooses. The alleged incompetent person, if accused of a serious crime, is usually referred to the forensic hospital for further management.

Criminal responsibility or the plea of "not guilty by reason of insanity" generally is initiated by the defense in a petition to the court presenting some preliminary rationale. Many jurisdictions have an independent panel of mental health experts who perform the evaluation and report their findings to the court, while others refer these evaluations to the forensic hospital.

To be excused of criminal behavior, a defendant must evidence severe illness, which must be linked clearly to the offenses themselves in accordance with the legal framework supplied in the local community's "test" for "insanity." In this context, "insanity" is exclusively a legal term describing that situation of illness severe enough to satisfy the requirements of the locally accepted "test." In most of the United States, one of the following tests is required for a finding of insanity.

The M'Naghten test, formulated in 1843, has been the traditional one borrowed from English law and in use in more than half of the jurisdictions in the United States:[18]

> Every man is to be presumed to be sane, and . . . to establish a defense on the ground of insanity, it must be clearly proved that, at the time of the committing of the act, the party accused was labouring under such a defect of reason, from disease of the mind, as not to know the nature and quality of the act he was doing; or if he did know it, that he did not know he was doing what was wrong.[19]

In the 20th century, many states and the federal courts adopted the recommendation of the American Law Institute in the Model Penal Code. This formulation is usually denoted by the initials ALI:

> 1. A person is not responsible for criminal conduct if at the time of such conduct as a result of mental disease or defect he lacks substantial capacity to appreciate the criminality of his conduct or to conform his conduct to the requirements of the law.
> 2. As noted in the Article, the terms "mental disease or defect" do not include an abnormality manifested only by repeated criminal or otherwise antisocial conduct.[20]

While there are several variations on the precise wording of the tests from state to state and there are a few alternative tests which have been employed, the two cited above are the most widely used. Under the ALI test, expert witnesses are usually permitted greater latitude in presenting their reasoning than is possible under the more specific rubric of M'Naghten. A thorough discussion comparing the meanings which have been attached to these statements is beyond the scope of this chapter. Such analyses are available in several reference works.[21-24]

Although statutes clearly define legal insanity, both physicians and lawyers frequently misinterpret the issues. For example, some psychiatrists argue that if the defendant is severely mentally ill, it would be advantageous to hospitalize. The purpose of the insanity defense, however, is to excuse; there are other mechanisms to seek hospitalization for mentally ill prisoners.

> An arsonist with bipolar disorder entered a plea of insanity based upon a manic episode diagnosed by one of the authors. When first

apprehended, he had denied the offense, attributing the fire to a cigarette carelessly thrown into a wastebasket. However, he had taken his dog out of the house, as well as documents, including insurance policies, and had waited until his wife went to her job to toss the cigarette. When confronted by the fire marshall, who said that the fire had started in several areas of the house, he confessed. He then acknowledged that his fire-setting was against the law. One of the forensic psychiatrists found the defendant legally sane based upon these and other facts, in spite of the unequivocal clinical evidence of mental illness.

Other types of evaluations which may be sought from the forensic hospital include: diminished capacity, competency to understand Miranda warnings, competency for execution, death penalty mitigation, pre-sentence evaluation, sexual psychopath evaluation, dangerousness, etc. The current state of the law nationwide is regularly reviewed in the *Mental and Physical Disability Law Reporter*[25] issued since 1976 by the American Bar Association Commission on the Mentally Disabled. Virtually all forensic evaluations have some definition in local statute or regulation. When such guidance does not exist, the forensic hospital must request clarification from the court, or the Attorney General, or the requesting attorney, before undertaking the examination.

A major function of forensic hospitals is the comprehensive inpatient treatment of dangerous incompetents, insanity acquittees, mentally ill patients transferred from correctional institutions and detention centers, and those whose mental illness manifests in such a violent and aggressive manner that treatment is impossible in a less restrictive setting. Such treatment includes most traditional mental hospital modalities, but often there is emphasis on educational and vocational rehabilitation and control of behavioral expression of symptoms. Those facilities which house dangerous incompetents usually operate specialized programs which prepare patients for the intricacies of courtroom proceedings as an adjunct to their general treatment. Many forensic hospitals transfer their patients to less restrictive hospitals when aggressive symptoms have subsided, but others accept responsibility for outpatient care and follow-up.

The Clifton T. Perkins Hospital Center operates a halfway house for forensic patients at a satellite location as well as a substantial aftercare mechanism. This has been called the "five year conditional release" and constitutes a unique resource.[26] The community's representatives are notified when the patient leaves the security area for the first time, and the judge must approve all conditional release plans prior to any implementation. Insanity acquittees are afforded several opportunities for hearings on their need for continued confinement, and the hospital's opinion is represented by legal counsel. At any time during the conditional release should it appear that the aftercare plan is in danger, the patient may be taken into custody by "body attachment" and returned to the hospital. If there is good cause, the five years of monitored follow-up may be extended indefinitely.

Other duties for the forensic hospital may include education of mental health professionals in forensic psychiatry, consultation to other mental health clinics and hospitals, education of those in the criminal justice system about mental health law and practice, participation in the process of drafting law and regulation, and public relations.

ARCHITECTURE AND MILIEU

This is a long-term place. What binds people here, both patients and staff?

You might say that it is the sally port, those electric steel doors, and the masonry walls and the barred windows and the guards. When we all started working here we were massively disconcerted by being locked in. We feared that through some mysterious force of a higher power, we wouldn't be let out. In our fantasies, we thought that the entrapment would be effected by the locks and tempered steel in the windows. . . .

This fear of entrapment is an intrapsychic phenomenon. Freud's maxim was that every fear corresponds to a former wish which was now repressed. Did we inwardly desire maximum security and its attendant loss of liberty? Whenever visitors go through those gates into maximum security some invariably find humor in suggesting that members of the party may not all be released to go home again. They jokingly accuse us of warming up empty beds with unsuspecting visitors whom we hold for a variety of reasons. These jokes reflect anxiety over conflicted feelings: the fear of being locked in, and the wish for confinement. . . .

Freud attributed a heightening of the sense of guilt to a thwarted gratification of aggressive drives. It really is intriguing, when you think about it. The patients are brought here wrapped up in chains like Marley's ghost and ultimately find themselves on a wide open unit where they stay of their own volition and finally gradually leave as free men; our staff members arrive freely, with trepidation lock themselves in, and ultimately find separation from the facility a difficult and often painful move. The management of aggressive drives, either gratified through behavior or thwarted and attended by feelings of guilt, becomes a shared focus. Voluntarily and involuntarily we commit ourselves to grapple with the violence and potential destructiveness which are within us all. . . .

There is a story that the original concept for a maximum security mental facility placed the structure on Smith Island in the Chesapeake Bay. The planners of that day evidently underestimated the clout of the Eastern Shore delegation in Annapolis. Jessup was the next best idea—a Devil's Island on dry land. It was to be the place of last referral. It was not anticipated that many committed to Perkins would find their way out. When, in the early days, some did find an unauthorized way out, the wall was raised 10 feet to its present 30-foot height. The notorious cell block under ward 7 still stands, a reminder of the dungeon mentality that contributed to the design of the fortress-like structure of the old building. . . .

At the original dedication, however, the place was hailed as a humanitarian step in the management of those few mentally ill persons whose illnesses manifested in violent and aggressive acts. Open air porches, a spacious gymnasium, and large dayrooms were among the positive features. The heating system embedded in the masonry, with no radiators or ducts, was innovative but destined to become a colossal headache. . . .

The new building reflects openness to the public with large windows, open courtyards, artwork, landscaping, and improved public space. The physical intrusion of security apparatus is minimized, yet many contemporary monitoring capabilities have been built in. This openness means that the community will be directly aware not only of our successes, but also of our problems. The days of reticence are over. . . .[27]

The forensic hospital must provide a physical environment which minimizes the likelihood of patient escape, which enables safe and secure day-to-day activities for staff and patients, and which is hospitable and humane. Meeting these somewhat disparate objectives challenges the creativity, sensitivity, and professional knowledge of design groups, which may include mental health professionals, architects, engineers, and security experts. Details of structural design are weighed against each program requirement: security, safety, humane functioning for psychiatric treatment. These structural and program goals, furthermore, must be met within the limited resources usually provided by communities with conflicted feelings about the populations to be served. Most such institutions are identified as "maximum security." Traditionally, this designation means masonry construction of walls, roofs and decks, detention windows and screens, relatively impenetrable perimeter, and access and egress monitored through a single, guarded, double-doored "sally port."

The security perimeter may consist of a wall, fence, or the skin of the building itself. Control of movement across the defined perimeter rests in the sally port, which must itself be physically secure. In some hospitals, the sally port construction is virtually impregnable. No one passes through the sally port without positive identification and proper authorization. A cardinal responsibility of the forensic hospital is the secure containment of those committed there. The close supervision of all traffic afforded the facility by a well operated sally port ensures proper custody.

Uninterrupted operation of the sally port is the duty of the security department of most forensic hospitals. In contrast to traditional psychiatric hospitals, forensic facilities have a well developed, uniformed security force responsible not only for the sally port, but also for corridor security, riot and hostage control, transportation, perimeter surveillance, often fire safety, and monitoring of any specialized security apparatus the facility may deploy. This department may require police academy training for its officers, in addition to their general in-house orientation. In some hospitals, security officers are assigned military rank similar to a police force. The relationship of the security department to the clinical departments of the facility is usually problematic. The needs of custody and security do not always mesh with the needs of the treatment programs for flexibility. Both needs are vital, however, and can only be achieved through close collaboration among the hospital's departments. Neglect of either set of needs and responsibilities may be disastrous.

A survey of forensic hospitals throughout the country revealed that none permitted weapons within the perimeter.[28] Most prohibit any armed staff. Frequently, patients are brought to the facility by armed guards who must check their weapons at the sally port. Contraband includes weapons, knives, razors, and other metallic objects that may be fashioned into dangerous implements. Such items are controlled by sensitively calibrated metal detectors through which patients and visitors must pass. In many facilities, staff also is cleared for entry by the same process.

> Three "shanks" were confiscated from a patient within a week. He made each of them with a large straightened paper clip and used rags from clothing as the handle.

> W. B. was transferred periodically from prison to the hospital. He would usually bring a razor blade hidden in his pharynx.

It is an open question whether weapons promote secure transport, but most forensic hospitals which undertake this obligation instead use restraints applied to the patient's extremities to provide a physical deterrent. Another area in which controversy exists is the physical location of staff offices. In some facilities, all personnel spend their entire day within the perimeter, while in others offices are on both sides. Often the structure of the building housing the unit, rather than any preordained program plan, determines this question. The quality of the institutional program is enhanced by a high volume of staff traffic in all parts of the facility during as many shifts as possible.

Within the facility, movement of patients and staff may be relatively similar to that in other psychiatric hospitals. Some patients may be permitted to sign out of their units and move unescorted, others may be secluded, while many may be permitted movement only in a supervised group. Some facilities rely more heavily on internal locked doors than do others. The sally port renders attempts by patients to get staff keys relatively futile. No staff member carries a key which would permit exit from the secure perimeter. There are many methods and gadgets which enhance internal security, including paging systems with microphonic monitors, radio telecommunication, telephone alarm mechanisms, television monitors, electrically supervised and operated door locks, personal security systems, motion detectors, and sharp-eyed staff who remain sensitive to security issues. Design of security systems for custody facilities has become technologically sophisticated and many consultants populate the field, but there is no substitute for a competent, sensitive, alert, and caring hospital staff.

A particular method of maintaining safety is the "shakedown." Borrowed from detention facilities, this operation is usually conducted by security personnel. A defined ward area or the entire facility is carefully searched while the patients are retained in a particular area. The search is thorough and time-consuming; it is unannounced and, with luck, unexpected. The "contraband" sought includes weapons, illicit drugs, hoarded prescription drugs, money (usually not permitted in forensic hospitals), matches (wall-mounted lighters are available), and other items identified at the facility as potentially hazardous.

Increasingly, forensic hospitals are developing the capability to provide less restrictive environments than the maximum security facility characterized above. For example, the pre-release unit at Perkins, located outside the perimeter, is always unlocked, and the patients are granted free movement. They hold jobs in the community and have weekend home visits. However, this unit is only available to patients adjudicated "not criminally responsible by reason of insanity." Patients transferred from prison remain within the perimeter until they are ready for return; civil transfers return to their facility of origin. Some facilities identify themselves as medium security. Such a designation suggests locked-door units without sally port control and lighter-duty construction of the building. These characterizations may have more definition in prison construction than in the design of forensic psychiatric hospitals.

Whatever the level of security, the forensic hospital must strive to provide as humane a ward environment as possible. Modern materials and lighting can create lively and inviting program and residential space without compromising security. Planning for renovation of the maximum security area at Clifton T. Perkins Hospital Center envisions increased patient privacy, opportunities for small group meetings, and no more than four patients in each bedroom. Coinless telephones which reverse charges permit 24-hour access. The living quarters in the new medium security building at Perkins are decorated with functional furniture, colorful bedspreads, and cheerful art-work. A kitchenette and a laundry room equipped with washing machine and dryer are available on each 20-bed ward. These efforts enhance patient dignity and, therefore, will augment the power and effectiveness of the therapeutic program.

PROGRAMMING

> Two dualities of clinical work often lead to misunderstandings between medicine and law. They are the notion of ambivalence and the notion of alliance. These two clinical entities have one thing in common that contrasts them with the adversary system. The adversary system has one separate representative (attorney) presenting *each* side of the case, a total of two people. In contrast, the "two sides" of both ambivalence and alliance reside within the *same* person.[79]

Referrals to forensic hospitals are usually prearranged and admissions should be scheduled according to priorities based on medical need. Usually patients referred by physicians in pretrial detention facilities or commitments by local emergency room physicians of those arrested by the police receive preference. Less pressing are the requests for transfer of patients from other hospitals or from prisons, as these facilities generally have better treatment capabilities than jails or police lockups. Patients committed for court-ordered evaluation generally are the least pressing medically, but in many jurisdictions competency evaluation orders are employed more frequently to gain access to treatment services than to answer forensic questions.

Admissions to forensic hospitals are partially under court control. There is, however, variability from state to state in the degree to which medical control may be exerted. Wherever possible, procedures should favor an admission sequence determined by medical needs, strict adherence to licensed or program capacity, prompt removal of patients who no longer require inpatient services, and expedited evaluation of inappropriate admissions. To this end, some states have initiated community-based outpatient forensic evaluations to minimize unnecessary usage of hospital beds. The forensic hospital must not become the annex of the detention center, nor should it be permitted to succumb to inappropriate demands of the criminal justice system.

Until individuals arrive at the hospital, they are under the custody of the transporting agency. A critical first step in the admissions process is the validation of the documents accompanying the patient. Are the civil certificates properly completed? Is the court order signed? Do the identifying documents correspond with the papers authorizing the admission? In each jurisdiction, the relevant questions may vary, but in forensic settings there is no room for error in this process of verifying the propriety of the admission. In many instances, the remedy for breach of process is to discharge the patient into the community or to return seriously ill individuals to correctional settings lacking treatment resources.

The exchange of custody of the patient occurs in a secure location. The sally port is usually selected as the site where hospital staff accepts responsibility for the care and safety of the patient. At this phase of management, a structural barrier must exist to prevent escape. At no time in the admissions process should staff become the only barrier in a pathway out of physical custody. Patients must not be tempted to behave in any way which could result in injury. Therefore, shackles and other physical restraints are not removed before the first sally port door. However, it is equally imperative that the notion of care, humanity, and treatment orientation be communicated expeditiously. For this reason, removal of physical restraints by the transporting officials under the direction of hospital nursing personnel is recommended as soon as possible. After crossing the sally port, the patient enters the security area and is taken to the admission suite. The message of hospitality should already have been conveyed by the staff and the hospital environment. The admissions process either can be one of the most volatile operations in the patient's care or can set a positive atmosphere for the balance of the patient's course in the hospital. In a forensic hospital, the management of this process is of paramount concern.

During the admission phase, the patient is physically searched, showered, examined, advised of rights, and furnished with the hospital patient's manual. The patient's possessions are inventoried and stored. Hospital clothes are issued and basic data are collected. Initial observations and reports of the transporting officers are recorded. The patient is prepared for assignment to the admissions ward. Calm and experienced staff members who can relate well and inspire confidence are assigned to handle these procedures.

After the patient's admission, a comprehensive evaluation follows. This usually consists of a psychiatric admission workup; a physical examination; psychological, nursing, and social work assessments; laboratory tests, and other examinations as indicated by either the patient's condition or the nature of the court order. Unique, however, to the forensic hospital, at all junctures of the evaluation, is the availability of the results to outside agents. Therefore, the patient should be advised repeatedly of the limits of confidentiality of the particular evaluation process. The evaluation is generally available to the judge, the defense attorney, and the opposing counsel. Other unique aspects of the evaluation are the need to obtain police reports, legal histories, and "rap sheets," and to meet the specific time constraints imposed by statute. All records of prior medical and psychiatric treatment and hospitalization are to be scrutinized. While such records might be of limited clinical usefulness to a physician treating a current illness, the evaluator's failure to fully review or otherwise account for past medical records can lead to humiliating cross-examination in court and the appearance of carelessness, no matter how irrelevant the records may have been to the opinions expressed.

The forensic psychiatric examination differs from the non-forensic in several fundamental aspects. First, before any interview is begun, the patient is advised that a report will be rendered to the court and attorneys. Second, the objective of the evaluation is to answer very narrowly defined questions of competency or criminal responsibility rather than to define treatment goals. Third, the examination must be completed within specified timeframes. Fourth, in the case of responsibility, the evaluation has the specific goal of determining the patient's state of mind at a time in the past when the crime allegedly occurred. The patient's behaviors, activities, functioning, relationships, and occupational performance at a time in the past must be discovered by an investigative process, drawing on many sources, and a coherent psychological formulation must emerge by reconstruction. Reports by the defendant's family, eyewitnesses, the victim, coworkers and others are as relevant and revealing as the mental status examination itself. Subsequently, a formal staff conference takes place at which such reports are reviewed, the patient is interviewed, the staff deliberates, and an opinion is rendered to the court. This conference culminates the evaluation. A written summary of the conference will reveal the findings of those legally empowered to render opinions, but the final letter to court will reflect the majority opinion, which will become the hospital's "official" position. The language used to express the evaluator's findings is directed towards lay fact-finders rather than towards mental health professionals and must be clear and understandable.[30]

Although the final forensic evaluation report is usually the product of a multidisciplinary collaboration, the mechanism by which a forensic hospital communicates its findings is formalized and usually the responsibility of one individual. Consistency, clarity, comprehensiveness, and conformity with statutory requirements and language are the hallmarks of the forensic hospital report. All legally required questions must be addressed in terms that are legally sufficient. Ambiguity must be eliminated. In order to insure the quality of the format of its correspondence, the forensic hospital carefully constructs the sequence of its letters to the court and adheres to that format unswervingly.

Treatment within a secure setting preserves many of the aspects of traditional psychiatric programming. In the past, it was apparent that inpatient treatment of the legally insane was considered futile. The experience at Perkins and other modern hospitals dictates otherwise. In spite of the twofold goal of amelioration of illness and protection of society, the resistance and aggressiveness of the clientele, and the restrictiveness of the institutional setting, substantive treatment activities flourish and clinical progress occurs. As in other situations where patients may be involuntarily treated, forensic hospitals must cope with "due-process" hearings, "medication review" panels, "least restrictive" alternatives, ombudsmen and advocates, as well as a variety of judicial and nonjudicial hearings on continued treatment, forced treatment, and "dangerousness." Individualized treatment planning, treatment team collaboration, and increasing levels of individual freedom of movement are features shared with non-forensic inpatient programs.

The program structure at Perkins is designed to exert a favorable influence throughout patients' stays. Patients are assigned team leaders with whom they interact on a daily basis. The presence of all team members on the ward tends to strengthen patients' confidence in the stability of their milieu. Chemotherapy remains a significant cornerstone of clinical treatment, as most patients' diagnoses are in the schizophrenic spectrum. To avoid hoarding and facilitate compliance monitoring, administration of medication by oral concentrate is preferred on maximum security wards. Individual and group therapies are furnished by any member of the multidisciplinary professional staff who has been privileged by the medical staff and approved by the clinical director. Choice of a particular therapist is based upon clinical indications and the staff member's availability. The main type of psychotherapy offered is supportive rather than analytic and is directed toward strengthening defenses rather than personality reconstruction. Significant therapeutic tasks include the development of insight and awareness of the illness and its destructive potential, recognition of signs of relapse, and realistic assessment of future career options.

Group therapies focus on here-and-now interactions and are directed towards improved reality-testing and behavioral awareness and modification through group validation. Specialized or homogeneous group therapies focus on patients who share certain commonalities, including sexual offenders, passive males, aggressive males, physically sluggish males, incompetents, convicted felons transferred from prison, etc. These groups generally have specific goals and may employ didactic methods as well.

Family therapy is increasingly utilized. Studies at Perkins have suggested that the presence of a family support network promotes favorable outcome when measured by criminal recidivism.[31] Patients in a maximum security hospital often experience a sense of isolation engendered by their family's emotional and physical distance. Often they are met with outright rejection, particularly when their violence was directed at family members. Efforts to bridge this gap are often clinically rewarding.

Most of the treatment modalities used at Perkins are consistent with general psychiatric hospital programming. Nevertheless, the maximum security facility retains certain unique characteristics. Most of its patients have committed acts of violence and have the potential to repeat such behavior. It is critically important to retain for treatment particularly those patients whose violence is associated with substantial mental illness. Management of their violent propensities may be facilitated by treatment efforts addressing the patient's psychiatric condition. Initially, the hospital supplies external controls to compensate for the patient's internal disorganization. The tight environment, rehearsing of the rules and regulations, antipsychotic medication, the presence of a security force, an alert and sensitized staff, and a formidable seclusion room are all features which enhance the patient's sense of externally sufficient control and which may serve to reduce tension. The use of seclusion, restraints, involuntary medication, and security staff intervention is, as in any hospital, controlled by written policies and procedures. Patients are aware of their right to refuse treatment and frequently they refuse psychotropic medication. In emergent situations, the physician may override the patient's refusal for up to 72 hours, but otherwise, a clinical review panel is assembled which may institute or recommend forcing medication against the patient's will. Such decisions are based upon considerations of the patient's dangerousness to self or others. In some cases external guardians may be sought through the court as alternative decision-makers about treatment issues.

Additionally, the assessment of "dangerousness" assumes increased significance for the clinical staff of the forensic hospital. One of the institution's most important responsibilities in treating mentally disordered offenders is recommending their discharge from the hospital. Professional judgment about their dangerousness or degree of unpredictability is a critical clinical function. While many studies have shown that mental health personnel do not accurately predict dangerous acts,[32,33] assessment of dangerousness may be conceptualized as more indicative of a potentiality than predictive of an event. Most forensic hospitals have evolved a system by which the patient's environment is gradually expanded and his behavioral options increased. In the patient's movement from a tightly monitored admissions unit to a less severely restricted residential unit, both the patient and the staff of the hospital are afforded increasingly open opportunities for the discovery of each other's degree of predictability. In this manner the sense of danger becomes modified by actual experience shared by patient and staff.

Acts of violence within the hospital are not infrequent. In addition to clinical management, review and analysis of such incidents, it has been the policy of Perkins to report to the State Police assaultive behavior of significance. Although sometimes frustrated by the limited priority assigned to intramural problems by the police, staff nevertheless believe that a police investigation tends to diminish violence within the institution and promote a clear message that assaultiveness is not condoned. Patients found "not criminally responsible" in relation to a certain criminal act are thereby reminded that they remain responsible for their behavior otherwise.

W. B., a 36-year-old male, was admitted pursuant to physician's certificates from the prison. During the admission psychiatric examination, Mr. B. severely battered the doctor, who required sutures and was subsequently unable to return to work for three weeks. The physician pressed charges. Mr. B. was brought to trial, convicted, and sentenced to three additional years in prison consecutive to the time he was currently serving.

The degree of remission of illness and reduction in violent potential which the professional staff of a forensic hospital accepts as sufficient for a patient's release to the community is substantial.[34] The risk of premature discharge militates against a liberal discharge policy. In fact, there is increasing recognition of the need for closely supervised outpatiency for this class of mentally ill patients, as illustrated by the creation of the "psychiatric security review board" in Oregon.[35,36]

Another unique aspect of the treatment program is the need for secure escort of patients outside the facility. Forensic hospitals have developed procedures for the transportation of patients to courts, other specialty treatment facilities, and occasionally funerals of close family members. These methods utilize physical restraints and avoid the use of sidearms or other weapons. Usually the patient is escorted by both security and nursing personnel. It is helpful to maintain radio contact between the hospital and transport unit. Whenever a forensic patient is off-grounds, at least two staff members should be in attendance. The time of greatest risk for escape and potential harm to the community or the patient is during movement or treatment outside the security area of the hospital.

Another critical element of forensic hospital programming is the development of procedures governing the control of internal disturbances or riots. The facility must also elaborate a procedure for the management of hostage situations. There should be mechanisms for media information and the identification of a public information office when necessary. Direct communication linkages with the police and fire department are recommended. All such mechanisms must be rehearsed, evaluated, and refined regularly. The institution must have the capability of responding to serious trouble while simultaneously maintaining reasonable care and custody. A particular area of difficulty is evacuation of patients. While all hospitals call fire drills periodically on each shift, few remove patients from the building. The forensic hospital is usually hampered in the evacuation process by the very elements of security that interdict elopement. Therefore, total timed evacuations of both patients and personnel are to be carried out, analyzed, and perfected. Forensic facilities characteristically provide a secure outdoor space, well removed from the hospital structure, which can accommodate all patients and staff in the event of fire or other disaster. Few facilities have developed workable mechanisms for the removal of patients geographically in the event of an external disaster, although this risk is not inconceivable. Preparedness for a variety of crises is an ever present demand weighing particularly heavily upon the forensic hospital.

FUTURE TRENDS

Performing forensic mental evaluations of violent sexual offenders is demanding and at times terrifying work. The emotional stresses on the examiner in collecting the data, confronting and evaluating the accused, facing the tension of the courtroom, and working in forsaken dungeons are only rivalled by the strain of containing the extreme countertransference forces engendered. The offenses are sordid and repugnant; the defendants are often aggressive and hostile. One's own inner emotional forces become powerfully aroused and threatening. The clinician, trained to attempt empathizing with his patient, may experience self-revulsion. It is important, therefore, that those in the field work together, share their experience, and provide group support. The importance of some institutional setting, such as a hospital, court clinic, or university clinic, providing multidisciplinary resources cannot be overemphasized in this context. The work, while trying, absorbs clinicians of many backgrounds in its challenge. The boundaries of knowledge in the behavioral sciences are closely scrutinized and public policy is shaped as mental health workers explore this interface with the law.[37]

Increasingly, forensic services are conceptualized not as facility-based, but rather as statewide programs. The court-ordered evaluations, which formerly occupied a substantial portion of the hospitals' energies, are rendered locally or regionally in outpatient settings. Forensic hospitals have become more treatment oriented; instead of being the hub, they have become one of the spokes in a comprehensive and coherent array of state forensic services.

As the forensic facility's mission has changed, the relative influence of security and therapy on program design has found a new balance. Administrators have turned towards the Joint Commission on Accreditation of Hospitals for standards. Additionally, they have worked toward modification of standards in order to accommodate the unique aspects of forensic programming, such as the partial control of admissions and discharges by the court.

Part of the impetus for these advances has been increased public advocacy for patients' rights and also deinstitutionalization of patients from general psychiatric hospitals. Whether coincidental or not, the demand by the criminal justice system for mental health services has grown substantially in many jurisdictions.[38] A new responsibility of the forensic hospital will be to identify those who more properly should be served in non-forensic programs and assist the courts in diverting these patients to other treatment agencies. Forensic psychiatrists will participate in drafting legislation and articulating regulations to facilitate professionally acceptable treatment in the least restrictive settings possible.

An area which will receive more attention is professional liability. The patients in forensic hospital are often experienced in many aspects of the legal system; "jailhouse lawyers" abound. The professional decisions often have enormous consequences for the individual patients, who are frequently extremely litigious. Not only are staff members more exposed to malpractice litigation, but administrators are also vulnerable to suits suggesting misconduct in their supervisory obligations. These pressures will encourage communities to offer enhanced support to the professional staff and leadership of forensic hospitals in coping with this increased liability exposure.

In the past, outside review of procedures and practices of forensic hospitals was largely nonexistent. The advocacy which has permeated all mental hospitals has moved into the forensic institution as well. As a result, patient grievance systems are being implemented and staff members are being identified as in-house patient advocates. These trends are amplified by legal service organizations sanctioned to establish a presence within the hospitals. Any tendency of a forensic hospital to slip towards nontherapeutic or inhumane practices will be vigorously challenged and publicized.

Ethical dilemmas abound in forensic practice, but nowhere are they more vexing than in association with the community's execution of the death penalty. The recent Supreme Court ruling in *Ford v. Wainwright* potentially creates a new category of patients "incompetent to be executed."[39-41] Are they to be treated and restored to "competency"? Do they have a "right to refuse" treatment? How often may they be found incompetent? Who will do the psychiatric evaluations? Where? These are the challenges for the near future. As our knowledge increases, the ethical quandries will multiply further.

In this new climate, a well-trained clinical staff will become essential for institutional survival. Forensic hospitals will develop careful mechanisms to check the credentials of all professional staff. An orderly and formalized process will be instituted to assign staff privileges. Specialized topics such as forensic evaluation, management of the assaultive patient, fire safety, etc., will become the focus of reemphasized inservice staff training efforts. Around the country, post-residency fellowships in forensic psychiatry are increasing in number. The American Academy of Psychiatry and the Law, an organization of forensic psychiatrists established in 1969, has not only promoted the development of these post-doctoral programs, but also supported the creation of a specialty board in the field. Forensic subspecialty components are forming in psychology, social work, and psychiatric nursing. All these activities will produce more committed and competent professionals to continue in the exciting and pioneering work at the professional interface between law and psychiatry.

REFERENCES

1. Allderidge PH: Criminal insanity: Bethlehem to Broadmoor. Proc R Soc Med 1974; 67:897-904
2. Webster's New World Dictionary. New York, Simon & Schuster, 1980
3. Slovenko R: Psychiatry and Law. Boston, Little, Brown, 1973, p. 111
4. Mikkelson EJ: The Bridgewater 100: an analysis of admissions to a hospital for the criminally insane. Psychiatr Q 1980; 52:190-200
5. Baxstrom v. Herold, 383 US 107, 1966
6. Steadman HJ, Keveles G: The community adjustment and criminal activity of the Baxstrom patients. Am J Psychiatry 1972; 129:304-310
7. Slovenko R: Psychiatry and Law. Boston, Little, Brown, 1973, p. 110
8. Rawls W: Cold Storage. New York, Simon & Schuster, 1980
9. State Mental Health Forensic Directors (SMHFD), a division of National Association of State Mental Health Program Directors (NASMHPD), Washington, DC
10. American Bar Association: First Tentative Draft Criminal Justice Mental Health Standards. Washington, DC, 1983
11. Spodak M, Silver SB, Wright C: Criminality of discharged insanity acquittees: fifteen year experience in Maryland reviewed. Bull Am Acad Psychiatry Law 1984; 12:373-382
12. Goldmeier J et al: A halfway house for mentally ill offenders. Am J Psychiatry 1977; 134:45-49
13. Allderidge PH: Criminal insanity: Bethlehem to Broadmoor. Proc R Soc Med 1974; 67:897
14. McGarry L et al: Handbook, Competency to Stand Trial and Mental Illness. Rockville, Md, NIMH, 1973
15. Hill v. State, 35 Md App 98, 369 A 2d 98, 1977
16. Raithel v. State, 280 Md 291, 372 A 2d 1069, 1977
17. Dusky v. United States 362 US 402, 1960
18. Stone AA: Mental Health & Law: A System in Transition. New York, Jason Aronson, 1976
19. Daniel M'Naghten's Case, 10 Clark & Fin 200, 8 Eng Reprint 718, 1843
20. American Law Institute, Model Penal Code, Proposed Official Draft, sec. 4.01, 1962
21. Silver SB: Criminal responsibility: a psychiatric point of view, in Violent Behavior, Vol 1. Edited by Hertzberg L, et al, New York, Spectrum, 1985
22. Sauer RH, Mullens P: The insanity defense: M'Naughten vs Ali. Bull Am Acad Psychiatry Law 1976; 11:73-75
23. Silver SB, Spodak MK: Dissection of the prongs of A. L. I. Bull Am Acad Psychiatry Law 1983; 11:383-391
24. Finagrette H, Hasse AF: Mental disabilities and Criminal Responsibility. Berkeley, University of California Press, 1979

25. Mental and Physical Disability Law Reporter. Publisher, Commission on the Mentally Disabled, American Bar Association, Washington, DC
26. Weiner BA: Not guilty by reason of insanity: a sane approach. Chicago-Kent Law Review 1980; 56:1057–1085
27. Silver SB: Reflections. Delivered at the dedication of the Medium Security Building, Clifton T Perkins Hospital Center, Jessup, Maryland, 1985
28. Kerr CA, Roth JA: A Study of Facilities and Programs for Mentally Disordered Offenders. Washington, WESTAT Corporation, 1983
29. Gutheil TG, Magraw R: Ambivalence, alliance, and advocacy: misunderstood dualities and psychiatry and law. Bull Am Acad Psychiatry Law 1984; 12:51–58
30. Silver SB, Spodak M: Forensic mental evaluation of the violent sexual offender, in The Sexual Aggressor. Edited by Greer JG, Stuart IR. New York, Van Nostrand Reinhold, 1983
31. Madden DJ: A followup study of sixty-five mentally ill offenders on convalescent leave. Unpublished, 1978
32. American Psychiatric Association: Clinical Aspects of the Violent Individual. Washington, DC, 1974
33. Monahan J: The Clinical Prediction of Violent Behavior. Rockville, Md, NIMH, 1981
34. Silver, SB: Treatment and aftercare for insanity acquittees in Maryland. Testimony before the Subcommittee on Criminal Law of the Committee on the Judiciary, United States Senate, USGPO. Washington, 1983, Serial No. J-97-122:374–383
35. Bloom JL, Bloom JD: Disposition of insanity defense cases in Oregon. Bull Am Acad Psychiatry Law 1981; 9:93–99
36. Roth L et al: Insanity Defense Work Group, American Psychiatric Association Statement on the Insanity Defense. Am J Psychiatry 1983; 140:681–688
37. Silver SB, Spodak MK: op. cit., p. 60–61
38. Steadman H et al: Explaining the increased crime rate of mental patients: the changing clientele of state hospitals. Am J Psychiatry 1978; 135:816–820
39. *Ford v. Wainwright*, 477 US XX, 91 L Ed 2d 335, 106 S Ct XX, (No. 85-5542), 1986
40. Salguero RG: Medical ethics and competency to be executed. Yale Law J 1986; 196:167–186
41. Radelet ML, Barnard GW: Ethics and the psychiatric determination of competency to be executed. Bull Am Acad Psychiatry Law 1986; 14:37–53

II
The Admissions Process

5
The Psychiatric Emergency Room

Andrew Edmund Slaby
Mary Eileen McNamara

Nowhere in the trajectory of psychiatric care is as much expertise immediately demanded and required as in the practice of emergency psychiatry. For many individuals, it is the first contact with psychiatry and the contact determines their subsequent trajectory of care. For many nonpsychiatric physicians, it is the most or only visible component of the psychiatric care system. Emergency psychiatric service may be a source of help and relief to patients and general nonpsychiatric staff alike or a cause of great frustration and disappointment. For the medical community at large, and psychiatric community in specific (including psychiatric hospitals, community mental health centers and private clinicians), the quality of emergency psychiatric care either promotes harmony and cooperation or causes disruption and ill-will.

Recent social and economic changes have enhanced the importance of emergency psychiatric care. Deinstitutionalization and shorter hospital stays in general have increased the population of chronically psychotic patients in the community requiring service. Limited availability of psychiatric beds and pressures to avoid hospitalization when possible increase demands on emergency personnel for thorough evaluation and outpatient crisis-oriented

---

Mr. Ari Solomon helped in identifying literature relevant to this chapter.

treatment. Finally, increased personal and medical awareness of the importance of psychological well-being and the medico-legal implication of neglecting such issues have increased emergency psychiatric referrals. Ideally, an emergency treatment area is designed to allow evaluation and care of patients in an atmosphere that calms psychological pain and enhances a patient's sense of dignity, while at the same time providing competent medical intervention and protecting against threats of violence.

In practice, psychiatric ER's differ widely in structure and offered services. A disconcerting number of "emergency services" in psychiatry consist solely of an on-call social worker or nurse either stationed in a hospital or available via telephone, who evaluates referrals in any available nook and cranny of the emergency room. In some instances an emergency room physician untrained in psychiatry is available for "back up," while in many free-standing psychiatric hospitals a psychiatric resident, independent of any real attending supervision and without rapid access to medical assistance, "supervises" emergency services. The potential for error, mismanagement and catastrophe in such systems is evident, and such disasters are not rare. In the past, psychiatric emergency services could "bury their mistakes," as patients and families were reluctant to admit to psychiatric care, and as the general cultural view of psychiatry was that little could be done at best. Such views are happily changing, and with this change there has also been increased public and legal insistence on competent care, as the rising number of malpractice suits attests.

STRUCTURAL REQUIREMENTS

Ideally, an emergency treatment area is designed to allow evaluation and care of patients and their families in an atmosphere that contributes to the calming of psychological pain and enhances patients' sense of dignity. Because the optimum circumstances for interviewing depressed and anxious patients differ from those required for restraint of violent patients, at least two emergency psychiatric rooms are necessary: an interview room and a seclusion room. Even given such, there is always uncertainty as to problems presented by new patients. In approximately 60% of patients who are or will become violent, it is immediately obvious that restraints are required.[1] In the other 40%, violence erupts only after evaluation has begun. Therefore, interview rooms and seclusion rooms do have common requirements. Both rooms should be free of anything patients may use to cause harm to self or others. Rooms should have no breakable glass. Pictures, ashtrays and windows should be composed of plexiglass or similar plastic-like substances. Cords and ropes (including wires for lamps and telephone cords) should be of minimum length. Medications and sharp objects such as needles are stored elsewhere, as are objects prone to theft, such as prescription pads. In general, emergency psychiatric rooms are as barren as possible. Creative use of color and fabric promotes a sense of calm and provides an ambience that promotes respect of patients and staff alike.

Two doors are recommended for every room. If there is only one exit, it can be blocked by a patient in the event of an assault upon a clinician. If to avoid this a clinician sits by the door (a strategy that may not work anyway), patients may become more agitated and feel trapped themselves. Two doors opening outward solves both problems by allowing escape of both. Doors should be able to be unlocked from either side. One or more alarm buttons placed in each room enhance the safety of a clinician who may be abruptly assaulted. Rooms should be located to allow other staff and security guard access if required.

Maximum confidentiality of information provided by patients and other informants is provided by care to acoustics in construction of walls, doors, and floor coverings. Rooms are optimally designed to allow several people to be seated comfortably. Evaluations may require that a family of six or a similar number of police, clergy, or hospital personnel are seen together. Sofas are less likely to become weapons or assaultive trajectories than chairs; therefore, the former are preferred to the latter.

Seclusion rooms, where safety of patients and clinicians is of paramount importance, have more elaborate requirements. Restraints of proper quality and specifications must be available. Leather restraints are the preferred mode of physical control.[2] Posey belts and velcro limb restraints are ineffective with the combative patient. Patients may become easily entangled in jacket binders and improvised restraints of gauze, elastic bandages and sheeting. When used on struggling patients, cloth binding becomes twisted and can lead to limb ischemia and strangulation.

Emergency staff must be educated in appropriate indications for and application of physical restraints without injury to either patient or clinician. Physical restraints are required where there is risk of imminent physical harm from explosive behavior and/or where pharmacological methods are either ineffective or contraindicated. Patients may be appropriate for restraints but not for seclusion. Violent patients with concomitant medical problems, such as combative elderly patients with renal failure, require restraint to prevent them from harming themselves accidentally, but should not be out of range of observation since immediate intervention may be required. All areas where patients are restrained or in seclusion should be in staff view. Records must be kept of the rationale for restraints and precautions taken. This includes frequent monitoring of vital signs. Just as a patient's potential for a behavioral emergency may not be immediately obvious on admission, potential exists for the emergence of an unexpected medical catastrophe. Examples include unheralded first myocardial infarctions in middle-aged men, the onset of coma and hypotension from unreported overdoses, and hypoglycemia from missed meals in unknown diabetics.

Restraints should be frequently checked for integrity and rotated on a regular schedule. Necessity for continued restraint should be reevaluated and documented frequently.

Any emergency psychiatric service, whether in a public, general, or private psychiatric hospital, or in an HMO, should have equipment available to institute cardiopulmonary resuscitation and other emergency measures. This includes at minimum a stethoscope, oxygen and Ambu bag, a sphygmomanometer, an IV setup with several different kinds of intravenous solutions, a cardiac monitor and/or EKG, and emergency medications such as parenteral glucose (D5O). All personnel should be trained in cardiopulmonary resuscitation and regular drills should be scheduled. Appropriate methods to summon further assistance, such as an ambulance to a private psychiatric hospital or the "CPR team" to the psychiatric section of a general emergency room, should be known to all.

Medications for psychiatric emergencies should be available. This includes medication for dystonic reactions such as Cogentin, Benadryl, or Symmetrel, and a stock of neuroleptics for emergency use. Optimally, representatives of both high potency agents such as Navane and Haldol and low potency sedating agents such as Thorazine or Mellaril are included. Antianxiety agents to calm acute panic are also desirable. Short-acting drugs allowing more precise titration and lessening the danger of unwitting overdose are desired. These would include Ativan and Xanax.

It is an administrative decision whether the emergency psychiatry service provides other medications. Those available vary from setting to setting. Health maintenance organizations provide medications in emergency settings for clients who have run out of a prescription. General hospitals may wish to provide medications to destitute patients. Others refer patients to 24-hour pharmacies. Other health care facilities may require that the clinician or agency that is following the patient long-term be the only source of prescriptions, both to provide continuity of care as well as to guard against the occasional patient who "shops" from emergency service to emergency service for medications.

Administrative decisions should also be made about whether to provide holding beds for extended evaluations. Holding beds for 24 to 72 hours reduces cost of care by minimizing need for further hospitalization but places demands on an emergency service for meals, staffing, and room.

STAFFING

Ideal staffing for an emergency psychiatric service is contingent upon its agenda and its patient population. Large inner-city emergency rooms see a high number of patients with alcohol and drug abuse, schizophrenia and other psychotic disorders, referred by police and often violent. State psychiatric hospitals, which are often at some distance from major cities, most commonly see chronic patients referred and triaged by local mental health centers. The general hospital emergency rooms of suburbia and smaller towns may see a very diverse patient population of teenagers with substance abuse and/or depression, alcoholic executives, cocaine users, geriatric patients who have attempted suicide, rape victims, young adults with new-onset schizophrenia or manic psychosis, and families in crisis because of unplanned pregnancy, financial disaster, and a legion of other problems.

Moreover, psychiatric emergency rooms see a broader spectrum of patients than desirable because of the confusion that exists in the general public as to the province of psychiatry.

> A 45-year-old schizophrenic, mildly retarded woman presented to the free-standing emergency room of a psychiatric hospital. When interviewed by the resident, she said, "My doctor said if I have any problems come here. So I brought my son here 'cause he sounds funny." The resident ran out to the unattended waiting room where she found the patient's son, an 11-year-old asthmatic, cyanotic and in bronchospasm.

Well-meaning social service agencies without access to medical assistance may make inappropriate referrals.

> One of the authors (M.E.M.) was asked to see a 65-year-old grandmother because "she was acting strangely and probably had a relapse of schizophrenia." When the pleasant gray-haired lady and her anxious daughter were interviewed, they were asked what the problem had been and the daughter replied, "Well, the right side of her face drooped, she couldn't use one arm and she talked all garbled." Grandmother was admitted to the general hospital for Coumadin.

Psychiatric services are not immune to inappropriate referrals from other services as well (known as "dumps" in the patois of the ER). Unfortunately, once a patient has received a psychiatric diagnosis, medical investigation and acumen may cease as if psychiatric disease confers some immunity to other illness. It has been the authors' unhappy experience to diagnose severe hyponatremia, herpes encephalitis, angina, stroke, pneumonia and long-bone fracture in patients after "medical clearance." In addition, in any emergency room daily stress and tension often produce adversarial group dynamics between various disciplines of medicine, which then impact upon the triage and disposition of patients. Overworked and overburdened residents suspect residents in other disciplines of dumping patients to the other specialties in order to reduce the workload. That this suspicion is justified, both for psychiatry and other disciplines, is more common than attending physicians and administrators wish to believe. Hospitals may also be guilty of "dumping" indigent patients to other hospitals.

Appropriate staffing is determined by population served. General hospital emergency services receive a great number of alcoholic and drug-abusing patients. In some institutions, these patients are deemed the province of psychiatry. In others, they are assigned to medical personnel with psychiatric consultation. HMO's see a larger population of the "working well" presenting with depression or family crises. Private psychiatric hospitals may choose to see only previously evaluated inpatients.

Staff, regardless of disciplinary training and setting, have certain common requirements. Emergency psychiatric clinicians should be skilled in rapid assessment of both individual patients and the patients' families and social supports. Knowledge of indications for consultation, for hospitalization, and for use of restraints is required for all personnel. Explicit protocols for these issues serve to guide consistent care despite differences in training. All involved staff must have talent in composing clear and intelligent notes. Emergency psychiatric evaluations are often used to develop treatment plans, to facilitate referrals, and to evaluate a person's behavior at the time seen in a court of law.

The multidisciplinary team approach, when available, provides the broadest coverage. With the team approach, history may be obtained by any of the members if a standardized data base is used to provide consistent information gathering. Specific diagnostic evaluation and psychopharmacologic intervention are performed by a psychiatrist or by a nurse practitioner under a psychiatrist's supervision. Psychiatric nurses administer medications, monitor vital signs and restraints, and monitor possible emergence of complications of treatment, such as extra pyramidal side effects of neuroleptics. Appropriately trained social workers and psychologists provide supportive crisis psychotherapy. Social workers effect appropriate community disposition.

Trainees from various disciplines benefit greatly from the unique exposure that emergency work provides. Trainees by their very role require supervision, which by the stressful and sometimes unpredictable nature of emergency work is more rigorous and consistent in the ER than in other settings.

All emergency clinicians need access to legal consultation for issues of refusal of treatment and competency, as well as regarding confidentiality and its Tarasoffian exceptions. Access to consultation to other specialties (principally internal medicine, neurology, and surgery) is required. Administrative consultation occasionally is necessary, as in the instance of disasters.

Access to security personnel is mandatory for emergency psychiatric clinicians. In the tumult of an inner-city emergency service, security's physical presence is a 24-hour requirement. In all locations, security must be readily available to restrain patients and protect clinicians and other patients from attack. In some locations security guards are chosen and trained directly by the psychiatric staff. In others, security guards are provided by the general hospital administration or hired from private agencies, such as Pinkertons or Wells Fargo. In all cases, the psychiatric staff are responsible for the appropriate and efficient function of security in their department. Supervision and training of security guards by the psychiatric personnel, where indicated, provide safety for patients and medico-legal protection of the staff.

Maintaining quality staff and staff morale is difficult.[3] Friction between specialists is engendered by patients who frustrate attempts to care and cure. Anxiety is engendered by the nature of patients' problems, especially suicide, homicide, and undiagnosed medical emergencies. Emergency work in general may not be valued by an institution. This is especially true where nonpsychiatric personnel are unaware of psychiatry's special demands and stresses. Disposition for psychiatric patients is more limited than for other specialties, and the possibility for legal problems with the violent, depressed, impulsive, or psychotic patients is high.

Staff efficiency is enhanced and turnover reduced by a high degree of coordination, a firm level of accountability within a defined structure, and strong leadership. Protocols guide consistent care. Regular conferences prepare clinicians to meet complex clinical problems. Management of difficult patients creates hope and enforces esprit de corps. Required vacations, minimizing changes in shifts, and reductions in the work week prevent exhaustion. Enhancing clinical safety, technical assistance, and some attention to individual needs of personnel create an atmosphere of concern and unity.

PATIENT POPULATION

Emergency room populations change, reflecting changing patterns of behavior in society. For example, suicide attempts among adolescents and cocaine-related disorders, which were once rare, are now common problems confronting psychiatrists. The move to deinstitutionalize chronic patients that commenced in the 60s has resulted in a larger number of patients with chronic psychosis presenting to the emergency room. Drug abuse follows trends, and where previously only inner-city emergency services received patients with narcotic abuse, such drugs are now a nationwide problem.

Individuals using emergency rooms are more likely to be single, younger, without social supports, schizophrenic, alcoholic or otherwise substance abusive, and indigent.[2,4] The closer individuals live to a hospital, the more likely they are to use the emergency service, so location and changing demographic characteristics of a hospital's surroundings are reflected in the patient population.

Patients may be self-referred or may have been referred by other specialties. In part, referral patients reflect the opinions of the local medical community and the culture as to the agenda of psychiatry. In some areas, for example, substance abuse is handled directly by separate, independent rehabilitation programs, while in others such problems are considered the province of psychiatry. Depending on the skill of an emergency psychiatric service and on its liaison with the medical community, the emergency psychiatric service is viewed either as a disposition for unwanted patients or a resource for support and care. Communication of the emergency psychiatric service with the rest of the emergency personnel, confidential care of medical staff's own psychiatric problems, and availability in general crises have an impact on how and which patients are referred. For example, if psychiatric clinicians are viewed as distant, critical, and uncooperative, patients who desperately need psychiatric help for depression or family crisis may be thought too nice to be referred to "those guys" and hence fail to receive treatment.

A problem that faces all emergency services is that of the repeater patient. Repeaters tend to be single, male, unemployed, without insurance, and often diagnosed as schizophrenic or personality disordered.[4,5] Such patients fail to utilize appropriate community resources for the long-term care that they need; they are unable or unwilling to accept prior recommendations for referral or placement. Such patients who may visit the emergency room daily, are a source of frustration to clinicians.

The psychiatric emergency service is a barometer of gaps in the health care system. Over the years, emergency psychiatric services have evolved as a focus of social support and ongoing treatment of patients. With the reduction in the rate of inpatient episodes, outpatient visits have increased twelve-fold.[6] It is mainly the disorganized, often psychotic patient who utilizes the ER for "primary care."[4] Such a patient's condition may also be complicated by malnutrition, infection, and thermal injuries as well. An example is a 50-year-old chronic schizophrenic woman living a marginal existence in the streets. Her chronic psychosis makes her fearful of agencies that can help her, but the fact that she is not acutely dangerous to self or others makes her not certifiable to a hospital. Even if she were certifiable, she might be discharged back to the street in less than a week.

CRISIS INTERVENTION

Crisis-oriented therapy aims to restore functioning, minimize impairment, and facilitate growth. Crisis occurs when there is a disruption of usual function. A crisis can be predominantly medical, such as a life-threatening myocardial infarction, or predominantly psychiatric, such as an acute psychotic episode. A crisis can also be a disruption in a broader pattern, such as marital dysfunction. The mode of resolution of such crises determines whether a biologic, psychologic, or social system improves function or is permanently impaired. Crises are opportunity for change, both for good or ill.

Successful crisis resolution demands a variety of therapeutic skills. What may appear to be an insurmountable crisis or therapeutic impasse is resolved if resources both in the patient and in the patient's social community matrix are mobilized. Assessment of the exact nature of a crisis requires both cross-sectional and longitudinal evaluation of the patient. Families and friends provide valuable information that patients are unable themselves to provide, as illustrated in the following clinical vignette.

> A 39-year-old man presents with a manic episode to the psychiatric emergency room. The patient has flights of ideas, elation and restlessness, and is unable to provide much coherent history. His wife and children state that the patient always experiences difficulties with anniversaries and birthdays. His fortieth birthday is tomorrow. The family also reports that the patient has consistently responded in multiple similar episodes to low doses of phenothiazines and has never required hospitalization. Further, they report that because of rapidity of response, no one has presented the idea of lithium maintenance. They note, however, that the patient and his family have suffered financial depletion, employment disruption, and personal embarrassment attendant to the mania.

These data provide a basis for a treatment plan. The patient is prescribed a neuroleptic for amelioration of acute symptoms. Referral is made for lithium maintenance and for supportive psychotherapy to mollify the stresses of birthdays and anniversaries.

At other times, family and friends may be identified as major sources of difficulty patients are experiencing. Crisis resolution may demand clarification and articulation of problems felt by all.

Families may be a source of anxiety to both patients and emergency clinicians. In times of stress, any person may tend to be more defensive, curt and short of temper. Moreover, patients' families often have a great amount of diagnosed or undiagnosed psychopathology. Even for a healthy family, guilt may militate against a smooth working relationship when time and resources are limited. Great patience, endurance, and a tolerance for anger are required of a clinician if a working alliance is to be formed. The same difficulties that arise in psychotherapy arise in the emergency room and the same clinical skills are required. These include abilities to identify transference and countertransference and projection, and to distinguish between realistic and neurotic "resistance."

DISPOSITION

Crises afford people opportunity to become aware of their resources and hidden strengths. Crisis-oriented therapy enhances this awareness and serves to direct energy to resolving crises. The nature of the disposition plays a major role in whether patients will continue the process of growth and recovery. Familiarity with medical and social resources within and beyond the emergency setting is required.

Some patients may be managed by brief crisis-oriented therapy with one or two follow-up visits. Instances include management of some behavioral changes induced by drugs such as PCP, and family ventilation following news of unexpected death or other loss. Most patients, however, require referral to other treatment programs for further care. Emergency clinicians require a working knowledge of public and private resources in their area. Social agencies, school and church-related programs, community health centers, halfway houses, hospitals, and private therapists provide a spectrum of referrals.

Referrals vary according to patient need and desire and by what is possible in a given locale. For example, a clinician may believe that an anxious man will benefit from marital therapy as well as medication, but the patient refuses one or both recommendations. Acting-out teenagers benefit from hospitalization, but adolescent psychiatric units are often not available and existing psychiatric units unsuitable. Lack of funds and inadequate insurance sometimes necessitate referral to distant public facilities or otherwise compromise dispositions. Limitations exist in most communities.

Hospitalization is the last resort for patients. Clinicians forget the social stigma of psychiatric hospitalization still exists in some communities, no matter how cruel and irrational. Liabilities of hospitalization include expense, loss of time at school and work, separation of patients from their social supports in the community, and the insidious effects of institutionalization that develop even in brief hospitalizations.

Need for hospitalization does not depend solely upon the nature of the patient's illness. The context in which the illness occurs also plays a role in the decision to hospitalize. A moderately suicidal patient who has supportive family and friends may do well with supervised outpatient care, whereas mildly suicidal, divorced and friendless patients may require hospitalization.

Not hospitalizing patients usually requires more effort on the part of an emergency psychiatric staff. For example, patients with chronic psychoses may be managed as outpatients. This requires, however, that emergency staff are aware of and contact agencies in the community that are capable of such management, convey the needed information to the agency, and ideally, confirm that appointments have been kept. If patients are not hospitalized, responsibility for supporting the patients and their families evolves on emergency clinicians until appropriate disposition has been found or the crisis resolved. Studies [2] indicate that success of placement in a disposition is enhanced when clinicians personally link patients with treatment. Follow-through is significantly diminished when patients are simply provided with names of psychiatric clinicians or treatment centers.

In some instances, hospitalization is required. Severely suicidal and homicidal patients, severely psychotic patients, and demented patients without community supports are examples where hospitalization is necessary. It is a good policy in such instances to maintain a list of hospitals, the services provided and the financial or insurance coverage required. This allows patients and clinicians a number of treatment alternatives from which to choose.

At times, patients must be certified against their will. Regulations of states vary as to when certification is necessary. In general, the spirit of these regulations is to protect both patient and society from harm. It can be as harmful to fail to certify a patient as to certify inappropriately. Although certification of patients against their protestations is painful for clinicians, the possibility of suicide or homicide leaves no ethical choice.

Not all destructive behavior is the result of psychosis. Many individuals who have committed a violent act should be referred to legal authorities. Psychiatric illness does not underlie all forms of violence; more importantly, psychiatry does not have the solution for all causes of destructive behavior. We cannot afford to pretend that we do, as it vitiates our integrity as psychiatrists and undercuts the credibility of what psychiatry as a scientific medical subspecialty can offer.

TRANSPORTATION

Emergency room staff are responsible for the safe and effective transport of patients to their disposition. This is true for all patients, certified or otherwise. Psychotic, alcoholic or otherwise compromised patients may not be certifiable, but if they become involved in a vehicular accident after leaving the emergency setting, medico-legal action may ensue.

Patients, certified or otherwise, should not be released from the emergency room until they are suitable to travel. For alcoholics and other substance abusers, this involves time to "dry out." For psychotic patients, medication is offered. Clinicians should know how and with whom a patient plans to leave the emergency room and determine as best possible the suitability of the plan.

Patients who are sufficiently disturbed and require certification should only be transferred to other facilities by ambulance. Other severely disturbed but voluntary patients should also be transported by professional services. Family and friends may be unprepared to deal with problems that may arise en route.

Patients should never be deceived about their destination. Family or friends may tell a patient that they are going to see a nonpsychiatric physician. The emergency staff should not collude with this deception because it undermines physician credibility and infantilizes patients.

Emergency staff should make every effort to assure that transportation of patients is uneventful. Suicidal and homicidal patients, once certified, should be searched for concealed weapons and drugs. When medication is administered in the emergency room time must be allowed for observation and management of side effects before the patient leaves. Dystonic reactions and anaphylactic shock are more effectively and safely treated in a hospital than in an ambulance.

Ambulance drivers should be informed of potential difficulties. Violent patients require restraints and/or extra staffing in the ambulance. Ambulance services may stipulate for liability reasons that all patients be restrained regardless of potential violence. If patients are to be restrained, they should be informed in advance to avert an eruption in the ambulance. Family and friends are sometimes of value in calming patients. In other instances, it agitates and embarrasses patients to have loved ones see them in restraints.

Medications are provided to be used in transportation, dependent on the level of expertise of ambulance staff. It is helpful to have women accompany female patients transported by male crew. Delusional patients may fantasize and sociopathic patients fabricate stories of sexual abuse. The presence of female attendants affords protection for both patients and crew.

STRESSES UNIQUE TO EMERGENCY PSYCHIATRIC PRACTICE

Emergency psychiatric work is fraught with stress. New clinicians find themselves anxious, depressed, and angry. Some experience a pervasive sense of uncertainty. Experienced clinicians suffer the same feelings. Both find themselves scanning obituaries for the names of patients whom they have recently evaluated and returned to the community.

In addition to the realities of patients' problems, a number of social forces interact to form the "climate" in which emergency services operate.[7] Some of these forces can be modified to reduce stress and burnout. Other stresses can only be understood. Emergency work demands quick decisions regarding diagnosis, treatment, and disposition, with the additional demands to manage violent and threatening behavior in the most expedient and safe way possible. There is no easy way to learn this. Nor is there any substitute for experience. Inservice education, continuing education courses and reading (in crisis-oriented therapy, diagnostic psychiatry and psychopharmacology) help to maintain expertise. Hospital supported educational programs serve to convey to clinicians a sense of commitment to quality care of patients and to staff enrichment and good morale. Textbooks describe clearly delineated problems grouped under chapter headings. Unfortunately, patients rarely present so neatly. The element of uncertainty as to the problem the next patient will present with, and the ambiguity of information upon which clinicians must base their decisions are continuing sources of anxiety.[2,7]

Good working relationships with triage and referral sources alleviate some stress. Knowledge that patients have been appropriately screened and have received medical or surgical clearance reduces clinician anxiety. Conversely, poor relationships with referral sources lead to problems for patients and clinicians alike. Even in the best of circumstances, however, patients are occasionally inappropriately triaged into psychiatry, as illustrated below.

> A 45-year-old woman was seen in the emergency room complaining of anxiety and shortness of breath. She had a history of chronic schizophrenia with four prior hospitalizations. She was triaged to psychiatry, where she became rapidly cyanotic, hypotensive, and died. She had on autopsy a massive pulmonary embolus.

Inappropriate triage is not unique to psychiatry. All good specialists require a state of art knowledge of differential diagnosis. Cardiologists must discern angina from esophagitis; surgeons appendicitis from pelvic inflammatory disease. Psychiatrists must be able to distinguish psychiatric disease from its possible mimics. Continuing education, inservice seminars, case conferences, and quality assurance reviews support this goal and ameliorate clinician stress.

The number of patients presenting to emergency rooms varies from hour to hour. Nothing guarantees a service will not be inundated. Clinicians must be pragmatic and able to enlist the aid of other personnel when necessary. A systemized plan to implement in the event of overflow, as well as for disasters, reduces stress.

Another great source of stress to emergency clinicians and a key factor in determining disposition is patients' inability to finance treatment. Stress is reduced if clinicians have good liaisons with local psychiatric centers. Nonetheless, the number of beds in such hospitals are finite and often full, or patients may be without appropriate financial coverage to be eligible. Failing such resources, it may be necessary to send a patient to a remote or poorly staffed hospital. In such circumstances, clinicians are placed in the unfortunate situation of having to rationalize this state of affairs to themselves, patients, or families. Guilty explanations at four in the morning do not improve self-esteem or disposition.

BURNOUT

The occupational hazard of all emergency clinicians is burnout. A dismaying list of stresses contributes. These include voluminous paperwork, hostile patients, low pay, long hours, doubting nurses, negativistic admission officers, persistent threats of violence, role blurring, lack of supervision, insufficient training, and social and professional prejudice. Burnout results both from stress and from inability to accommodate to and recover from stress. When a clinician or an administration is limited in ability to reduce stresses, more attention should be given to those factors that mitigate stress and facilitate adaptation. These interventions include debriefing sessions[8] supportive resources for clinicians, a calm and private clinical atmosphere, and rapport with other personnel.[7]

Some stress on an emergency service accrues from simple fatigue. Psychiatry in particular is dependent upon clinicians' abilities to detect subtle issues and nuances. This ability is severely impaired when clinicians are exhausted, tense and irritable. It is unreasonable to assume that any individual can perform at peak, or even acceptable efficiency through a lengthy work shift. Trainees and others should not be assigned a 24-hour shift. Administrators and directors of emergency services should limit emergency room work to 8–12-hour shifts. For all staff, vacations and other time-off should be not only available but mandatory.

It is painfully obvious in some cases that emergency psychiatric intervention will have little or no effect on the trajectory of a patient's illness. The alcoholic with recurrent emergency room presentations while intoxicated, the paranoid schizophrenic who refuses medications, the borderline who triangulates the emergency room with the private therapist, and many other help-seeking, help-refusing noncompliant patients frustrate psychiatric clinicians. Anger emerges as clinicians realize they are helpless in the face of obvious need for treatment. The same reflection that assists psychotherapists with issues of transference and countertransference is helpful in the emergency room, regardless of the disparity of the situations.

REFERENCES

1. Telintelo S, Kuhlman TL, Winger C: A study of the use of restraint in a psychiatric emergency room. Hosp Community Psychiatry 1983; 34:164-165
2. Slaby AE, Lieb J, Tancredi LR: The Handbook of Psychiatric Emergencies, 3rd ed. New York, Medical Examination Publishing Company, 1985
3. McPherson DE: Teaching and research in emergency psychiatry. Can J Psychiatry 1984; 29:50-54
4. Bassuck, E: The impact of deinstitutionalization on the general hospital psychiatric emergency ward. Hosp Community Psychiatry 1980; 31:623-627
5. Nurius PS: Emergency psychiatric services: a study of changing utilization patterns and issues. Int J Psychiatry Med 1983-84; 13:239-254
6. Goldman H, Adams N, Tanbe C: Deinstitutionalization: the data demythologized. Hosp Community Psychiatry 1983; 34:129-134
7. Nurius PS: Stress: a pervasive dilemma in psychiatric emergency care. Compr Psychiatry 1984; 25:345-354
8. Hoffman JA, Forssmann-Falck R: Emergency psychiatry training: the new old problem. Gen Hosp Psychiatry 1984; 6:143-146

6

The Admissions Process

Barry Rudnick

Admission to a psychiatric hospital constitutes an experience that is emotionally quite different from entry to a medical or surgical facility. Many patients have at some point visited a conventional medical hospital, but know little about a psychiatric institution. And the amorphous nature of mental illness itself heightens the patient's perception of the admission process as frightening and cryptic. Because many patients are admitted at the insistence of their families and referring clinicians, hospital personnel often find themselves in the position of admitting patients who do not wish to be there at all and who wish to leave, fearing permanent incarceration. Addressing a patient's anxieties and fantasies about admission thus constitutes a large amount of the "business" an admission's officer must transact as he arranges for the patient to enter the hospital.

The reasons for a patient's admission vary widely. In reviewing the phenomenon of hospital admissions from the emergency room, Feigelson et al.[1] found the severity of a patient's illness to be an important variable. But other factors were also crucial, and these included such parameters as the ER physician's level of experience or the existence of a crisis intervention program within a particular hospital. Gerson and Bassuk[2] studied the subject of psychiatric emergencies, focusing on several parameters associated with hospitalization. They found that dangerousness, the severity of psychopathology, and the absence of social supports play a role in the decision to hospitalize. But the level of training is also important: Hospitalization referrals decrease in frequency as the clinician's level of experience increases. Studies regarding the nature of the patient-therapist relationship and its effect on hospitalization were also reviewed by the authors, but the results were unclear.

The smoothness of the admissions process is influenced by many objective and subjective factors. Solomon[3] found that the attitudes of individuals who accompanied the patient to be most important; patients who were accompanied by persons in favor of hospitalization were most likely to be admitted. Holmes and Solomon[4] studied the theoretical factors affecting the admissions officer's decision to admit a patient. These factors included such variables as the admitting staff's perception of the patient's psychiatric condition and attitudes toward mental illness. The authors found that such "soft" variables were important for both first-time admissions and readmissions.

The matter of the patient's entry into the hospital has been studied by Vera,[5] who states that "all too often, professionals surrender the responsibility for creating a true therapeutic contract in the face of administrative pressures or ritualism, or simply by minimizing the impact of the first encounter between patient and professional." Vera emphasizes the nature of the early contact between staff and patient, a factor which would appear to play a large role in the retention of the patient within the facility. Steinglass and coworkers[6] have also drawn attention to this variable in reviewing the parameters which reflect discharge against medical advice (AMA); those authors point out that patients more prone to AMA discharges generally tend to view the hospital not as a place for sustained psychological help, but as a temporary resource for short-term help. This expectation, however, is difficult to clearly elicit from prospective admissions even when they are personally interviewed, for many patients are not very sophisticated about hospitalization and view the psychiatric institution much the same way that they view a conventional hospital.

The admissions officer often finds himself spending more time with the family of a patient than with the patient himself. Much support must be offered, and it is useful to give both parties a glimpse of the hospital; many facilities offer tours guided by former patients or volunteers. A variety of pre-admission interviews are helpful in matching expectation with reality. But the best of plans may still fail.

> A 25-year-old woman from a prominent family was considered for transfer from one private hospital to another. Doctors at the first facility stated that the patient needed long-term care for the treatment of her personality disorder; they had been only minimally successful in their attempts and the family wished for another hospital to treat their daughter. Family members saw the patient as "depressed" and were distraught over a recent abortion she had undergone. The patient

herself denied any psychological difficulties and insisted that she did not need any inpatient care. Because she had been suicidal in the recent past, an involuntary hospitalization was considered, but the patient was from another state and legal difficulties arose concerning transfer. Ultimately, the patient arrived on a voluntary basis and promptly submitted a three-day notice to leave.

This case illustrates problems in motivation and expectation. Patients admitted to a psychiatric hospital often lack introspection and have a marginal desire for change; families may contrive these admissions and exert considerable influence on both the patient and the hospital itself. A patient may agree to admission but rapidly change his mind once he arrives on the ward and sees other disturbed patients. The presence of a locked door also serves to alarm newly admitted patients. Issues of privacy become dominant, since patients rarely have single rooms, nor are they treated in any special manner. All these issues must be addressed by staff early in the course of admission. Usually, ward or hall meetings in the mornings welcome newcomers to the hospital and address many such concerns. Still, the patient must come to grips with his fears. The situation is similar to earlier life experiences, such as school or summer camp, where anxieties and lonelinesses are handled through acquaintances and friendships. Those patients who utilize the hospital best are individuals who can somehow early integrate their difficulties with the milieu and see some reason or hope for staying and working on their problems.

Perhaps most useful in coping with these early admission anxieties is the "three-day notice," an artifact whereby the patient agrees that he will submit a written notice of intent to leave but delay the actual departure for 72 hours. The delay is not legally binding, but it does give the staff time to discuss discharge with him. Usually, staff and other patients successfully persuade him to remain. Most patients who submit such notices are ambivalent about leaving anyhow; for a freshly admitted patient, the availability of this "notice" arrangement serves to assuage concerns about incarceration which arise upon admission.

Since a psychiatric hospital has a fixed number of beds occupied by patients with various diagnoses, the institution has limits on the diagnostic variety of patients it can accept. Thus the admissions officer must balance the needs of a prospective admission with preservation of the psychosocial milieu. For example, it may not be possible to admit a manipulative borderline patient because the only vacancy is on a ward already containing three other such patients. Or, a unit may be unable to receive a suicidally depressed patient because it already has on it other such patients, and staff do not have the time required to "special" yet another patient on close observation. Physical limits quickly become the focus for broader clinical and political concerns within the institution. To a large extent, the admissions officer must "sell" the admission to the hospital staff, treading delicate boundaries around staff's fear of certain behaviors such as suicide or violence, insurance coverage, legal issues, and clinical appropriateness. The following is an example of this complexity.

> A 30-year-old heavy drug abuser with the recent onset of a drug-induced psychosis was considered for admission to a chemical dependency unit. The unit had a philosophy of actively confronting its patients and generally accepted individuals who were reasonably motivated for change. Thus a psychotic patient would clearly not fit into its structure and might be worsened by the group confrontation. But the ward for the treatment of psychotic patients was filled with very disturbed patients and staff could not handle an individual who might require active detoxification. The admissions officer himself was currently under mandate from the administration to accept patients with suitable insurance, but the hospital had some staff shortages and a holiday weekend was approaching.

This case illustrates the forces impinging on the admissions process. Such forces wax and wane but always shape the admissions policy and make it one of flux.

Although the newly admitted patient is quickly transported from the admissions office to the ward or unit where he will reside, the process itself is a more laborious task. Hartlage[7] has stated that "an absolute minimum of 21 hours is spent in routine administrative and nursing activities associated with the admission of a given patient." A large component of this time revolves around the necessary paperwork concerning the patient and his illness. And the need for certain paperwork to be in order requires that an admissions office become somewhat bureaucratic. The office must review all involuntary certificates to ascertain that the patient's admission is truly justified and documented. But outside clinicians may certify patients as a means of making a quick disposition and never elucidate the underlying issues pertaining to dangerousness; reasons listed on certificates may include such phrases as "patient is nonfunctional" or "patient may become dangerous" or "patient is incompetent to handle his affairs."

> An outside clinician discussed with the admissions officer the suitability of referring a patient whom he was treating. It was agreed that the patient was suitable, but no decision was made about the timing of the actual admission. The patient appeared at the hospital several days

later, having been sent by ambulance. There were no vacant beds. The patient had been sent as an involuntary admission, but the certificate merely indicated "chronic suicidality" as the reason for incarceration.

In the above case, the reason listed on the certification would never withstand the subsequent scrutiny of any hearing officer. This illustrates the point that the admissions officer must begin anew and reevaluate each patient's suitability for hospitalization, bearing in mind his own hospital's criteria for admission. Misunderstandings can easily arise in this process, whereby referring physicians and families simply expect the patient to be admitted without question. An experienced admissions officer learns to rigorously evaluate all admissions by telephone and to adopt a very literal posture regarding the actual reasons for certification and admission. A high index of suspicion is required. To a large extent, the admissions process is an adversarial one; this is often not appreciated by the referring clinician.

A patient's financial condition is another critical factor in admission. Homeless patients and social emergencies constitute a certain number of admissions within the public hospital but play less of a role within private hospitals. Occasionally, a private hospital will be referred an indigent patient with limited insurance who may be eligible for a limited stay. For example, an unemployed and chronic alcoholic may have some Medicare insurance. Certain such patients may benefit from a short stay which stabilizes them medically, but others are often not treatable on a short-term basis nor amenable to psychotherapeutic intervention. Yet to obtain a certificate of need, the hospital must often have some provision for the care of an indigent population; thus some private facilities have grants-in-aid or other financial means to extend the care of some patients beyond expiration of insurance.

The determination of a patient's economic status shapes his entry into the hospital and determines the length of his stay. It also shapes the type of treatment he will receive. Some patients have insurance policies which cover a year or more of intensive inpatient care, while others may have coverage for only a week of symptomatic treatment which excludes individual psychotherapy. All this must be clarified prior to admission, making the process quite complicated and difficult to explain to the patient and his family. Many patients are unaware of their psychiatric health care coverage, although political action groups such as the National Alliance of the Mentally Ill are bringing about changes in this area and informing their membership of hospital benefits. Also, some diagnostic groups, such as alcoholics or drug-dependent patients, can even manipulate their insurance benefits to advantage, entering and leaving the hospital in such a way as to obtain maximum coverage. In this era of deinstitutionalization of public health care, an interesting paradox has arisen whereby some patients entering the public hospital are found to have insurance and turned back to the private sector.

Legal issues occupy much time in the admissions process. In some states, it is policy to offer every patient a voluntary admission even if the patient is too psychotic to fully understand the nature of any admission. Later, if the patient wishes to leave and is perceived at that point to be dangerous, he can be certified. The goal of admission is to make each entry to the hospital a voluntary one to the extent it is possible and to preserve awareness on the part of patients. Yet even when patients are told in detail about the admissions process, they may fail to comprehend or remember the event. Olin and Olin[8] studied the consent process in 100 newly admitted psychiatric patients and found that few recalled the terms of the admissions contract when interviewed directly after admission itself; ten days later, when calmer, a greater number recalled details about the admissions procedures.

Disclosure laws, civil rights issues, and court matters are all involved in the process of admission. Patients must be told that they have the right to an attorney, the right to a hearing, the right to make telephone calls, and other personal rights. Forms acknowledging these rights must be signed by the admitting physician. Failure to do so incurs legal risk, as illustrated by the following example.

> A 30-year-old man with a history of bipolar affective disorder was involuntarily admitted after a manic episode. He was correctly certified by the referring general hospital and admitted to the private facility by the on-duty resident at night. But the physician did not document the reading of the patient's rights within the medical record. Thus, at the hearing the patient was released by the hearing officer. The patient immediately became involved in a criminal act within the community.

In the above case, the hospital could incur liability because it had failed to properly retain the patient. An involuntary admission must proceed according to protocol, and no phase of it must escape administrative scrutiny.

Institutional transfers are another administratively difficult task for admissions personnel. Such transfers form an important source of referrals but are often compromised by clinical dilemmas.

> A 75-year-old woman was referred from a general hospital because of depression and a history of an overdose. When the admissions

officer was informed that the patient had pneumonia, he indicated that transfer must await medical clearance of her condition. The hospital nonetheless transferred her the following morning.

A 30-year-old alcoholic appeared at a general hospital emergency room in an intoxicated state. He told staff that he might overdose. The staff thus certified him for involuntary admission and notified the private hospital admissions officer who agreed to accept the patient. No mention was made of his intoxicated status, however, and when he appeared the next morning, he was sober and remorseful, steadfastly denying suicidal ideation or depression.

In these instances, patients were sent in haste or without proper screening. Emergency room staff may wish to "clear house" and hence certify patients who are later found inappropriate for admission.

Other kinds of institutional transfers involve arranged admissions from facilities already caring for the patient, though unsuccessfully.

A 30-year-old borderline patient became hopelessly enmeshed in the milieu of a highly regarded private hospital where she demonstrated such severe "acting-out" behavior that staff deemed her no longer treatable. Transfer to a new facility was seen as possibly affording her a fresh start with new staff who might better manage her case. The second hospital agreed to accept the patient and, alerted to her manipulativeness from the start, engaged in successful work with her.

Cases such as this often represent the burnout of staff who have cared for difficult patients over long periods of time. Transfers, if well planned, can be beneficial in some instances. In other cases, statements of hopelessness by one hospital may spur a rival facility to take on the patient, though a wary admissions officer may realize that his institution has in fact little to offer the patient.

In summary, the admissions process is similar to the psychotherapeutic process in the sense that it involves attention to unspoken issues, to behavior, and to an awareness of "countertransference" factors that impinge on the officer. Anger, dismay, and hope are all common affects encountered in the work of bringing patients into the hospital for treatment. And while economic factors may exert some influence on diagnoses and lengths of stay, recurring clinical concerns still continue to shape the nature of the admissions process.

REFERENCES

1. Feigelson E, David E, Mackinnon R, et al: The decision to hospitalize. Am J Psychiatry 1978; 135:354-357
2. Gerson S, Bassuk E: Psychiatric emergencies: an overview. Am J Psychiatry 1980; 137:1-11
3. Solomon P: The admissions process in two state psychiatric hospitals. Hosp Community Psychiatry 1981; 32:405-408
4. Holmes W, Solomon P: Criteria used in first admissions and readmissions to psychiatric hospitals. Social Science and Medicine 1980; 14:55-59
5. Vera MI: On the therapeutic aspects of psychiatric admissions. Social Work In Health Care 1980; 5:361-367
6. Steinglass P, Grantham CE, Hertzman M: Predicting which patients will be discharged against medical advice. Am J Psychiatry 1980; 137:1385-1389
7. Hartlage LC: Concept in psychiatric hospital admissions. Social Science 1970; 4:675-676
8. Olin GB, Olin HS: Informed consent in voluntary mental hospital admissions. Am J Psychiatry 1975; 132:938-941

III
Hospitalization

7
The Diagnostic Process

Bruce Leopold
John R. Lion

Patients admitted to an inpatient service arrive with a diagnosis. The diagnosis reflects their history and previous label, or their mood, or their behavior; in a number of cases, the admitting and discharge diagnoses are different. Hospitalization often helps clarify the diagnosis, primarily because the patient is seen by many people over a period of time. In addition, the hospitalization answers the questions of why, at this point in time, the patient is being admitted to the facility. These reasons may shed light on the diagnosis by clarifying, say, the recurrent mood swings previously not noted or by underscoring the contribution of the patient's borderline personality or certain antisocial propensities.

Much has been written about *DSM-III* and the attempt of the profession to define nonetiologic, phenomenologic entities seen by all clinicians.[1-5] The various axis notations in *DSM-III* are important means to establish different diagnostic dimensions of the patient. Most workers within the hospital come to appreciate that a diagnosis tells little about therapeutic effort, hopefulness or hopelessness, or the profound characterologic issues surrounding the patient. Neither does the diagnosis explain psychopathy or convey the suicidal despair sometimes seen in severe marital discord. *DSM-III* helps the insurance company but may do less justice to the therapist and hospital staff working with an extremely rebellious adolescent whose ferocious limit-testing creates extraordinary turmoil on a ward. Medical diagnosis, by contrast, may seem more often to depict the disease process and its appropriate treatment.

> A severely alcoholic woman, still actively drinking in her early sixties, was admitted in a depressed state following a suicidal gesture. Her insurance specifically excluded treatment for alcoholism, and there were no private funds. Both grown children confirmed her alcoholism. One agreed with the treatment team's assessment that her depression had to be considered quite secondary. The other argued strenuously that the alcoholism should be downplayed in the medical documentation and stated: "You see how depressed my mother is!" This child actually threatened to sue the treating clinician if alcoholism were listed as the principal diagnosis.

This case illustrates the simultaneous importance and irrelevance of the diagnosis, for the issue at hand is not the alcoholism of the patient but the manipulativeness of a daughter. "Stretching" the diagnosis is currently referred to as "DRG creep," wherein a more reimbursable entity is substituted for another, thereby allowing the patient to stay longer in the hospital.

The admitting clinician is wise to question the diagnosis each time he sees a rehospitalized patient, for new facets of illness may become apparent with each clinical scrutiny.[6,7] Sometimes, the new information sheds light on deeper intrapsychic processes that defy easy diagnostic statements.[8]

> A woman in her early twenties had, in retrospect, developed endogenous depression in childhood, leading to adverse consequences on her self-confidence and object relations through several developmental phases. A hypomanic switch in her mid-teens was initially greeted by the patient and her family as a boon, as she became extroverted and involved in life. Within two or three years, however, her illness progressed to frank mania, commencing a series of short-term hospitalizations that culminated in a year-long one. Upon discharge, the bipolar process was acknowledged by all parties, but despite placement in a halfway house and involvement in state-of-the-art therapy, she did poorly, quitting her volunteer job, engaging in autistic daydreams of happiness and petty quarrels with her peers and counselors. Eventually she spoke of suicide and was rehospitalized. Upon further diagnostic investigation, she was able to acknowledge profound demoralization of an unexpected sort: "My illness is a horrible punishment for something I must have done in the past, although I don't know what." Unknown to all, the patient was wrestling with a personal "diagnostic"

problem: Why had she been so afflicted, and was there any point in trying to achieve as stable and gratifying a life as possible?

This patient's anguish led to her hospitalization, but to say that she was depressed in the traditional textbook sense was inadequate, if not inaccurate. Many patients are hospitalized because social support systems fail, leading them to flounder, or because they decompensate through drinking or not taking medication, but the diagnosis stays the same, and the question becomes one of understanding the readmission. As the patient becomes increasingly symptomatic, a wife, parent, or employer indicates to the patient that he is "ill" and sets in motion the admission; the diagnosis, however, has been evident all along, and the hospitalization reflects social reactions, not diagnostic complexities of the type seen in medicine where complications of illness (i.e., post-cancer-radiation pneumonitis) lead to rehospitalization.

The parents of a ten years' post-head-trauma victim brought their 20-year-old son to the hospital as an ostensible late afternoon "walk-in," stating he had unexpectedly driven to their house after a violent argument with his handicapped wife. Since he had come in crisis seeking help, they reasoned it was wise to "strike while the iron was hot." Following admission, a phone call to the patient's former psychiatrist revealed that the parents had in fact seriously spoiled him over the years. In the latest incident, the patient had gone to a store, made a small purchase, and provocatively walked out without paying. Later, the father had gone and "made good." The relevant diagnosis for this admission was the parents' ambivalent inability to set limits with their brain-damaged son. They had impulsively flown the patient many miles hoping to place him in a long-term inpatient behavior modification program — which the patient would have nothing of, quickly signing himself out of the hospital.

Here an antisocial act in an organic personality disorder led to a crisis, and the parents' poorly conceived response (their "illness" and not the patient's) led to the admission.

A married, unemployed woman in her mid-twenties was admitted with a history suggestive of a borderline personality disorder. She had been in individual and marital therapy for a number of months without much improvement. Close questioning revealed that the therapist, with the husband's support, had been pressing the patient to deal with her frigidity directly, by simply having intercourse with her husband.

She could not and would not do this, leading to increasing frustration on all sides. Diplomatically, she was advised to change therapists, which she did. She also eventually left her husband. Follow-up revealed cessation of self-mutilation and gainful employment.

Here the admission was prompted by a poorly advised therapeutic intervention. The personality diagnosis might have been correct, but the immediate precipitants (the "admitting diagnosis") pertained more to anxiety and a psychosocial crisis than to the characterologic issues.

Adolescent turmoil may be far more virulent and potentially destructive for a patient than even the most severe nonsuicidal depression. Alternately, some forms of insidious depression appear before the clinician in a more obscure form, barely diagnosable, suggestive more of character pathology.

A high school senior was hospitalized to the great surprise of all who knew him following a night spent in the family garden with a loaded shotgun intermittently pressed to his temple. On first accounting, his family was viewed as vigorous, prosperous, and as close and happy as one could reasonably wish for. The patient himself was healthy, attractive, and overall rather mature and normal. By history and clinical exam, he met the criteria for neither major depression nor dysthymic disorder. No hypomanic episodes were uncovered. The smaller perturbations in his recent life were reviewed; he described an initial episode four months prior involving the relatively abrupt onset of difficulty falling asleep and early morning awakening, then anorexia, followed ten days later by dysphoria and negative thinking, all clearing spontaneously after another week. He then remained asymptomatic until, following a minor injury that sidelined him from the sport of the season and his breaking partially off from the girlfriend he'd become disillusioned with, he noted the rapid onset of more serious dysphoria and pessimism. His parents left for the weekend, and he rapidly became suicidal.

The patient in this case probably had an incipient, endogenous depressive illness, but the melancholic symptoms were so subtle that the diagnosis was made with difficulty. The lack of a reasonable precipitant for the glaring suicidal behavior confused the clinician, for the precipitant sharply influences not only the disease process but also the clinician's view of the disease; without a reasonable explanation for suicidal behavior, the diagnosis may be ascribed to manipulation or illicit drug use. An exhaustive diagnostic inquiry with emphasis on possible brain dysfunction did little to clarify matters.

In the end, the probable family history of affective disease led the clinician to suspect biochemical depression in its usually atypical adolescent form.

A bipolar spinster in her early forties, who lived with her divorced and retired mother, was admitted in an agitated state with physical disarray atypical for her usual manic bouts. Two weeks prior, while evidently euthymic, she had spoken of something being amiss with mother. Although the admission diagnosis was recurrent mania, it turned out that:

1. she wasn't manic;
2. something *was* wrong with mother (a totally unexpected initial psychotic episode);
3. because of her own Axis II difficulties (avoidant/dependent), she had been unable to take effective executive action and get her mother evaluated;
4. instead, she gradually panicked and took extra pills to calm herself;
5. becoming lithium-toxic (blood level = 2.06!);
6. resulting in her unusual, wide-eyed, tremulous presentation.

Here some detective work was involved in arriving at the correct diagnosis. What makes the case more complex is the fact that it became apparent to staff that the patient knew about the narrow toxic-therapeutic ratio of lithium and yet "forgot" and took too many pills. It was surmised that she wished to make herself sick and remove herself from the mother's increasing psychosis. The powerful role of unconscious elements in the patient's psychopathology shaped the ultimate diagnosis, but the diagnosis in this case — a toxic state — hardly does justice to the dynamics.

The moment of admission is an important window into the diagnostic complexity of illness. The patient rarely arrives alone, and observations about family interactions, blame and guilt, and the effects of symptoms on the various parties help the clinician formulate the chain of events in his mind. "Depression" may be sadness in the presence of the spouse; alone, on the ward, the patient's mood may brighten. Or, conversely, it may become worse as a function of the homesickness arising from his dependent personality. Few diagnoses in medicine are as interpersonally dependent as psychiatric ones.

A young man in his mid-twenties, moderately retarded from birth, was brought for admission by his parents because of serious assaultive behavior at his relatively new residential placement. The initial history given, the mother remained quiet while the father dwelt at length upon the several medications the son had received and the succession of clinicians employed without benefit. When mother's comments were sought, after some hesitation she described the stress of the patient's handicap on their family, and related how in her judgment her husband had seriously spoiled the patient. It became apparent that the well-meaning father had devoted his recent life to volunteer work with the handicapped. He was now director of the very residential program the son was in and was unwittingly sabotaging the staff's efforts to give the patient the limits he'd never received at home.

This case illustrates the "family diagnosis," commonplace with the admission of children, adolescents, and geriatric patients. Each member has a "story," and each is enmeshed within the patient's own illness. Separating and identifying these contributing elements is part of the diagnostic process.

A father brought his college-student son, recently somewhat assaultive, for admission with both involuntary commitment certificates and a judge's order for evaluation. The son's evident grandiosity, combined with a sociopathic manipulativeness, suggested hypomania as well as a personality disorder. The son quickly signed a voluntary admission form, thereby vitiating the certificates. The admitting clinician, anticipating the patient's subsequent submission of a "three-day notice" of intent to leave, asked the father to sign a "permission to certify" hospital form. The father replied that he would but then left the hospital without doing so, to the annoyance of the staff. The patient eventually eloped from the hospital and was not returned by the family.

Here the family's cowardice or manipulativeness sheds immediate light on the possible diagnosis of an antisocial personality; and so, the power of the family looms large. Families can successfully disguise and hide or distort the real behavior of the patient. Diagnosis in psychiatry often involves uncovering such deceptions which have pathologically unraveled the integrity of the family.

The first few days in the hospital give important clues to the diagnosis. A rapid clearing of aggression, disorganization and confusion may be suggestive of substance abuse; the clinician may arrive the next day to find the patient bright and cheerful, barely recognizable from the day before. Some patients admitted with a history of serious anxiety and depression perk up within a few days, making the diagnosis seem less like an endogenous process. The observations nursing staff make are crucial, and major contributions are sometimes made by the least skilled staff on the ward.

A woman in her early seventies, three years a widow, now living with a *day-time* hired companion, became depressed for the first time after the death of a close friend from a progressive neurologic disease. Several psychiatric hospitalizations, chemotherapy trials, and day treatment involvements followed without much benefit. She was admitted to a different facility, where initially certain historical and interpersonal observations suggested a reactive/characterologic basis for her prepsychotic major depression. Continued chemotherapy efforts led to bothersome side effects but no clear mood improvement. Then, brief nocturnal episodes of confusion were noted by the *night* nursing staff; neurologic and psychometric assessment revealed strong evidence for an early dementing process superimposed on generalized mild cortical atrophy. A review of her history indicated a stepwise downhill course that had been obscured by suggestive psychodynamics. Peripherally "silent" or lacunar multi-infarct dementia with depression was the discharge diagnosis, and the psychological treatment efforts were greatly curtailed.

In this case the observation by some night shift nursing staff that the patient was confused reshaped the diagnosis. In the area of behavior disorders, perceptions by staff are particularly valuable. Less senior staff may be able to befriend the patient more effectively. Splitting on a ward may be sensed by staff and discussed at their meetings, thus elucidating a diagnosis, such as a borderline personality. Occupational and recreational therapists may observe dependency, hostility, or psychopathy.

Medical illness may coexist with psychiatric disease affecting the patient's symptoms and diagnosis. Here the clinician must think in "two dimensions," as it were, the worlds of psychosocial stress or pathology and metabolic derangement.

A woman in her mid-twenties, without prior psychiatric history, employed, and soon to be married, was admitted as a transfer from another psychiatric hospital with the diagnosis of acute schizophrenic episode. Several days before, her family had taken her in a grossly psychotic state to an emergency room, where she had been medically evaluated. Close clinical assessment in the second psychiatric facility revealed some atypical, delirious-seeming features to her psychosis. A reading of the poorly legible original handwritten ER note referred to a serious headache she'd developed a few days before. A spinal tap was done (though in retrospect, perhaps an emergency brain CT scan should have come first) and the fluid hand-carried to the general hospital lab, where a marked pleocytosis was found. Immediate transfer to a neurology service was made; herpes simplex encephalitis was subsequently identified.

In this case, medical consultation helped ultimately make the appropriate diagnosis.[9-11] But not all cases can be diagnosed by laboratory tests; in the field of alcoholism and drug abuse, a great deal of diagnostic inquiry proceeds on the basis of intuition and suspicion. The ability of the clinician to be highly suspect of his patient may help, but sometimes even this is not sufficient to make the correct diagnosis.

A man in his early forties, with well-documented chronic pain syndrome, iatrogenic narcotics dependence, and delayed posttraumatic stress disorder, was admitted following the onset of severe recurrent psychogenic amnesia. To the staff's surprise, his wife was an occult narcotics abuser, and it was her stealing his oxycodone and then lying to him about it that had occasioned the rage his amnesia defended against.

Drug-dependent patients pose special problems in diagnostic evaluation within a hospital, and drug discontinuation may be an important process in the diagnostic process. Some psychotic patients may also benefit from scrutiny during a drug-free state, without the cover of antipsychotic agents, which obscure the nature of the deranged cognition. This requires staff who are tolerant to the procedure and a milieu that can handle patients who are medication-free.

Confrontation of the patient's behavior and discussion of his diagnosis within the hospital during a ward or hall meeting are often illuminating. The mere naming of the disease process is in itself demystifying, and the reaction of other patients may catalyze the patient's efforts at acceptance and recovery.

A man was told during a hall meeting that staff considered the correct diagnosis in his case to be alcoholism. The patient was quite vehemently opposed to this "label" and berated staff, accusing them of "ruining" his life. His anger was commented upon by other patients, who had previously noted his tendency to be accusatory and demanding. Another patient, an alcoholic, then talked about his own denial.

Some patients react strongly to diagnostic labels while others seem almost indifferent to them or cynical about the terms, perhaps reflecting limitations imposed by the disorder itself.

A young schizophrenic patient was informed about his diagnosis but reacted with inappropriate grinning and remained withdrawn the remainder of the ward meeting, much as he had done during the previous weeks of his hospitalization.

A patient's ability to grapple with his diagnosis is an important step to mastery of illness. Patients often consult the patient library for books or may procure other reading materials directly from nursing or medical sources.

A borderline woman asked her physician for information concerning the term "borderline." She had learned about her diagnosis from nursing staff, and the term was discussed at a hall meeting. She was anxious about the term and stated that she felt very "sick" when she realized that she was categorized as a patient with this illness. The patient had been hospitalized previously and had a long history of self-mutilation and substance abuse together with poor object relationships. Her physician gave her the section on borderline personality in the *DSM-III* to review. The patient studied the section overnight and reported the next day that she felt relieved by the fact that so many of her symptoms and behaviors had actually been classified and described under one heading; previously, she was convinced that she had a bizarre mental disease which no one could describe or treat.

The diagnosis of mental illness, intricate and with varying prognosis, can initially be frightening to patients who learn about it. Yet, the diagnosis usually appears on insurance forms, and patients eventually must be told something of their disease. Such disclosure may augment the treatment process.

Overall, the diagnostic process in psychiatry sometimes bears little resemblance to that in medicine, and formal diagnoses do not always reveal the psychosocial complexities of etiology or treatment. Hospitalization remains a time-honored way of clarifying complex diagnostic pictures, its value resting in slow observation of the patient, his family, and his interaction with the milieu.

REFERENCES

1. Spitzer RL et al: Clinical criteria for psychiatric diagnosis and DSM-III. Am J Psychiatry 1975; 132:1187-1192
2. Spitzer RL: The diagnostic status of homosexuality in DSM-III: a reformulation of the issues. Am J Psychiatry 1981; 138:210-215

3. Lipkowitz MH et al: Diagnosing schizophrenia in 1980—a survey of U.S. psychiatrists. Am J Psychiatry 1983; 140:52–55
4. Klerman GL et al: A debate on DSM-III. Am J Psychiatry 1984; 141:539–553
5. Bayer R et al: Neurosis, psychodynamics and DSM-III—a history of the controversy. Arch Gen Psychiatry 1985; 42:187–196
6. Strauss JS et al: The course of psychiatric disorder, III—longitudinal principles. Am J Psychiatry 1985; 142:289–296
7. Keller MB et al: "Double Depression": Two-Year Follow-up. Am J Psychiatry 1983; 140:689–694
8. Akiskal HS: Dysthymic disorder: psychopathology of proposed chronic depressive subtypes. Am J Psychiatry 1983; 140:11–20
9. Advances in Clinical Decision-Making—the Role of the Biopsychiatric Laboratory. J Clin Psychiat, 47 (Suppl) ('86)
10. Beresford TP et al: CT scanning in psychiatric inpatients—clinical yield. Psychosomatics 1986; 27:105
11. Weinberger DR: Brain disease and psychiatric illness—when should a psychiatrist order a CAT scan? Am J Psychiatry 1984; 141:1521–6

8
Milieu Therapy

Wolfe N. Adler

Milieu therapy has been the subject of many scholarly treatises and has been studied by a diverse group of scientific investigators, including anthropologists, sociologists, psychiatrists, psychologists and professional nurses. Yet it is difficult to find an account of what actually transpires on psychiatric units today. This chapter is an attempt to begin to redress that deficiency.

TWO MODELS OF MILIEU THERAPY

There are two essentially antithetical models for conceptualizing the role of the psychiatric milieu – the *medical milieu model*, which views the milieu as nothing more than a backdrop for inpatient psychiatric care, and the *psychosocial milieu model*, which views the milieu as a therapeutic instrument in its own right.

The Medical Milieu Model

Milieu therapy, according to this model, is conceptualized as a more or less passive, basically adjunctive treatment modality, the two primary functions of which are: to ensure the safety of patients (as well as staff), and to provide the necessary atmosphere wherein specific active treatment interventions, such as individual psychotherapy and pharmacotherapy, may be effectively rendered to the patient. This approach closely approximates that of medical or surgical floors of general hospitals and is based upon the assumption that psychiatric patients, like their medical counterparts, suffer from specific diseases, of single or simple etiologies, for which specific treatment approaches are best applied.

This model emphasizes physician authority and autonomy. The essential role of the milieu staff is to provide moral support and encouragement to patients in order to render them optimally receptive to the ministrations of the doctor. As in the following example, patients may pass through the milieu experience, essentially untouched by the social environment, except for individual bedside-type interactions with nursing staff who reaffirm, support, and augment the attending doctor's therapeutic approach.

> A 59-year-old unemployed accountant is admitted because of suicidal ideation, hopelessness, and severe psychomotor retardation. Since he has not responded previously to antidepressant medication, he is scheduled to begin ECT within three days of admission. Nursing staff assist the physician in counseling the patient about the nature of the problem and what to expect from treatment, express optimism that his suffering will be alleviated, and encourage patience. When the patient asks how soon he will be taken off "suicidal precautions," he is told that it will depend on how soon he begins to respond to his ECT treatments. He is encouraged to discuss this concern with his doctor. The patient's depression responds well to eight ECT's and after an uneventful course in hospital he is discharged on the 28th day.

Patients who enjoy a good recovery within this kind of social milieu usually have considerable personality assets, a good premorbid adjustment, solid social supports, and a well-functioning family system. Their illnesses tend to be more purely biological in etiology, such as a drug-induced depression in an endogenously predisposed individual, or to be precipitated by severe psychosocial stressors, such as being fired or losing a loved one.

The Psychosocial Milieu Model

An impressive literature has evolved that provides testimony for the idea that the social system of the milieu can have a significant impact, both positive and negative, upon the rapidity, form and extent of the patient's recovery. Innumerable sociological studies and anecdotal reports have underscored the fact that patients do poorly in hospital environments which neglect their dignity, or their need for a balance between calm-restoring privacy and social involvement, or their susceptibility to the sometime subtle, oftentimes obvious, effect of the behavior of others. Stanton and Schwartz's classic study[1] of the social system of a psychiatric hospital showed vividly how patients' psychopathology can be magnified by unidentified pathogenic interactions within the patient group and between patients and staff. While their findings focused on the negative effects of a mismanaged milieu, subsequent investigators and milieu therapy clinicians have experimented with ways of mobilizing the therapeutic potential of the milieu.

A major breakthrough was made by Maxwell Jones,[2] whose work with personality disordered patients in a psychiatric unit at the Belmont Hospital in England in the early 1950s became the main inspiration for much of the subsequent development of the practice of milieu therapy. Many of his concepts are still held as articles of faith by most milieu therapists, e.g., that adaptive functioning is fostered by patients' taking responsibility not only for their own individual well-being but also for that of others, and that decisions are arrived at best when patients and staff collaborate as equals and in as democratic a fashion as possible. So influential was Jones' thinking that the name he gave to his approach, "the therapeutic community," came to be used synonymously with milieu therapy. One of his most important innovations, the community meeting, is today almost universally employed as a major instrument for the fostering of collaboration between patients and staff. However, his insistence upon strict democratic forms, which was taken by some of his followers to the extreme of having decisions made by vote, is rarely heeded today. Since the typical patient population being treated on psychiatric units today is, compared to Jones', much more heterogeneous, with a generally lower level of cognitive and interpersonal functioning, staff need to operate in a more active and authoritative mode. Moreover, advances in psychopharmacology and other specific therapeutic modalities, e.g., individual and group psychotherapy, have made it increasingly necessary for professional judgment to be exercised in treatment planning.

When the clinical knowledge and skills of staff are not actively utilized, mob psychology can become activated and chaos can ensue, as in the following example:

> A patient announces at a community meeting that money has been stolen from her wallet and asks the staff to tell her what can be done about it. A nurse responds by asking the patients if they have any thoughts. When staff are pressed by other patients to explain what needs to be done, the patients are told that this is a community problem and a plan of action should be developed by all concerned. A patient who has been on the fringes of the group and has irritated many by his oafish and sadistic remarks reproaches the group for making a mountain out of a molehill. Another patient remembers seeing him standing in the doorway of the victim's room. Several patients agree that he is the most likely culprit. He shoves an ashtray

onto the floor and storms out of the meeting. The patient group then clamors for his transfer to another facility. Despite staff's doubts about the culpability of the indicted patient, the transfer was made.

The psychosocial model of milieu therapy differs from the medical model in the following important ways:

1. It views the psychiatric ward as an open and complex system in which interacting elements, i.e., individual patients and staff members, are continuously affecting each other.
2. Nonphysician treatment team members and patients are potentially potent therapeutic agents.

FUNCTIONS OF THE THERAPEUTIC MILIEU

Control

Safety is an overriding concern in the management of the milieu. The hospital has a fundamental duty to protect the patients and staff from physical harm. Many patients enter the hospital in an acute state of excitement and panic. Others tend to become aggressive in reaction to frustrating or frightening events or because of poor impulse control, paranoid hypersensitivity, or antisocial tendencies. Even though assaults upon patients occur rarely, it is by no means uncommon for patients to feel unusually vulnerable to physical assault. This fear commonly derives from the belief that there is an association between mental illness and violence. Moreover, most patients suffer from a pervasive sense of impotence and inadequacy, which causes them to feel defenseless in the face of provocative, verbally aggressive, or rude behavior.

Patients can only feel secure when they believe in the milieu's ability to prevent and control acts of violence. To this end, strict rules and clear expectations are of paramount importance. Explicit and meaningful sanctions against aggressiveness, or even mere threats of aggression, must be unhesitatingly applied, especially after "talking the patient down" and helping the patient put the anger into words do not work. When all else fails the use of a seclusion room or physical restraints may be required.

Insulation and Asylum

Usually patients are admitted to a hospital because a serious strain has occurred between the patient and his normal social environment. Efforts by the patient and significant others to cope with each other have failed. The patient, no longer able to tolerate them or to be tolerated, ends up being exiled to a psychiatric hospital.

At the time of admission, a male patient might, for example, be panicking over incestuous impulses threatening to get out of control, in which case being prevented from having contact with his children will alleviate his fearfulness and enable him to regain his equilibrium. Or a depressed and desperate young woman might have been making impossible demands on her family for attention and sympathy, until their frustration reaches a pitch of hostility which they no longer can control. A brief respite from their incessant squabbling, i.e., an enforced separation and armistice of only a few days, can help settle things down. More longstanding and deeply entrenched strains may require a more protracted period of limited contact. These respites can be accomplished by limiting visiting hours, banning visits for a period of time, or having staff monitor visits.

Social Reintegration

The ultimate purpose of the control exerted by the milieu program over the patient's contact with significant others is the eventual reintegration of the patient back into the family, community, and work setting. This goal guides much of the exploration and discussion at community meetings, small group meetings, and one-to-one patient-staff interactions. Patients are continuously challenged to identify and alter those behaviors and beliefs that give rise to subjective distress and disturbances in their relations with others. This problem-solving approach is thoroughly collaborative in nature, with patients being helped by both staff and other patients. Some milieu programs also use structured discharge-planning group sessions, where the practical orientation focuses on such details as how to find an apartment, interview for a job, make use of transportation, and engage in an aftercare program.

When patients and staff join forces to direct a patient's attention away from reality-avoiding symptoms and towards the task of reengaging with the real challenges of living, the resultant peer pressure can incite the patient to begin reintegrating herself with the world outside the hospital.

> A 28-year-old nurse becomes highly distraught, suicidal, and somatically preoccupied after learning that her alcoholic mother has cancer. She quits her job impulsively, stays in bed for several weeks, and is admitted to the hospital. Her presenting complaint is that she is physically ill. She denies being upset by her mother's illness or the loss of her job. She is confronted repeatedly by nursing staff about her avoidance of the real issues. Several patients offer examples to her of

how they have used symptoms to avoid unpleasant realities and to keep from succumbing to the pain of grief. At a discharge-planning meeting the group reads and evaluates advertisements for nursing positions in the classified section of a local newspaper. One patient offers to go with the patient to an employment interview, whereupon the patient asks for and receives permission to go the next day, alone.

Patient-Role Induction

The assumption of the sick role is a double-edged sword. Some patients succumb all too readily to pain or emotional distress in order to obtain relief from normal role expectations, to gain sympathy, or to act out in rebellion. Too much eagerness on the part of staff to take over for patients those tasks and responsibilities which they can do for themselves perpetuates sick behavior and prolongs treatment.

It is, nonetheless, extremely important for psychiatric patients to accept the fact that they are suffering from an illness. Denial of illness is the foremost obstacle to the successful implementation of psychiatric treatment. Unfortunately, it is usually those patients who need treatment the most, such as the psychotically disordered and substance abusers, who are most strongly defended against the idea that they are ill and in need of treatment.

Many patients need to be vigorously confronted about their denial. It is very useful to enlist the assistance of patients in this effort, since many patients are inclined to see the staff's views concerning mental illness as being self-serving. The approach taken needs to be tempered and guided by the recognition that the resistance to being classified as mentally ill and the opposition to treatment are oftentimes deeply entrenched and multidetermined. Many patients equate having a mental disorder with being insane and thus fear being socially stigmatized and becoming a social outcast. The dread of mental illness is also associated with other fears, especially loss of one's individuality, of control over one's life, and of one's credibility. Many patients fear being kept in a psychiatric hospital for the rest of their lives. Many have irrational fears of psychiatric medications and of being forced to submit to procedures that would alter them in some fundamental way. Patients with severe cognitive deficits may not be able to readily comprehend information given them. Persistent efforts by staff are required to educate them about their illnesses.

The milieu program needs to strike a very delicate balance between the view that problematic ideas and behaviors are due to mental illness and the view that people are themselves responsible for their actions. Inappropriate behaviors should never be shrugged off or glossed over as merely manifestations of an illness. Patients need to be encouraged to see themselves as capable of acquiring more and more voluntary control over their behavior and as needing to take responsibility for their actions.

Many patients, especially those who are chronically delusional, tend to be highly distrustful of staff, but they sometimes respond to the blandishments of their peers. In the following vignette a patient who had obstinately rejected staff's repeated efforts to get him to take medication eventually becomes cooperative and responds to the sincere and persistent pleas of a peer.

> A 32-year-old male patient with a long history of repeated hospitalizations because of seclusive and bizarre behavior is admitted after getting into a physical brawl with his brother. At his first community meeting he insists that the man he fought was really the devil and that he himself is being marked for execution because of his psychic powers. He is plied with questions about his strange beliefs and mentions in passing that he stopped taking his neuroleptic medication two weeks earlier. A female patient who had met him on the same ward during a previous admission and had taken a liking to him offers to accompany him whenever he needs to go to the window where medication is dispensed. He suddenly becomes remorseful for the trouble he caused his family and vows never to go off his meds again. He laughs, probably because he knows that he is not likely to keep that promise. His female friend breaks into tears and says, "You keep this up and you will end up killing someone someday." After several days of being the focus of his friend's admonitions, the patient relents and becomes impeccably compliant for the remainder of his stay.

Structure

Psychiatric decompensations, whether of psychotic proportions or not, are always associated with a breakdown in adaptational structures. Sleep and eating patterns are usually disrupted, time becomes formless, and goal-directed behaviors disappear, to be replaced by inactivity or misdirected and impulsive relief-seeking.

Upon this state of internal disorganization, order needs to be superimposed. Time needs to be structured, routines developed, activities organized, rules of behavior backed up by consequences. To this end the patient's day needs to be thoroughly scheduled. There should be a consistent time for awakening, taking care of personal hygiene, meals, therapy sessions, meetings, activity therapies, resting, leisure activities, and retiring. Meetings should start punctually and end on time. Attendance should be made mandatory. Therapeutic activities should be scheduled days in advance. Specific times should be set aside for doctor's appointments and visits from relatives and friends.

Rules of conduct need to be explicitly communicated, with a firm expectation that they will be observed. Reasonable sanctions need to be administered when all else fails.

> A confused, autistically withdrawn patient is found smoking in a nonsmoking area. When she fails to heed the exhortations of staff and patients, she is placed on cigarette restriction for several hours. Cigarettes are then doled out to her one at a time. When this fails, she is restricted to the smoking area and is rewarded with a cigarette every half-hour for abiding by this restriction.

Although some abnormal behaviors, such as delusional speech, are best ignored, most should lead to socially appropriate, natural responses. The rules of the milieu program should be designed to simulate, as much as possible, those of normal society.

> At a community meeting a middle-aged male patient who has been consistently rude and caustic in his behavior asks to be allowed to sign out for walks with another patient. A nurse reminds the group of the rule that no patient can be forced to escort another patient, and asks if there are any volunteers. None comes forward. Several patients say that they don't feel comfortable being with him because he is so often belligerent. His request fails for lack of a willingness of others to accept the responsibility of escorting him.

Support

For purposes of this discussion, support refers specifically to efforts to increase each patient's sense of well-being and self-esteem. Supportive interventions include praise, assurance and advice. Ordinarily, unless deterred by obnoxious or menacing behavior, people are naturally inclined to be supportive towards others, especially those who are troubled. The giving of praise or assurance does not require special training or a postgraduate education. Therefore, professionals tend not to see these interventions as a legitimate part of their therapeutic armamentarium. Consequently, the therapeutic potential of these supportive techniques has been traditionally understated in the professional literature on psychotherapy and other psychosocial therapies. Obviously, when praise is offered insincerely, or as a seductive ploy, or when reassurance is given prematurely, the clinician's credibility and effectiveness can be seriously undermined.

Milieu Therapy

Regardless of the merits of the case against supportive interventions in formal psychotherapy, they play a very important role in milieu therapy. Milieu clinicians, rather than engaging in maneuvers to "protect the transference," need to be always forthright and available. Especially for the kinds of patients one finds in psychiatric hospitals, clinical aloofness and non-directiveness will only give rise to bewilderment and mistrust. Psychodynamic interpretations are usually beside the point and should never replace straightforward observations, explanations, or suggestions:

> A profoundly thought-disordered patient walks into the nurses station and says to his therapist, "The woman of my dreams is the Whore Babylon." The therapist replies, "I wonder if you are saying that your attraction to your mother has been upsetting you lately." A nurse, standing by, intervenes with: "Now, Bill you know you are not supposed to come into the nurses station. You've done so well until now in giving us our privacy in here. Could you continue doing that?" The patient gives his therapist a disgusted look, says "Thanks" to the nurse, and promptly leaves.

Knowing when and how to offer praise and reassurance in a therapeutically effective manner requires clinical wisdom and skill. It is indeed no simple matter to buoy up the spirits of a hopelessly despondent and self-abasing depressed patient. Similarly, patients with borderline personality disorders are given to misinterpreting the intentions of others and can react to positive remarks by feeling insulted or humiliated. However, in our experience, even when patients seem to shrink from praise, they privately savor it.

Gratitude is another supportive response, and one that can almost always be safely and usefully given, when deserved.

> A 42-year-old woman whose husband ran off with another woman two months earlier becomes abjectly depressed and actively suicidal. After three days of being virtually mute and unapproachable she angrily reproaches the nursing staff at a community meeting for putting too much pressure on another patient to talk. A nurse responds, "Thanks, I think we needed that." Later that day she is seen quietly conversing with her silent friend and earns a wink from a nurse passing by. During the next three weeks she turns her attentions to other patients and is given the title "Mother Earth." The day before she is discharged she obtains a volunteer job at another hospital.

The more regressed and asocial the patient, the more important it is to take advantage of the reinforcing and motivating effect of praise. This technique is especially important on token economy wards.

Involvement

Another interesting therapeutic dimension of the milieu is what Gunderson[3] calls "involvement." This refers to the active collaboration by patients in solving each other's problems. Without exception, acutely upset patients are intensely self-preoccupied, and chronically disordered patients tend to live in a world of their own. Drawing their attention away from themselves can appreciably lessen their anxiety and sense of isolation, as well as affording them the opportunity to practice and be rewarded for prosocial behavior. This involvement by patients in their fellows' treatment enhances their own involvement in their own therapy and undermines the tendency to perceive staff as patronizing know-it-alls. Patients are, thereby, acculturated into the value system of the milieu; they assimilate its beliefs and enjoy a greater sense of belonging.[4] Besides, patients often have much of value to say to one another, and to staff as well, as the following vignette of a community meeting dramatically illustrates:

> News of the suicide of a recently discharged patient sends a shock wave through the milieu. An emergency meeting is called. In a trembling voice the patient's doctor starts the meeting by reporting what he knows about the circumstances of the patient's death. A patient observes: "Doctor A, you are taking this pretty hard, harder than I expected." Another patient chimes in: "Doctors have feelings too; we are *all* distraught over this." Another patient: "I never thought I could feel like this about someone I hardly know." Next patient: "I'm angry (at the patient who has suicided), and now I know what my social worker meant about anger being legitimate even if it isn't fair." Next patient: "Suicide is not sweet."

Problem-solving

Two levels of problem-solving go on continuously and simultaneously in a therapeutic milieu: that of the individual, and that of the group. The former focuses upon the individual's intrapsychic dynamics, interpersonal disabilities, and practical problems of living. These issues are best dealt with either in small groups or in one-to-one interactions.

At the other level the focus is on the day-to-day life of the ward and the interpersonal difficulties that inevitably arise. These issues are frequently addressed at full-scale community meetings. For example: What should be done about the patient who is threatening another patient? Should the unit door be locked? Can mealtimes be extended, bedtime postponed? Who is going to escort whom? When should suicide precautions be lifted? Is the seclusion room really necessary? Can't the process of signing-out be made easier? How can the seclusive patient be drawn out or should he be left alone? What should be done about the patient who uses the phone irresponsibly? When can visitors come outside of the usual visiting hours? Are staff being fair? What can be done about the group's apathy? Why can't all the patients go home for Christmas?

Most psychiatric patients have lost confidence in their ability to solve problems, particularly their own. One of the most important tasks of the milieu is to restore patients' faith in their ability to overcome their difficulties through an act of striving to find solutions. When patients discover, as in the community meeting about to be recounted, that a seemingly insurmountable problem of group apathy becomes resolved once the right combination of helpful suggestions is achieved, faith in active problem-solving is strongly reinforced:

> At a community meeting the head nurse points out that every year the ward gets decorated for Halloween. She asks for volunteers. No one responds. She comments sadly, "We are all so depressed this morning." A patient says, "We're just not interested." Another patient joins in: "This isn't fair. Why should we have to even bother with this?" Another nurse says, "Fairness is in the eyes of the beholder." A patient retorts, "Then why don't you decorate it yourself?" Another patient suggests that her roommate is an artist who might help with the overall design of the decorations. The roommate says she is better at drawing. Another patient offers to cut out paper, but claims to be no good at drawing. By the end of the day the entire ward is strung with smiling pumpkins.

Acquisition of Insight

It is a matter of some controversy as to whether the milieu should be the locus for the acquisition of insight into the unconscious dynamics underlying the patient's conscious thoughts, feelings and behavior. Some clinicians feel that this uncovering process should be saved for individual psychotherapy or formal group therapy. They fear that insight occurring outside of therapy may not make it to therapy, that patients are prone to act out their negative transference to the therapist by taking their problems to someone else, or that insight occurring outside of therapy is valueless because it cannot be worked through. Interestingly, similar misgivings were invoked when group therapy was first introduced as a competitive alternative to individual psychotherapy.

Nonetheless, the milieu oftentimes affords unique opportunities for the emergence of valuable insights.

> A 34-year-old woman who requested admission because of growing panic over her hostile feelings toward her three-year-old daughter becomes enraged when her request to have her daughter visit is turned down. When the head nurse reminds her of the ward rule against small children visiting, the patient screams, "I will kill anyone who gets in the way of me and my daughter." Another patient reminds her that she came to the hospital because she was having similar murderous feelings toward her daughter. This comment is followed by a prolonged and stunned silence. A male patient who had previously taken her side in the argument says, "Oh, I didn't know that. Then who has your daughter been getting in between?" A nurse asks, "Has your husband been visiting?" Another patient replies "No, she's said that he doesn't have time because he has to stay home with the child." At this point the angry mother breaks down and cries, and receives a consoling arm around her shoulder from her male protector.

Education

Psychoeducation, or illness education, is becoming increasingly recognized as a necessary ingredient in each patient's overall treatment program. Stimulated by the advent of the informed consent doctrine, as well as by the prevalence of noncompliance to medication regimens, psychiatric milieus are increasingly utilizing educational techniques aimed at providing patients with the basic facts concerning their illnesses. What are the signs and symptoms of the illness? What are the known causes, if there are any? Is the illness inheritable? What is its usual course? What treatments are available? What drugs are effective? How do they work? What are their side effects? How long do they need to be taken?

Illness education is still in its infancy as a developing systematic therapeutic intervention, although it is already clear that combining didactic presentations with group discussions is a useful strategy. As in other types of learning, repetition is mandatory. Heretofore, doctors have naively assumed that since patients routinely misunderstand or forget much of what they are told about their illness, they lack the capability of assimilating this kind of information. But clinicians themselves need to be repeatedly exposed to the same information before it is mastered. Illness education can be a highly

Milieu Therapy

effective approach to counteracting the patient's denial and opposition to treatment.

LEVELS OF SUPERVISION AND FREEDOM

Most milieu programs have worked out a system for titrating the amount of staff supervision needed by each patient. These systems are known by various names, e.g., "privilege," "permission," "step," and "responsibility" systems. At our hospital the latter terminology is used because it captures the central criteria for determining the amount of supervision needed, i.e., how much responsibility is the patient capable of taking for him or herself.

The number of different responsibility levels differs from milieu to milieu because of differences in average length-of-stay, mix of patients, the degree to which the unit is self-contained, and the treatment philosophy of the program.

Short-term units tend to have fewer levels, since the fewer the steps, the more rapid the progress up the responsibility ladder. Patients in these programs are encouraged to move out of the hospital quickly, and need to have the opportunity to "try out their wings" at the earliest possible time, such as by leaving the unit on their own on walks or for personal errands and by making visits home. Long-term programs tend to allow patients increasing liberties at a more deliberate speed and may have a graded system of as many as eight different responsibility levels.

Personality disordered patients, especially those in intermediate and long-term programs, may need the greatest number of steps because of their impulsivity and their tendency to test the limits of social toleration and physical safety.

Many free-standing psychiatric hospitals have central dining rooms and offer many therapeutic activities off the unit. They, therefore, tend to have more elaborate systems of graded responsibility levels, since patients frequently have to move about within the hospital's buildings and upon the surrounding grounds.

The mission or philosophy of the program determines in large measure how readily patients are given increased liberties. Some programs place a much greater emphasis on patient autonomy than others. Programs that emphasize supportive approaches and place improvement of self-esteem high up on their list of therapeutic goals are likely to be more liberal in allocating liberties to patients. On the other hand, programs that emphasize structure and involvement, and are more tailored towards reshaping the patient's behavior, tend to have a more rigorous and complex system of responsibility levels.

One example of a system of responsibility levels is as follows:

Intensive Special Observation: This level provides the most intensive staff supervision. It is used for acutely suicidal, self-mutilating or aggressive patients. The patient never leaves the unit and is constantly in view of staff 24 hours a day. For some patients, staff may need to be within arm's reach of the patient at all times.

Special Observation: The patient is checked by a member of the nursing staff approximately every 15 minutes. The intervals between checks should be irregular enough that the patient cannot anticipate when the next check will take place. The patient is considered a moderately high risk for causing injury to self, but is not considered imminently dangerous. Or the patient may be medically unstable enough to require this level of supervision. The patient may go off the unit but only in the company of a staff member.

Staff Escort: The patient is observed no less often than every half-hour and may go off the unit with a group of no more than six patients in the company of a staff member. The patient may be at risk for wandering off, deliberately eloping, engaging in antisocial behavior, acting bizarrely, or experiencing an intolerable level of anxiety.

Patient Escort: The patient may leave the unit on a staff-approved sign-out to a destination within the hospital but must be in the company of another patient who is both willing to do the escorting and is on patient escort or a higher level of responsibility. The patient can behave properly under conditions which support the patient's motivation to conform his behavior to reasonable expectations.

Unescorted Privileges: The patient may leave the unit unaccompanied with staff's permission for a specified time and purpose. The patient is moving steadily towards discharge and is able to behave effectively without being under the direct scrutiny and supervision of others.

Ideally responsibility levels are assigned after input from both clinical staff and patients. Most hospitals require them to be documented and authorized by a doctor, in the same way medication orders are. Token economy programs may require patients to earn a certain number of points or tokens in order to either maintain their level or achieve a higher level of responsibility. Some programs require patients to obtain the approval of a minimum number of milieu staff, and patients may be required to submit and defend their requests for a higher responsibility level at a community meeting.

A 29-year-old unemployed man who is hearing voices that he attributes to the devil and which are commanding him to kill himself is immediately, upon admission, place on intensive special observation. A week later the voices are accusatory, no longer commanding, but he still admits to feeling hopeless. He is placed on special observation. Over the next few days his mood brightens and he begins to engage in brief interactions with others. He is then placed on staff escort. Within the next two weeks his mood continues to improve and he no longer demands to be released from the hospital. He is placed on patient escort. On his first accompanied trip off the ward he runs away from his patient escort and several hours later is brought back to the hospital by his parents. He is placed back on staff escort. Over the next month he demonstrates insight into his problems and recognition of his need for further treatment. He is reinstated on patient escort and after two incident-free weeks is given unescorted privileges and begins to make visits home.

THE PSYCHIATRIC TREATMENT TEAM

If a team can be defined as a group of individuals who possess different skills and carry out different roles but whose efforts are coordinated towards the achievement of a common goal, then the psychiatric treatment team is a classical example. A typical treatment team consists of one or more psychiatrists, clinical psychologists, professional and paraprofessional nurses, activity therapists, and social workers. Most milieu programs use a matrix organization, with authority overlapping the program leadership and the clinical departments represented by the various professional disciplines. Generally, the coordination of the work of members of the treatment team is carried out under the direction of a unit chief, who is usually a psychiatrist. The head nurse, thus, would be responsible to both the unit chief and a nursing supervisor. Similarly, other disciplines would have dual reporting responsibilities. Each member contributes input into the evaluation of the patient, participates in the treatment planning process, and plays a unique role in the actual care delivered to the patient. These contributions vary according to the special expertise of each discipline and the particular psychological and interpersonal skills of each individual team member.

In milieu programs that overemphasize egalitarianism within the patient-staff group, disciplinary boundaries are less clear, and there is a tendency for staff's professional skills to decay. Roles become confused, responsibilities are ill-defined, and the decision-making process may be vague and cumbersome. Moreover, the opinions of the most clinically judicious staff may not prevail over those of staff who are more verbally facile or more intent on having things their own way.

In the vignette that follows, the clinical care of a difficult patient is mismanaged because the staff have not developed a clear sense of their respective roles and responsibilities. As a result, the opinions of patients and staff are given equal weight, regardless of disparities in expertise, and an expedient, inhumane and nontherapeutic solution is implemented:

> Ward A is in turmoil after being bombarded day and night by the incessant harangues of a recently admitted manic patient. A community meeting is held. The patient group implores the patient's psychiatrist to increase his medication. He responds by indicating that he will discuss that option further with the treatment team later that day. A nurse asks the patients what they can do to help. The patients insist that the manic patient be put in the seclusion room. A vote is taken and all of the patients, along with half of the staff, vote for seclusion, whereupon he is immediately placed in the seclusion room. Another patient insists that they go on with the agenda of the meeting so that her sign-out can be discussed, leaving no time to process what just happened.
>
> Later that day at the staff meeting the psychiatrist asks the treatment team to decide on the medication question. The social worker offers the opinion that the patient is suffering not from a manic episode but a catatonic excitement and should be switched from lithium to a neuroleptic. The sentiment of the group remains in favor of an increase in lithium, but the decision is postponed until the following morning so that the opinions of the evening and night shift can be gathered. Meanwhile the patient remains in seclusion and out of control.

Most milieu programs today are hierarchically organized, with clear roles and responsibilities that are often formalized in written job descriptions. Within this type of team structure, it is always clear who is responsible for making the ultimate decision, and each discipline is able to make full use of its particular knowledge base and special skills. However, the team needs to be constantly alert to the possible intrusion of professional bias and rivalry upon the decision-making process. Psychiatrists might unduly favor the use of medications and conceptualize the patient's difficulties as being entirely comprehensible within the context of the diagnostic criteria of *DSM-III-R*. Others are also apt to see things only from the vantage point of their own disciplines. To counteract these tendencies there must be both enlightened leadership and responsible followership. The ethos of the team must include a respect for the uniqueness of the contributions of each discipline, a recognition of the importance of good group morale, and an appreciation of the special and unique personality assets and liabilities of individual members.

The same manic patient is administratively transferred the next day to Ward B and a different treatment team. At a treatment team meeting that day the staff share what they have heard about the patient. The social worker comments that the patient's parents seem appropriately concerned but feel exhausted. She asks the doctor what she plans to do. The doctor replies that she will increase the patient's lithium and asks the head nurse if she thinks the patient can be maintained out of seclusion for the time being. The head nurse asks her staff if they think they could give it a try and they agree to take the patient out of seclusion.

The next morning the head nurse informs the patients at the community meeting that the manic patient has just started receiving heavier doses of medication and that the staff has decided to try to keep him out of seclusion. She asks the patients to try not to feed into the manic patient's need for attention.

THE COMMUNITY MEETING

The community meeting's potential for good and harm has been portrayed in many of the preceding vignettes. While the overall management of the milieu and smaller one-to-one interactions among patients and staff both contribute greatly to the overall therapeutic effect of the milieu, the community meeting usually looms, symbolically at least, as the keystone of the milieu approach.

It is critically important that the purpose of the community meeting be clearly defined. One of its most important functions is to provide an organizing vehicle for communication and the resolution of problems arising in the day-to-day life of the ward.

It is useful to have several different kinds of community meetings. One meeting should be exclusively devoted to patient requests for sign-outs and changes in responsibility levels. Another meeting should be used to plan group activities, and another to discuss interpersonal problems on the ward. Emergency community meetings need to be called when a serious incident occurs, such as an attempted suicide or the confiscation of a cache of marijuana. In addition to giving the staff the opportunity to assess each patient's reaction to the incident, these meetings afford the group the opportunity to ventilate and to develop a plan for preventing future similar occurrences.

Because of their large and heterogeneous membership, community meetings have a tendency to become chaotic. Frequent silences signal that the purpose of the meeting has been lost sight of. Formal responsibility for running the meeting is oftentimes delegated to patients. Staff may assign or allow the patient group to elect the chairperson. Nevertheless, the staff must maintain the responsibility for seeing to it that the group stays on its task. "Leading from behind" is a special skill that milieu staff often employ at these meetings. The chairperson should have a set agenda, announce it at the beginning of the meeting, and keep the group on schedule throughout the entire duration of the meeting.

As distinguished from formal group therapy, the discourse at community meetings should take place on the level of practical problem-solving. When interpersonal conflicts need to be addressed, the focus needs to be less on what is going on in the meeting and more on what has gone before, between the conflicted members, and what ideally ought to go on after the meeting.

SPECIALIZED VERSUS GENERAL MILIEU PROGRAMS

The diversity of psychiatric disorders poses a particular problem for milieu programs. For example, chronic schizophrenic patients are prone to regress or at least become more withdrawn under the pressure of an overly stimulating and socially demanding milieu.[5] They cope poorly with the complexity and emotionally arousing aspects of community meetings and retreat further into apathy and autism.

Substance-abusing patients who are not severely impaired by psychiatric symptoms are better treated on a milieu of their own, one that heavily utilizes educational strategies, confrontation, and the AA philosophy.

Eating disordered patients usually can be treated on a general purpose unit but require intensive nursing supervision. Behavior modification and other nursing strategies specifically developed for these patients can be more efficiently delivered when all are placed on the same unit.

Borderline patients pose unusually difficult problems in milieu management. They can be highly impulsive and are very demanding of attention and special privileges. They often seem bent on foiling therapeutic interventions, and at the same time evoke powerful caring and protective responses.[6] In dealing with these patients staff are constantly at risk of falling prey to feelings of failure because of the inevitable frustration encountered in trying to alleviate their unremitting suicidal despair. Staff splitting, i.e., the division between staff who believe that patient is unusually needy and those who believe the patient is self-serving and untrustworthy, is a familiar phenomenon on psychiatric units. Because of the unusual ability of borderlines to use up the emotional resources of staff members, many milieu programs can only manage a small number of these patients at any given time. A more ambitious approach is to design a unit exclusively for the treatment of borderline personality disorders with staff especially trained in and selected for their abilities to therapeutically manage these patients.

Geriatric patients might also be best treated on a specialized unit. Their physical infirmities, cognitive deficits, and sensory impairments require special equipment and architectural modifications, as well as a specially trained staff.

In our experience, the inpatient treatment of adolescents and children can best be carried out on units that are limited to specific age groups.

CHARACTERISTICS OF THE MILIEU

A heuristically valuable way of examining the therapeutic characteristics of the milieu and comparing different milieus was devised by Rudolph Moos.[7] He and his colleagues had patients and staff use an ingenious rating scale, known as Ward Atmosphere Scale, which identifies and defines a number of the most salient characteristics of a psychiatric ward. Three of these characteristics — *involvement, support,* and *spontaneity* — reflect, respectively, the degree of patient involvement in the activities of the ward, the extent to which staff support patients and patients support each other, and the amount of behavioral spontaneity and emotional expressiveness staff and patients bring to their relationships. Programs which emphasize these characteristics tend to be more loosely structured, to have fewer rules and standard procedures, and to view psychiatric patients as being overly inhibited, dependent and frustrated. *Autonomy* is a milieu characteristic which reflects the degree to which patients are permitted to make decisions for themselves and are encouraged to take initiatives. Three other dimensions of the ward atmosphere as described by Moos (*practical orientation, personal problem orientation, anger and aggression*) might be conceived of as reflecting the therapeutic ideology of the ward. Finally, Moos delineates three important system maintenance dimensions of the milieu: *order and organization, program clarity, and staff control.*

THE FUTURE OF MILIEU THERAPY

The prospects for further development and refinement of milieu therapy are not bright. Third-party payers have long ago refused to recognize the specific therapeutic value of the milieu and refuse to pay for it per se. Hospital administrators, subsequently, have concentrated their attention upon resources that generate reimbursable care, such as laboratory and physician services, room and board. Ever-shortening lengths of hospital stay, due largely to arbitrary limits imposed by government agencies and third-party payers, have resulted in an increasing emphasis being placed on specific treatment modalities, particularly somatic therapies, at the expense of milieu therapy.

Psychiatric residency programs are required to provide residents with training in so many different areas that there is relatively little time left over for them to gain firsthand experience in the management of the milieu. It is hardly necessary any longer for a candidate to know anything about milieu therapy to become certified in psychiatry by the American Board of Psychiatry and Neurology.

Little in the way of careful scientific research has been or is currently being conducted in the field of milieu therapy. The only scientifically respectable study of the comparative effectiveness of different milieu systems was conducted in the mid '70s by Paul and Lentz,[8] who demonstrated conclusively that backward schizophrenics responded dramatically better to a highly organized and strictly conducted token economy approach than to a more traditional milieu approach.

Many of the techniques of milieu therapy developed in hospital settings have been successfully adapted to other treatment settings, e.g., halfway and quarterway houses, day hospitals and psychosocial rehabilitation centers. If access to inpatient psychiatric care continues to decline, the burden of the care of the mentally ill will fall increasingly to these alternative facilities, where further refinements and creative applications of milieu therapy are bound to occur.

REFERENCES

1. Stanton AH, Schwartz MS: The Mental Hospital. New York, Basic Books, 1954
2. Jones M: The Therapeutic Community. New York, Basic Books, 1953
3. Gunderson JG: An overview of modern milieu therapy, in Principles and Practice of Milieu Therapy. Edited by Gunderson JG, Will OA Jr, Mosher LR, New York/London, Jason Aronson, 1983
4. Almond R, Keniston K, Boltax S: Milieu therapeutic process. Arch Gen Psychiatry, 1969; 21:431-442
5. Van Putten T: Milieu therapy: contraindications? Arch Gen Psychiatry 1973; 29:640-643
6. Burnham DL: The special problem patient: victim or agent of splitting? Psychiatry 1966; 2:105-122
7. Moos RH: Evaluating Treatment Environments: A Social Ecological Approach. New York, Wiley, 1974
8. Paul GL, Lentz RJ: Psychosocial Treatment of Chronic Mental Patients: Milieu vs. Social Learning Programs. Cambridge, MA, Harvard University Press, 1977

9
Inpatient Psychotherapy

Melvin Prosen
Donald Ross

Outpatient psychotherapy is usually conducted in a one-to-one setting, focusing rather exclusively on the relationship between patient and therapist. In a hospital, this relationship is greatly diluted, and the therapeutic agenda revolves not only about the therapist but also about other "therapists" on a ward and the "life" of the ward to which the patient is assigned. Within a hospital, there are many people who render therapy in addition to the primary therapist; these include nursing staff, activities and recreation therapists, and even other patients within a group therapy setting.

In comparison to outpatient treatment, therapy within the hospital is a much more public event, open to scrutiny of others, and occurring amidst an open milieu. There is less privacy surrounding the individual treatment aspects of the therapy, for the therapist often reports some of the contents of the hour so as to alert staff to the patient's struggles, dynamics, and behaviors. In former years, there existed a therapist/administrator split, whereby daily privileges were handled by the latter and therapy could be "purer" and uncontaminated by the parameters mentioned above. But the movement away from a strict psychoanalytic model and towards a shorter stay for most patients has dictated a more comprehensive model of hospital intervention, with the therapist largely functioning as his own administrator and as a clinician fully involved in day-to-day care of the patient.

Hospitalization is a traumatic event for the patient and is usually accompanied by shame, guilt, and a sense of failure.[1] These feelings must be dealt with early in inpatient therapy. The first task for the therapist is to talk about the hospitalization itself, as well as the failures leading up to it, including the failure of outpatient treatment itself. No inpatient therapy can proceed until this occurs. On the other hand, staff, used to a flow of new admissions, may urge or coerce the patient to tell his "story" over and over again to various members of the health team. While this may appear cathartic, it does not respect the dignity of the patient who may prefer to talk privately with only one person; the patient may experience a worsening of symptoms as he feels overburdened from the need to reveal himself openly.

The psychotherapeutic task of dealing with issues surrounding hospitalization may occur in group therapy and individual therapy. The themes include the powerlessness of being in the hospital, lack of autonomy, the incarceration and its indeterminate endpoint, and lack of privacy. Some patients spend many days and weeks talking about these issues, to the exclusion of deeper material. Drug-abusing patients and alcoholic patients, for example, may spend all their time talking superficially within individual and group sessions about their illness. Others manage to cope with the trauma of hospitalization quickly and move on to intrapsychic issues.

The type of therapist assigned to the patient strongly influences the nature of the therapeutic relationship. The primary hospital therapist may be a senior attending or a medical student; levels of training may vary considerably. But in either case, the patient has an opportunity to see that therapist interact with other patients and with the staff as well. This creates skews in the transference and sharply influences how patient sees therapist and the therapy itself.[2] In some instances, the inexperience of the therapist may heighten this problem, as seen in the following cases.

> A 25-year-old female was admitted to the hospital after an overdose of antidepressants, which she took upon discovery that her husband was unfaithful. Early in her stay, she withdrew from other patients and felt resentful towards staff. She compared herself to the young, attractive resident assigned to her case, and found herself even more defective. Because the patient could not be mobilized, staff and patients began to chastise the resident for "not doing more." This created a situation whereby the therapist began to feel like the patient: useless and resentful. In supervision, the resident was able to get in touch with her own anger at staff allegations of ineffectiveness. This in turn helped her understand the patient's reactions, and she was able to mobilize the latter's anger in a productive manner, leading her to interact more on the ward.

> A 40-year-old man entered the hospital after losing his job and becoming paranoid. He assumed a hostile and provocative stance on

the ward and did not engage in activities. His young doctor was determined to work with him and hence adopted a position of advocacy, protecting him against the demands of the hospital staff. He also began to withhold data from other members of the treatment team until confronted by them, at which time he was able to see his behavior more clearly. He could then more effectively take on the role of therapist and challenge the patient when necessary.

These case examples illustrate the distortions that can occur in the patient-therapist relationship. They also illustrate the power of the transference and countertransference. Fortunately, the watchfulness of staff in both cases alerted the therapist to the problem. But sometimes this is not easy. A silent transference, for instance, is more difficult to deal with. In such instances, the patient views the therapist as ineffective, or omnipotent, or frightening. If such a patient has been in outpatient therapy previously, he may be already sensitized to the matter of transference and may eventually talk about the underlying feelings that give rise to the silence. But new patients who are inexperienced in the matter of therapy may have considerably less insight and may suffer with their feelings and perceptions, until such time as staff or therapist vigorously confront them. It is this fact—the confrontation—which makes inpatient therapy different from outpatient therapy. Outpatient therapeutic relationships are rarely disturbed by outside forces. But in inpatient work, there are many observers who comment on the nature of the patient-therapist relationship.[3]

A young borderline woman was admitted for depression stemming from a failed romance. She eagerly awaited her therapist's appearance each morning and emerged from sessions with him smiling. The therapist was dimly aware of her enthusiasm for him, until told by the nursing staff that the patient only talked about him and rarely about her former boyfriend. After awaking each morning she paced the halls, waiting for his arrival. Once aware of this reaction on her part, he confronted her with it.

A young borderline patient was admitted to the hospital because of suicidal ideation. As an outpatient she had a dependent and eroticized transference to her therapist, but perceived him as very "proper" and as someone who did not ever smile or laugh at the things she said. In the hospital, as she watched him interact with other patients and staff, she became enraged, commenting to staff that he seemed to do "just fine" with others and evidently "liked them better." On one occasion, she observed the therapist laughing with nursing staff and became very jealous. The doctor was alerted to her reactions and attempted to explore them in individual therapy with her. Although she resisted exploration, with nursing staff she became more relaxed and insightful and better able to understand some of her feelings and distortions as they pointed them out to her.

This case illustrates the corrective action possible by outside "therapists" who tell the primary therapist about the patient. Such occurrences often foster the impression that staff are "spying" on the patient, reporting all untoward behaviors to the therapist and curtailing the patient's dignity. In effect, inpatient therapy is often conducted in a fishbowl; the therapist must tread a delicate line between a private and public therapy. This "fishbowl" effect becomes very useful in dealing with difficult transferences, including those psychotic in nature. Borderline patients, for example, often engage in "splitting" behavior on the ward whereby they idealize one person and denigrate another. This stems from their basic inability to synthesize the good and bad in one person. In such situations, staff may easily realize what is occurring. One staff person may be the recipient of the patient's confidences, while another may be snubbed or avoided. Whether these differences are brought to the attention of the patient depends upon the progress in treatment; in some instances, the "split" is an inevitable part of the therapy and is left alone if a positive relationship exists with the therapist.

Inpatient therapy may involve individual sessions focusing on intrapsychic exploration or supportive sessions in which the patient's defenses are upheld and coping talents strengthened. Supportive therapy is more easily rendered by the team and is used in "crisis" work with impaired patients such as schizophrenics or those with severe personality disorders.[4] The interventions, even though quite simple, may be very effective.

A chronic schizophrenic patient was admitted because of poor drug compliance, leading to an exacerbation of his psychotic symptoms. He had little insight into his disease and avoided medications. In group therapy sessions, other patients confronted him about his multiple hospitalizations and urged him to take the prescribed medication, but he reacted with disinterest, stating that nothing mattered and that everyone was angry with him. Then another ill patient stated that apathy evoked anger and that "you bring about your own disapproval and you need to look at that." Another person asked the patient, "What would happen if you took your medication and never had to return to the hospital again?" The patient began to cry and told the group that he felt hopeless. The group responded by pointing out how he brought about his own hopelessness.

The group can be a very effective force in mobilizing support on a ward; this forms the basis for the use of self-help groups such as Alcoholics Anonymous. But insight can also be achieved, and often more persuasively than in a one-to-one setting. Even so, deeper issues may have to be dealt with alone with the therapist, though primed by the group.[5]

A woman struggling with anxiety and phobic concerns about harming her children listened to a group discussion of incest and became increasingly agitated. She excused herself from the group and went to her room, where staff attempted to intervene without success. Later that morning, in individual therapy, she revealed how she had been sexually abused by her stepfather. This led to a productive discussion about her phobic concerns.

What occurs on the ward fuels the content of the therapy hour later and vice versa; issues discussed in the privacy of a therapy later emerge on the ward or in group psychotherapy. Thus, a private discussion with a depressed patient about guilt over deficient mothering may translate into excessively maternal behavior on the ward with younger patients. Or a comment in group therapy about a patient's passivity may erupt within the individual sessions as a hurtful and angry outburst at a specific group therapy member, a remark which had not been expressed in the group itself.

Individual therapy is usually held twice or three times weekly in the hospital, but group therapy sessions may meet every day or even several times a day if one includes certain ward administrative meetings which inevitably have a therapeutic flavor. Institutions vary with regard to the importance they place on individual therapy. In some institutions, these treatments rapidly give way to other activities; in other locations, individual therapy is the most hallowed form of treatment. The latter philosophy is more typically seen in psychoanalytically oriented institutions.

The role of the hospital in bringing to light existing character pathology is an important one, particularly with individuals whose impulse ridden disorders necessitate controls on their aggressive urges and uninsightful behaviors. Rages against dependency and helplessness can be dealt with therapeutically, to the benefit of the patient.

An adolescent patient with antisocial propensities and aggression was admitted because of deteriorating social behavior with truancy and stealing. He initially refused to come into the hospital and entered only when legal actions was threatened. During the first 24 hours, his reaction to confinement on a locked ward was intense. He phoned his parents and girlfriend urgently and frequently, and cried copiously. He immediately signed a notice of intent to leave, then retracted it, and then signed another. He was furious with everyone and could not be consoled.

The outside therapist paid him a visit and sat with him in his room. When the patient fumed at his incarceration, the therapist questioned what he was so upset about — after all, it was a voluntary admission designed to avoid a far worse fate. The patient could not answer, but stated that he hated being locked up. The therapist suggested that the patient might derive some comfort in being protected from jail. The patient became silent, and the therapist then also suggested that the patient didn't like anybody coming near him; hospitalization most assuredly would involve other patients and staff trying to acquaint themselves with him. After this discussion, the patient quieted down and remained in the hospital; indeed, he ultimately became frightened of leaving when the time came for discharge.

This case illustrates the possibility of insight being achieved through a hospital-based psychotherapeutic encounter. Early in the hospitalization, it is not uncommon for patients such as the above to displace their hostilities onto staff, who then become the rejecting authorities. These patients then stimulate strong countertransference feelings on the part of staff who must deal with them and who feel repudiated. The way out of these dilemmas is not easy, but it is an important part of the psychotherapeutic endeavor. Later in the hospital course, patients with character pathology may listen to staff when they do not listen to their therapists, or they may benefit from peer group confrontations. Since authority structures are suspect, peer group approval is essential to hospital survival. Patients are more likely to be motivated to change if they can see their deviancies and respond to them. Some of this is conscious, but much is unconscious and a product of identification and socialization. The power of the hospital in promoting this socialization and maturation is immense.

Irrespective of philosophical orientation — i.e., biologic vs. analytic — no hospitalization really happens without some form of psychotherapeutic attention being paid to the patient. Individual therapy may or may not occur, or it may or may not be supplemented with group therapy or even psychodrama; at the very least, staff and adjunctive therapists inevitably help the patient with observation and feedback about maladaptive behaviors. Even if the hospitalization is for simple dose adjustment of a drug or for electroconvulsive therapy, some supportive work inevitably occurs. And the intensity and diversity of the therapeutic contacts make the hospitalization a richer clinical experience for the patient.

REFERENCES

1. Prosen M: Shame and Guilt Factors in Self Esteem Regulation. Paper presented at the Case Conferences of Sheppard Pratt Hospital, Towson, Maryland, May 1, 1985
2. Gill M: The analysis of transference, J Amer Psychoanal Assoc, supplement 1972; 27:263-288
3. Stanton A, Schwartz M: The Psychiatric Hospital. New York, Basic Books, 1954
4. Bloch S: What is Psychotherapy? London, Oxford Univ Press, 1982
5. Yalom ID: Inpatient Group Psychotherapy. New York, Basic Books, 1983

10
Inpatient Cognitive Behavior Therapy

James McGee

Except for those occasions where the patient is a clear "danger to self or others," hospitalization is rarely seen as the treatment of first choice for a psychiatric disorder. This seems to be particularly true in the current atmosphere of cost containment, DRG's, patient rights, deinstitutionalization, and the ideal of treating in "the least restrictive environment." Cognitive behavior therapy, because it derives from a social learning rather than "medical" model of mental illness, also comes to the psychiatric hospital with something of an antihospital tradition. The concept of "social breakdown syndrome"[1] has been identified by some cognitive behaviorists as an inevitable consequence of long-term inpatient psychiatric hospitalization. Furthermore, much of the research and practice of cognitive behavior therapy has been done by psychologists disenfranchised from and operating outside the mainstream of hospital psychiatry. Cognitive behavior therapists, if permitted to practice in a traditional, and usually psychodynamic, inpatient setting, have invariably been relegated to working with the most regressed and least responsive chronically psychotic patients. Ironically, it is out of this "shotgun" marriage of cognitive behavior therapists and regressed psychiatric inpatients that one of the most impressive achievements of the cognitive behavioral approach has developed, i.e., the "token economy."

Generally speaking, the cognitive behavioral therapies continue to enjoy a greater degree of acceptance by psychologists rather than psychiatrists. Nonetheless, these treatment approaches have become an integral part of the therapeutic repertoire of many psychiatric hospitals. In large measure, this is simply because the cognitive behavioral therapies "work." Not only do they produce positive change in patients, but also, because of their high degree of objectivity, specificity, outcome orientation, and time-limited nature, they readily lend themselves to accountability.

Accountability is the contemporary "buzz" word in health care in general and psychiatric care in particular. The cognitive behavioral approaches are by nature "accountable." The current demand for specificity in the documentation of psychiatric services, so repugnant to many psychodynamic clinicians, is both a welcome and already familiar way of doing business for the cognitive behaviorists.

The primary advantage to the cognitive behavior therapist in hospitalizing a prospective patient lies in the degree of environmental control available in an inpatient setting. In order for many of the most popular cognitive behavioral techniques, such as flooding, response prevention, token economy, etc., to be effective, total and precise control over environmental contingencies is essential. That high degree of environmental control, which is crucial to both the assessment and treatment of the patient, is normally available only in an inpatient psychiatric setting.

COGNITIVE BEHAVIOR THERAPY

Cognitive behavior therapy is a theoretical and technical approach to the alteration of deviant human behavior that involves the systematic application of principles of both cognitive and behavioral psychology. Cognitive behavior therapy is a relatively recent development in the history of the psychotherapies. An appreciation of it depends on some understanding of both the behavioral and cognitive schools of therapy.

Behavior Therapy

Behavior therapy has been defined as "treatment deducible from the sociopsychological model that aims to alter a person's behavior directly through the application of general psychological principles."[2] Joseph Wolpe,[3] a pioneer in the development of behavior therapy, describes it as "the use of experimentally established principles of learning for the purpose of changing unadaptive habits." The earliest reference to behavior therapy in the professional literature appeared in 1953 in a monograph written by Lindsley, Skinner and Solomon[4] which described the use of operant conditioning principles to alter behavior in regressed adult psychotics. There are presently at least a dozen or more definitions of behavior therapy, all of which share the following common features:

1. A focus on observable and directly measurable target behaviors;
2. An effort to establish causal relationships between antecedents, behavior and consequences, particularly through the use of a "Skinnerian" experimental analysis of behavior; and
3. An emphasis on operational definition of concepts so that they can be replicated experimentally.

Cognitive Therapy

Until recently, behavior theorists and therapists alike placed little if any emphasis on the relationship between thinking or cognition and behavior. It was not until the early 1970s, when Arnold F. Lazarus published his classic book entitled *Behavior Therapy and Beyond*,[5] that behavior therapists developed a respect for cognitive psychology. The particular brand of cognitive theory and therapy which became so appealing to behavior therapists was developed by Albert Ellis and Aaron Beck. Ellis and Beck proposed that thoughts, attitudes, belief systems, and values are acquired much in the same fashion as overt behaviors. For example, a child who repeatedly hears parents express the belief that "all dogs are dangerous" is likely to adopt that belief himself. In the future, then, this particular belief will influence the child's behavior in his dealing with dogs. The central issue here is that a maladaptive behavior, i.e., phobic avoidance of dogs, has been acquired in the absence of a concrete learning experience with the phobic object.

Cognitive therapy thus emphasizes the relationship between the way individuals feel and behave and the way they think. Put another way, human beings feel the way they feel and act the way they act because they think the way they think. Probably the clearest articulation of the principles which come under the rubric of cognitive theory and therapy was developed by Albert Ellis with his rational emotive therapy.[6] According to Ellis, as a result of various life experiences, individuals acquire both rational and irrational belief systems. When an individual operates on his rational belief systems, his feelings and behavior will invariably be healthy and adaptive; when the individual relies on his irrational belief systems, this produces maladaptive, self-defeating behavior and negative emotional states.

Origin of Cognitive-Behavior Therapy

A merger of the cognitive and the behavior therapies was first formally proposed by Albert Bandura in his *Principles of Behavior Modification*.[7] In that text Bandura developed a "social learning theory" that integrated the biomedical, intrapsychic, and environmental approaches to human behavior. According to cognitive behavior theory, human behavior, both adaptive and maladaptive, is the result of (a) biological factors; (b) psychological factors; and (c) environmental factors. It follows, then, that cognitive behavior therapies emphasize the interplay of the individual's biology, psychology, and environment, for purposes of both assessment and treatment. In cognitive behavior therapy, none of these three factors is seen to have primacy over the others. Instead, it is thought that the biological, psychological, and environmental aspects of one's behavior interact and even influence one another. Thus, on one occasion a person's behavior might largely be environmentally determined. Subsequently, however, the individual develops a number of belief systems about his own behavior which influence his behavior in the future regardless of environmental contingencies.

COGNITIVE BEHAVIORAL ASSESSMENT

Cognitive behavioral assessment is a process involving direct behavioral observation and data collection on overt behavior accompanied by a similar process aimed at identifying the beliefs, attitudes, and values that precede, accompany, and follow the occurrence of disturbed feeling states and behavior. The advantage of targeted cognitive behavioral assessment is that it provides data with a high level of specificity that have potential implications for treatment.

Goals of Cognitive Behavioral Assessment

The primary purposes of cognitive behavior assessment are:

1. To clearly identify the target behaviors and maladaptive feeling states and faulty cognitions which are to be increased or decreased in frequency or eliminated entirely;
2. To "select out" patients who may be more properly treated with other modalities, i.e., ECT, pharmacotherapy, insight-oriented therapy;
3. To identify any environmental factors which might elicit, prompt, reinforce, or support the cognitive, emotional, or behavioral targets;
4. To identify environmental factors that can be manipulated to alter the maladaptive feeling states, cognitions, or behaviors; and
5. To appraise the general potential of the patient to be able to respond positively to cognitive behavioral therapeutic interventions.

Like most forms of psychological evaluation, cognitive behavioral assessment begins with an interview with the patient and direct observation of his or her behavior. The interview is frequently supplemented by a variety of different types of questionnaires and surveys of the descriptive/self-report type. For the most part, there is relatively little use of traditional psychological assessment procedures such as intelligence or projective testing. In addition, cognitive behavior therapists frequently use in-vivo assessment procedures. These involve actually accompanying patients into various types of social situations where their problem behaviors, cognitions, or feeling states are most likely to emerge. This emphasis on in-vivo assessment is based at least partially on the fact that verbal reports of one's own behavior frequently leave much to be desired in terms of accuracy, specificity, reliability, and validity. In addition, the behavior of the patient observed in a clinical setting may not be particularly representative of his usual behavioral repetoire.

In those instances where the patient's hospitalization has been prompted by the presence of dysphoric feeling states, the assessment process begins with an attempt to precisely identify the nature, frequency, intensity, and duration of these feeling states. If, for example, the patient reports that he is depressed, then the cognitive behavior therapist would almost immediately attempt to ensure that the therapist and the patient have a common language to describe depressive symptomatology. The therapist would not assume that the patient's definition of depression is in accord with his own clinical understanding of depressive phenomena. In addition to acquiring a narrative description of the patient's symptoms of depression, the cognitive behavior therapist would also make inquiries about the intensity of the depressive symptoms and the frequency with which they occur. Questions would also be asked about the duration of the depressive episodes and the typology or qualitative nature of the depressive symptoms. The patient might at this point be instructed to begin keeping a daily diary related to the depressive symptomatology. The diary would permit the patient to make regular entries indicating the time and date of occurrences of depressive feelings and associated behaviors. The intensity of the depressive symptoms could be rated on a 10-point scale from mild feelings of sadness to extreme feelings of depression. Finally, the patient would be asked to record "external" and "internal" events which accompanied the depressive feelings. These would include "external" precipitants of depressive feelings, such as a rejection or criticism, and the occurrence of depressive cognitions, such as, "I am a worthless person." The assessment methodology for appraising depressive feelings described above can also be used when evaluating other dysphoric feeling states, such as anxiety, guilt, and pathological anger. Behavioral inventories and schedules such as the Fear Survey Schedule[8] or the Beck Depression Inventory[9] can be used to supplement the other aspects of this initial phase of cognitive behavioral assessment.

The second phase of evaluation involves identifying causal factors that underlie the dysphoric affective states. Perhaps the most comprehensive cognitive behavioral model useful for the second phase of assessment is Lazarus' "basic ID formulation."[10] "Basic ID" is a mnemonic for the seven modes or domains of human functioning which Lazarus feels need to be thoroughly evaluated in order to accurately identify the bases for disturbed feeling and behavioral states. The seven dimensions of "personality" subsumed under the basic ID mnemonic are:

1. Behavior
2. Affect (moods and emotions)
3. Sensation
4. Imagery
5. Cognition
6. Interpersonal relationships
7. "Drugs."

The D or drug modality includes, in addition to drugs (i.e., psychopharmacology), diet, exercise, nutrition, and any other medical/physical matters. The issue of "nature versus nurture" or the extent to which a patient's problems may be in part genetically determined is also considered under the D area. Lazarus maintains that the seven areas of human functioning are interactive; that is, alterations in one will affect the other six categories to one degree or another. However, he also feels that each area is sufficiently independent to require specific evaluation and treatment.

Table 1 is a "Modality Profile"[10] developed by Lazarus on a 40-year-old female patient with the presenting complaints "I drink too much and I worry too much." The patient as described by Lazarus is rather typical of the middle-aged female alcoholic who also suffers from a moderate degree of unipolar depression. Such patients are commonly found on the inpatient alcoholism units of psychiatric hospitals.

Role of Microcomputer in Cognitive Behavior Assessment

Many of the assessment procedures used by cognitive behavior therapists lend themselves readily to automation on today's relatively inexpensive microcomputers. Though conventional psychological testing is not widely used by cognitive behavior therapists, those tests that are employed are often available in a computerized form. For example, symptom checklists like the Beck Depression Inventory,[9] Fear Survey Schedule,[8] and the Symptom Checklist 90[11] all have software programs that are compatible with such standard microcomputers as the IBM PC and the Apple series. Much of cognitive behavior assessment involves counting and measuring behaviors

Table 1
Modality Profile

MODALITY	PROBLEM	PROPOSED TREATMENT
Behavior	Excessive drinking	Self-monitoring + Aversive imagery
	Carries out various compulsions	Response prevention
Affect	General anxiety	Relaxation training Positive imagery
	Bouts of depression	Positive reinforcement
	Holds back anger	Assertiveness training
Sensation	Tension headaches	Relaxation training
	Low back pain	Orthopedic exercises
Imagery	Scenes involving her mother's criticisms	Role playing + empty chair method
	Nightmares about failure (mostly work related)	Images of mastery
Cognition	Morbid thoughts	Thought stopping
	Categorical imperatives (shoulds, oughts, musts, etc.)	Rational emotive therapy
Interpersonal	Withdraws from many social situations	Social skills training (preferably in group)
	Quarrels with husband	Couples therapy
Drugs	Overweight	Self-monitoring/ self-control procedures
	Possible endogenous depression	Prescribe trial on antidepressant medication

according to frequency of occurrence, temporal duration, and intensity as measured on a linear scale. These types of measurements, along with longitudinal tracking of behaviors, are tasks that microcomputers can handle quite routinely. In the course of using a microcomputer to assess change in a particular patient, commercially available statistical software packages such as the SPSS are useful in determining the magnitude and statistical significance of change.

Microcomputers are also particularly useful in implementing ward-wide behavioral programs such as the time-honored token economy operant system, which will be described in greater detail later on in this chapter. In that setting microcomputers assist in the measurement of target behaviors, record the delivery of reinforcement, account for the ways in which patients purchase reinforcers in the token economy system, and measure change in both the individual and the ward-wide target behaviors. One unique application of microcomputers in assessment that may ultimately have a bearing on cognitive behavioral therapeutics has to do with the assessment of cognitive style. Weinman and his associates[12] report on a computerized assessment procedure for identifying various types of cognitive style that could be useful in both the evaluation and treatment of a patient using the cognitive therapies of Beck and Ellis.

Reinforcer Identification

Cognitive behavioral assessment also includes identifying reinforcers which can be used to influence the patient's behavior in a desired direction. There are two primary methods for identifying reinforcers. The first involves determining rewards valued by most individuals in the age range of the patient population under consideration. In an inpatient psychiatric setting, things like money and freedom to move about the hospital without supervision are good examples. The second method involves using the Premack principle,[13] which states that any high frequency behavior—or, in other words, anything that an individual does with regularity—is by its nature reinforcing. Schizophrenic patients, particularly those with negative symptoms, are notorious for their immobility. The fact that such a patient will sit or lie in bed for a long period of time, according to the Premack principle, means sitting or lying in bed could serve as a powerful reinforcer for other behaviors. If the same patient had a low frequency of socially appropriate speech, then appropriate speech could be increased in frequency by reinforcing it with "free periods" to lie down in bed. Table 2 lists reinforcers commonly used in psychiatric inpatient behavior change programs. These reinforcers can be commodities, privileges, and behaviors. What for one patient might be a target behavior, e.g., getting them to bathe more frequently, might for another patient be a potent reinforcer.

Generating effective reinforcers for certain patient types demands a great deal of creativity and imagination. With chronic schizophrenics with anhedonia, many normally reinforcing stimuli, events, and social situations are greeted with indifference or withdrawal. Finally, it should also be noted that in some instances reinforcers lose their potency over time. Thus, it is essen-

Table 2
Reinforcers—Inpatient Behavior Therapy Programs

Money	Writing material
Change in permission or responsibility level	Typewriter
Meals	Long walks
TV time	Taking classes at local college
Recordplayer	Bathing
Radio or Walkman	Showers
Talks with staff members	Shaving
Psychotherapy appointments	Access to toilet articles
Trips out of the hospital	Access to clothing
Visits with family or friends in hospital	Blankets
Visits to home	Comfortable bedding
Swimming	Decorations for room
Sports activities	Breakfast in bed
Card playing	Massage
Snacks	Use of musical instrument
Sodas	Hobby material and models
Private room	Sewing equipment
Naps during the day	Knitting material
Use of the phone	Smoking—pipe, cigars, or cigarettes
Newspaper	Art equipment
News magazines	Special exercise program
Other reading material	Photography equipment
Jewelry	Greenhouse or gardening activities
Trips to hospital snack shop	Joining staff table for meals
Trips to hospital store	Having all meals brought to room
Special hospital functions, i.e., dances, movies, etc.	

tial that the reinforcement side of a behavioral program be constantly monitored and adjusted.

Therapeutic Effects of Assessment

Evaluation of behavior through the use of frequency and intensity measures sometimes produces changes in the behavior that is being assessed. Occasionally, when nursing staff record antecedent and consequent activities of undesired behavior in a patient, certain things that staff might be unwittingly doing to elicit the undesired behavior are identified. Subsequently, staff make adjustments in their own behavior or in the inpatient milieu which bring about a change in the patient's behavior in the desired direction.

Self-Assessment and Monitoring

There are many occasions in an inpatient setting when it is desirable to have the patient participate in evaluation by engaging in self-monitoring activities. For example, a patient with some type of ritualistic behavior, such as compulsive handwashing, might be called upon to keep a running record of that behavior in order to establish a baseline. Obsessional patients can be induced to keep a frequency count of their obsessional thoughts and the number of times they engage in obsessional talk with other patients or staff members. Self-monitoring can be promoted by making the self-monitoring activity a target behavior as well as an assessment procedure. As a target behavior it is subject to reinforcement. The patient keeps a running record of a certain target behavior and is rewarded for the recordkeeping activity by receiving a reinforcer such as a cigarette, desired snack food, or free time to watch TV. The therapeutic effect of assessment can be particularly dramatic in instances of self-monitoring. The provocative patient made to keep a running record of the number of occasions when he is verbally abusive to others will frequently display a marked reduction in the very behavior that he has been asked to record. Self-monitoring, among other things, seems to create a type of "instant insight" or self-awareness about the monitored behavior.

Selection of Initial Target Behaviors

The ultimate success of the treatment program frequently rests upon the selection of the initial target behaviors. High-risk behaviors such as self-injury or assault on others must be attended to first. Beyond that, however, it is important to focus on target behaviors where there is a high probability of early successful change. Having both the treatment team and the patient "get off to a good start" with a successful treatment experience powerfully influences the subsequent enthusiasm of both parties. Another consideration in the selection of target behaviors relates to the phenomenon that change of one behavior frequently produces desired change in other behaviors as well. The physically unkempt patient with poor personal hygiene is often shunned on the ward. Additionally, the poor grooming of the patient has profound negative effects on self-esteem. When hygiene and personal appearance are improved through selective reinforcement, other desired social behaviors, such as increased attendance and participation in group therapeutic activities, frequently follow.

TECHNIQUES OF COGNITIVE BEHAVIOR THERAPY

Systematic Desensitization

Systematic desensitization or "reciprocal inhibition" is primarily used in the treatment of phobic anxiety states. "Reciprocal inhibition" involves creating in the phobic individual an autonomic state that competes with or prevents the presence of anxiety while simultaneously presenting the patient with gradually increasing doses of phobic stimulation.

Though systematic desensitization was initially developed to treat the classic phobic disorders, it has been applied to such conditions as obsessive-compulsive disorders and anorexia nervosa. With anorexia, for example, where the patient has a pattern of phobic anxiety and avoidance behavior related to food, eating, and weight gain, systematic desensitization procedures have been used successfully.

Flooding or Prolonged Exposure

Flooding and prolonged exposure are interchangeable terms used to describe a technique for the treatment of anxiety disorders based on the classical conditioning phenomenon of extinction. In flooding or exposure therapy, the patient is simply presented in-vivo with direct, prolonged exposure to the phobic object or situation. The patient has not previously been taught any relaxation methods. The preference of some therapists is to take the patient immediately into the most highly phobic situation that the patient can imagine. Some patients, of course, refuse to do this, thus requiring the therapist to go about the flooding more gradually using an in-vivo graded hierarchy. Because flooding can quickly produce dramatic results, it has become a preferred method for dealing with phobic disorders.

Response Prevention

Response prevention, closely allied to flooding and prolonged exposure, is typically used in conjunction with those techniques. Response prevention involves preventing the patient with an anxiety disorder from engaging in the avoidance behavior normally used as a way of avoiding or escaping from a fearful situation. Dirt-phobic obsessive compulsives, for instance, typically engage in undoing rituals such as handwashing as a way of managing their anxiety. A response prevention protocol would involve exposing the patient to the feared contamination but then "preventing" him from handwashing.

Assertiveness Training

Subsumed under the rubric of assertiveness training are a variety of cognitive behavioral strategies with the primary purpose of increasing social interpersonal assertiveness while simultaneously eliminating passivity, social deference, and withdrawal behavior. Assertiveness training is a blend of role-playing, behavioral rehearsal, and cognitive therapy techniques. Theoretically, it includes components of classical, operant, and imitation learning as well as cognitive acquisition.

Social Skills Training

Like assertiveness training, social skills training involves the use of a wide array of behavioral strategies designed to increase appropriate interpersonal behavior. Social skills training is used with patients whose deficiencies in social behavior are not limited to passivity and non-assertiveness but include a much broader range and variety of problems. It is highly educational in nature and is well suited for use in an inpatient setting.

Modeling and Imitation Learning Therapy

There are two categories of modeling and imitation learning therapy. The first is designed to enhance the acquisition of positive behaviors, while the second aims at the elimination of undesired behaviors, particularly fear, anxiety, and avoidance behavior. The typical therapy protocol involves demonstrating for the patient the desired behavior and then having the patient reproduce the behavior while being coached. An anxious patient, for example, is encouraged to observe and then imitate approach behavior in a model similar in age, sex, and general demeanor.

Operant Conditioning Based Procedures and the Token Economy

A system of response-contingent reward and punishment for the modification of maladaptive behavior is one of the most widely used cognitive behavioral strategies found in psychiatric inpatient settings. The clinical application of operant conditioning based procedures has produced some of the most dramatic achievements in the treatment of chronic psychotic patients. In a token economy system, patients receive reinforcement in the form of points or tokens for avoiding undesired or maladaptive behaviors while simultaneously engaging in socially appropriate prosocial behaviors.

Contingency Management

Contingency management is sometimes used with patients who are so regressed that they are unresponsive to token reinforcement and must receive direct reinforcement instead. With contingency management, naturally available reinforcers such as food, leisure time, or recreational time are provided immediately upon the display of a target behavior. It is common to begin profoundly regressed psychotic patients on the contingency management system and then later move them toward the token economy when their behavior reaches a higher level of functioning.

Contingency Contacting

In contingency contracting the patient and his or her treatment team generate a written contractual agreement which spells out in detail target behaviors, reinforcing consequences, and the relationship that exists between the two. Contingency contracting has the advantage of promoting full participation of the patient in treatment planning. It also is helpful in eliminating some of the debates and quibbling about reinforcement contingencies that can occur in less structured token economy systems. The fact that the patient participated in the development of the contract and signed it also seems to yield a higher degree of cooperation and compliance. A contingency contract might include an arrangement whereby a patient is given extra attention and contact with staff members in exchange for participating in some type of a work detail on the hall or attending a specific therapeutic activities.

Cognitive Behavioral Therapeutic Self-Instruction

Therapeutic self-instruction involves providing a patient with self-instructional scripts which have a regulatory influence over his own behavior. With the impulsive, borderline personality patient, self-instructional scripts designed to improve the quality of the patient's interpersonal relationships might include:

> Remember, you need to be careful in how you deal with other people. You have a tendency to be demanding and offensive to others. You also have a need to call negative attention to yourself at times. If you do these kinds of things you will offend others and they will reject you. That will result in your feeling very bad about yourself. You will be more successful in your interpersonal relationships if you go slowly and use good judgment.

At first self-instructions are spoken out loud in the presence of the therapist, who coaches the patient and provides encouragement. Later the self-instructions are done subvocally. The actual self-instructional scripts are developed by the therapist subsequent to an evaluation of the content of cognitions preceding, accompanying, and following a particular target behavior.

CLINICAL APPLICATION OF INPATIENT COGNITIVE BEHAVIOR THERAPY

Some of the most impressive applications of cognitive behavioral treatment approaches have been with schizophrenic patients. For that reason this section begins with a particularly detailed case study of a schizophrenic patient.

Schizophrenia

This young man was first admitted to a psychiatric hospital a few weeks before his 17th birthday. On admission, he was acutely psychotic — hallucinating, delusional, and assaultive. His acute disturbance subsided within a two-month period, primarily in response to substantial dosages of a neuroleptic. The patient's condition then gradually settled into the withdrawn, passive, detached, and uninvolved state characteristic of "negative"-symptom chronic schizophrenia with a relatively poor prognosis.

The first step in developing a cognitive behavioral therapy regimen for this patient involved a thorough assessment designed to determine the target behaviors that would be the focus on his treatment program. Nursing staff were instructed to keep a close tally of the patient's behavior along the following dimensions:

A. Self-care
  1. The time the patient got out of bed and the extent of staff effort to get him out of bed.
  2. Whether the patient attended the morning hall meeting.
  3. Does patient clean up his own room?
  4. Does patient attend to personal hygiene, for example, dressing neatly, combing his hair, brushing his teeth, bathing himself?
  5. Coming for medications voluntarily and cooperatively.
  6. Attending therapeutic and recreational activities.
  7. Participating in therapeutic and recreational activities.
  8. Patient's eating habits — attending meals in cafeteria and hoarding food in his room.
B. Staff relationships
  1. Requesting to be seen by a physician for some imagined somatic complaint.
  2. Interrupting nursing staff meetings.
  3. Ignoring nursing staff when they talk to him.
  4. Engaging in psychotic talk with staff or other patients, for example, perseveratively talking about delusions or hallucinatory experiences.

C. Interaction with other patients
   1. Frequency of appropriate social contacts with other patients.
   2. Frequency of inappropriate social contacts with other patients.
   3. Incidence of threatening or menacing gestures or verbalizations towards patients and staff.

The two main components of the patient's treatment under this behavioral regimen were:

1. Systematizing the availability of positive reinforcement contingent upon the display of prosocial and socially appropriate behaviors; and
2. Systematically ignoring or penalizing antisocial-maladaptive behavior.

A broad array of target behaviors was identified in two categories — behavioral excesses and behavioral deficits. Excesses included high frequency of inappropriate behaviors, such as talking to staff about delusions or interrupting nursing staff conferences. Behavioral deficits referred to behaviors that the patient was not performing, such as attending to personal hygiene or engaging in appropriate social interactions with other patients. Based on interviews with the patient and observations of his behavior, a list of reinforcers that would be used to promote desired behavior was also compiled. Additional reinforcers were added to this list on the basis of the Premack principle. High frequency behaviors, such as taking naps during the day, could be used to reinforce such low frequency behaviors as participating in therapeutic activities. (See Table 3 for a list of primary target behaviors used initially with this patient and Table 4 for a list of reinforcers.)

The specifics of the program were explained to the patient in the presence of nursing personnel. The patient was told that he would be given an opportunity to acquire a variety of privileges and commodities by getting up in the morning, going to the morning hall meeting, cleaning up his room, etc. To "prime the pump" the patient was given a demonstration of how the new system would operate. The patient was accompanied to his room, which was in its usual state of disarray. He was told that if he assisted the nurse in making his bed he would receive one token (one poker chip), which could be exchanged for a cigarette. The patient was instructed and encouraged to take up one side of the bedsheet and assist the nurse in straightening it out. He reluctantly cooperated and there was some slight improvement in the appearance of his bed. At that point, the nurse placed a poker chip in the patient's hand and he was given the opportunity to exchange that poker chip for one cigarette. He was reminded that this was how the new system would

Table 3
Target Behaviors

DESIRED BEHAVIORS	UNDESIRED BEHAVIORS
Gets up at 8 a.m. with one call	Making odd noises, uttering non sequiturs
Dresses appropriately	Making complaints of physical illness
Cleans room (dusts, sweeps, straightens furniture)	Annoying staff members
	Annoying patients
Makes bed	Interrupting the conversation of others
Attends morning group meeting	Talking about hallucinations
Bathes minimum 3 times per week	Delusional speech
Brushes teeth	Long speech latencies
Comes for medication on time	Staring at others
Attends first period therapeutic activity	Following others
Remains in therapeutic activity for full hour	Threatening behavior
Participates appropriately in therapeutic activity	Combative behavior

operate, i.e., in return for performing certain tasks he would receive tokens that could be exchanged for other things. The patient was then asked to pick up a pile of soiled clothing on the floor and deposit it in a clothes hamper. It was explained that if he would do that he would receive an additional token. After earning the token for that behavior, he was given an opportunity to exchange the token for a cup of coffee. In addition to the token, the patient received social reinforcement in the form of lavish praise for his cooperation. Pairing social and token reinforcement is done in an attempt to increase the patient's sensitivity to social praise and censure. You will note that, in an effort to stimulate the interest of the patient, achieving reinforcement was made extremely easy for him. Initially, in establishing an operant program, reinforcement should be easily acquired so the patient doesn't experience the system as a process of deprivation. The strategy of making it easy for the patient to acquire reinforcement is also based on the principle of "shaping" or reinforcement of successive approximations. Shaping refers to persistent reinforcement of behaviors that approximate the ultimate desired

Table 4
Reinforcers

Cigarettes	Reductions in neuroleptic medication
Coffee	Trips to town
Soda	Meeting with therapist
Evening snack	Talks with ward physician
Use of the TV	Taking naps
Use of stereo	Increases in permission level

criterion behavior while simultaneously not reinforcing (extinguishing) behaviors that do not approximate criteria performance.

During the first week of the program the patient received reinforcement for getting up and dressing and for cleaning his room and making his bed. Keeping the system simple in the beginning gave both the patient and his treatment team an opportunity to "break in" and develop a sense of how well or how poorly the patient would respond to contingent reinforcement. By the end of the second week, all the other target behaviors identified in Table 3 were being utilized and the patient's rate of performing desired behaviors was approximately 60% per day.

The token economy system emphasizes constant review of the treatment program to create a feedback loop in which the results of evaluation are translated into changes in the program. One point to emerge from that type of evaluation was that getting the patient up in the morning seemed to be of critical importance. On those days when he was successful at getting up and dressed many other positive things seemed to occur. Consequently, the three behaviors of getting up on time, getting dressed appropriately, and attending the morning hall meeting were chained together, so that all three behaviors were required in order for reinforcement to occur. The reinforcement for the successful completion of these three behaviors was five tokens. When the patient performed the getting up and dressed routine, all other desired behaviors displayed during the day were reinforced at a double rate. This bonus program was further refined so that two different types of tokens were used, white tokens and double-value red tokens. On those mornings that the patient performed the requisite morning behaviors he was placed on red tokens for the rest of the day; on those days when he slept in, he was on white tokens.

A subsequent review of the patient's behavior revealed that his most sought after backup reinforcer was cigarettes. Since the patient clearly invested more of his tokens in the purchase of cigarettes than any other thing, the price of cigarettes was doubled. In order for him to earn enough to purchase his daily quota of cigarettes, it became essential that he earn his way onto the double or red token system. (Note: Using cigarettes as a reinforcer *reduces* the frequency of smoking behavior. When cigarettes are available to patients noncontingently, they usually smoke at a higher rate.)

At the end of three weeks, the patient had made an almost complete turnabout, in the sense of achieving 100% performance of his target behaviors. He expressed satisfaction with the program and made suggestions about additional backup reinforcers that he wanted to earn. In response to this request, it was decided to give him an opportunity to go off the ward unaccompanied by a staff member. Access to a higher degree of freedom served as both a reinforcer and a target behavior: The patient could purchase permission to go about the hospital unaccompanied by a staff member; on those occasions when he purchased this privilege and performed it responsibly, he also earned tokens.

The program now began to focus on reducing the frequency of some of the patient's undesirable behaviors. In order to avoid having the program take on a punitive flavor, some of the undesirable behaviors were actually added to the list of backup reinforcers. Therefore, rather than presenting the patient with the notion that if he displayed what was regarded as an undesirable behavior he would be punished or fined, various forms of undesirable behavior were simply among the things available to the patient to purchase with tokens. This particular patient tended to be quite productive of hypochondriacal, physical complaints. In reality, the patient's physical health was remarkably good. Thus, added to the patient's list of backup reinforcers was "permission to talk to nursing staff and hall physician about physical ailments." Since the emphasis here was on reducing the high frequency of this behavior, a stiff price was attached to the behavior, namely 10 tokens. Other undesirable social behaviors, such as belching and emitting incomprehensible non sequiturs, were placed on what is known as an "extinction schedule." This involved having the staff and other patients on the unit completely ignore odd noises and non sequiturs.

Social and interpersonal skill training began with relatively simple behaviors occurring in the context of the patient's relationship with staff and other patients. The first goal was to have the patient verbally participate in the daily patient/staff hall meeting by making appropriate comments and asking questions. Since the patient was unwilling or, perhaps more likely, unable to spontaneously display appropriate verbal behavior in these hall meetings, it was decided to supply him with statements, comments, and questions that he could use in exchange for token reinforcement. It was expected that once the patient displayed some appropriate verbalizations in the meetings, they would receive social reinforcement from both staff and other patients. Under these conditions, his verbal behavior would possibly become a self-maintaining phenomena.

In individual and group social skills training sessions, various forms of social behavior were demonstrated for the patient. These included asking directions and the time of the day, greeting another person, and making small talk. After the social behavior was demonstrated for the patient, the patient was then encouraged to imitate the behavior and subsequently received feedback about how he was doing. In addition, he also received token reinforcement for cooperatively participating in the social skills training and also for learning the new social behaviors.

Initially, the patient received token reinforcement on a constant schedule. This meant that for every desired behavior that the patient emitted he was reinforced with a token. Research on operant conditioning with both human and nonhuman subjects demonstrates that a constant reinforcement schedule like this is the most effective training schedule.[14] The most effective reinforcement schedule for long-term maintenance of behaviors is "intermittent reinforcement," that is, response-contingent but only intermittently rather than immediately following every correct response. Translated into action, this meant that the patient was told that he would be observed by the staff for display of appropriate social behaviors. These appropriate social behaviors included having pleasant social interactions with other patients and staff on the hall. Periodically, when he was observed engaging in this type of appropriate social behavior, he would receive a bonus reinforcement of three tokens. He was instructed that since there was no way of determining when he might be observed doing this, it was to his advantage to do it quite frequently and he could count on periodically being observed and thus being reinforced. Under this arrangement there was a significant increase in appropriate social and verbal behaviors with staff and other patients.

An attempt was made to expand the patient's repertoire of social behavior by teaching him how to go out of the hospital into the local community. Again, the desired behavior, i.e., leaving the hospital, served as both a target behavior and a reinforcer. Each successful trip that he made into town was reinforced. On the other hand, from the patient's standpoint it was desirable to be able to do something like this, so he was willing to purchase the privilege. Since the patient had never gone into the community in the vicinity of the hospital, he had to be trained to do this. This included demonstrating and practicing how to use a bus and how to navigate around a local shopping center. In role-playing situations, the patient was taught how to deal with store clerks and other people whom he might encounter.

As the patient became more competent in social and verbal behavior, an effort was made to attack certain components of his schizophrenic thought disorder directly. Long speech latencies were dealt with by assigning the patient tasks like reading news magazines and newspapers and watching news programs and then requiring him to give detailed verbal accounts of what he had read and seen. While giving these verbal reports, his speech latencies were timed, and every time there was a pause in his speech beyond five seconds a kitchen timer would be started. If the pause lasted more than 45 seconds, the patient would be penalized one token. A shaping procedure was used so that in each subsequent session the length of latency permitted before a penalty was imposed was decreased slightly. In addition, during sessions in which there were no more than five penalized speech latencies the patient received a 10-token bonus. The patient received bonus reinforcement on an intermittent basis whenever he conversed with other patients or staff in an appropriate fashion and did not display any inordinately long speech latencies.

One somewhat unusual twist in the treatment program introduced at this point involved having the patient purchase reductions in his neuroleptic medication. The patient complained of side effects of the neuroleptic he was receiving, including dry mouth and sedation. He was told that for each week in which he achieved 100% performance in target behaviors he would be given a reduction of his neuroleptic medication by 5 mg. Using such a regimen the patient was able to reduce his medication by half prior to his discharge from the hospital.

The general treatment program described up to this point was kept in force for the remainder of the time that the patient was in the hospital. Self-monitoring, wherein the patient kept a record of his own behavior, was eventually broadened to the point where he kept all the records of performance of target behaviors and reinforcement. Once a day he would review his record with a member of his treatment team. Coupled with the self-monitoring program was a phasing towards a system of daily and eventually weekly reinforcement. Earning reinforcement on a weekly basis was roughly equivalent to earning a weekly wage rather than being immediately rewarded for each separate performance of a target behavior. At this time the patient also began a work therapy assignment in an upholstery shop. Each time the patient went to the work therapy assignment, he took with him a small card with a four-point rating scale printed on it. The points represented levels of performance on the job. Depending on the supervisor's ratings, the patient could receive from 25 cents to a dollar per hour of work.

After five months on the program, the patient was ready for discharge. He continued to have a pronounced and obvious thought disorder; however, he had, through the support of the specially structured environment, learned to cope with his schizophrenia and to function at a fairly high level in spite of it. The patient was discharged to a foster home, enrolled in a psychosocial rehabilitation program, and maintained on a moderate dose of neuroleptic medication. His outpatient treatment program continued to follow a cognitive behavioral model; this included reinforcing him with money on a weekly basis contingent upon his successful completion of various target behaviors.

Anxiety Disorders — Obsessive Compulsive

Cognitive behavior therapists conceptualize obsessive compulsive disorders as being composed of a matrix of phobic and avoidance behaviors. Obsessive compulsive patients experience phobic-like anxiety in response to situations such as real or imagined contamination by dirt or germs or because of mental events such as violent or sexual thoughts and fantasies. Compulsive behavior which follows anxious arousal in an obsessive compulsive disorder is seen as avoidance or escape behavior which serves the purpose of reducing the patient's anxiety. Cognitive-behavioral interventions with obsessive compulsive patients typically involve a combination of flooding or prolonged exposure to the phobic stimulus, response prevention, and finally, cognitive restructuring designed to correct the various misbeliefs which precede, accompany, and follow the obsessive compulsive symptoms. For those patients who cannot tolerate the anxiety generated by a flooding procedure, systematic desensitization or one of its variants can be used along with response prevention.

In the case of a 43-year-old obsessive compulsive woman with dirt and contamination phobias and handwashing compulsions, the following strategy was used. The patient was encouraged to soil her hands or "contaminate" them by touching prohibited things such as doorknobs, ashtrays, trash cans, etc. She was instructed to allow herself to become anxious and was assured that anxiety, while unpleasant to experience, would not otherwise harm her. Response prevention involved discouraging the patient from engaging in her "undoing" ritual. Thus, this patient was not permitted near a washroom for as many hours as was necessary for her anxiety to return to its base rate level. In addition, once she was permitted to go to a washroom, the time alloted to wash her hands was severely limited.

The approach taken with patients who have phobic anxiety to their own thoughts and imagery is quite similar. Patients with unacceptable violent or sexual fantasies are instructed to draw pictorial representations of them and describe them in detail into a tape recorder. Flooding involves having them look at the pictures they have created while simultaneously hearing the descriptions over the tape recorder and repeating over and over again their prohibited words or thoughts. Response prevention here involves discouraging patients from engaging in the undoing thoughts or behavior which normally follow their anxious arousal.

The cognitive restructuring of an obsessive compulsive patient focuses on explicit instruction in the illogicity of their thinking style and content related to obsessions and compulsive behavior.

Eating Disorders

Cognitive behavioral conceptualizations of anorexia nervosa and bulimia emphasize the notion that the symptoms of these disorders are acquired through processes of conditioning or learning. Cognitive behavior therapy interventions have largely focused on reduction of the phobic-like anxiety associated with eating and weight gain, along with "reinforcement" of behaviors incompatible with pathological dieting. Anorectic and bulimic patients are thought to have a wide range of conditioned fear responses to various food, eating, and weight gain stimuli that under normal conditions are affectively neutral. So, for example, when the anorectic patient sees food, thinks about food, or even prepares to enter a dining room, she experiences intense anxious arousal. Cognitive behavior therapists argue that these anxiety responses are both cognitively mediated and reflexive in nature and result from prior learning experiences. The avoidance and withdrawal behaviors so characteristic of anorectic patients when they are exposed to food or an eating situation are seen as operant. The reinforcement for this operant withdrawal is a reduction in the anxiety feelings that occur when the anorectic is confronted with food or other eating stimuli.

In addition, it is also posited that the starvation behavior of the anorectic receives social reinforcement to the extent that the anorectic's behavior serves as an effective and powerful form of influence over other members of her social environment, particularly her parents. The emaciated appearance of the starving anorectic does, of course, normally elicit high levels of caring attention. This attention, which is received contingent on the maladaptive behavior of self-imposed starvation, is seen as being a powerful motive for the maintenance of the behavior. Recently, the societal and cultural emphasis on slimness has been seen as a factor contributing to the current epidemic of eating disorders in this country. This cultural influence is most readily explained through principles of cognitive acquisition and imitation learning. The anorectic is viewed as falling under the influence of socially sanctioned "models" of extreme thinness in the media and through advertising. Indeed, it is a rather common clinical occurrence to have anorectic patients report that TV commercials and magazine ads promoting the cosmetic merits of slimness have had a powerful influence on their choice to engage in self-imposed starvation.

Cognitive behaviorally oriented inpatient treatment programs for eating disorders typically include some or all of these elements:

1. Deprivation: Access to such amenities as social contact, television, visits from friends and family, dayroom privileges, telephone calls, exercise, etc., is restricted.
2. Contingency management: Access to the above mentioned activities is linked to compliance with various aspects of the treatment plan.[15] For example, the patient may watch television when she has eaten so many meals or gained a predetermined amount of weight, etc. The

therapist may negotiate a treatment contract with the patient which spells out the specific system of reinforcements and reinforcement schedules.
3. Informational feedback: The prime cognitive intervention in the treatment program of an eating disordered patient involves providing the patient with precise and frequent informational feedback regarding the number of calories consumed and/or amount of weight gained or lost. Sometimes this feedback is monitored by the patient herself, under the supervision of the therapist, having the patient keep the charts and recording her own progress.
4. Negative reinforcement: Discharge from the hospital is made contingent upon achievement of stable weight gain.

Cognitive behavior therapy programs for the inpatient treatment of eating disordered patients are strongly geared towards two major goals: correcting the patient's various cognitive and perceptual distortions about eating and weight gain; and establishing and maintaining a medically acceptable body weight in the patient. Cognitive behavioral regimens have been shown to be particularly useful in the medical management and nutritional rehabilitation of eating disordered patients. Operant techniques, in particular, have been shown to be remarkably effective in achieving the critical first step of treatment, that of restoring weight.[16]

Borderline Personality Disorders

Perhaps no other group of patients presents the range of challenge and difficulty in management as those with a diagnosis of borderline personality disorder. Therapeutic interventions of any type, including cognitive behavioral approaches, are almost always met by these patients with a combination of resistance, suspicion, and hostility. On the one hand, cognitive behavioral strategies offer the advantage of not being regressogenic, i.e., they focus on and promote the more adaptive side of the patient. On the other hand, however, the explicit and direct nature of the techniques, which clearly attempt to bring about changes in the thinking, emotional reactivity, and behavior of the patient, can be seen by the borderline patient as provocative and highly threatening. For that reason, explicit operant reinforcement systems that reward and penalize the patient to bring about positive behavioral change rarely succeed with borderlines. Instead, the typical borderline personality disorder patient shows delight in sabotaging and defeating the most carefully thought-out operant reinforcement system.

Similarly, these patients reject the best efforts of the most exquisitely trained cognitive therapists. These patients invariably interpret the suggestion that certain aspects of their thinking may be illogical as a personal insult, attack, and criticism. They perceive the implied message of cognitive therapy, i.e., your thinking is in error and needs to be changed, as a direct attack on their intelligence, value, worth, and dignity as a human being. The direct cognitive approach is thus an insult to their already poor self-esteem. The other message of cognitive behavioral therapy, i.e., that one is capable of regulating one's own emotions and behavior, is also repugnant to most borderline personality disorder patients. As a group, these patients seem to share a basic assumption, namely either their emotional and behavioral difficulties are entirely inexplicable or, perhaps even more commonly, the responsibility for their feeling states and behavior belong to others. These patients equate responsibility with blame and thus go to great lengths to avoid accepting even a minimal degree of responsibility for what happens to them.

With these caveats in mind, the creative and imaginative cognitive behavior therapist is still able to adjust the cognitive behavioral approach to meet the special needs of borderline patients. Although, as mentioned earlier, explicit operant systems of reward and punishment do not usually work well with these patients, the judicious use of social reinforcement can bring about positive change. Borderline patients are exquisitely sensitive to the social response of others. Tempestuous episodes of emotional display and harmful behavior, such as delicate self-cutting and self-burning, are frequently motivated by an effort to get some type of attending or caring response from the treatment team and other patients in the environment. The cognitive behavioral model calls for putting that type of acting-out behavior on a strict extinction schedule. This means that as much as possible the provocative and emotionally sensational behavior of these patients should be ignored or treated with "benign neglect." In other words, the misbehavior of the patients should not be grounds for staff attention in the form of individual or group discussions of their psychodynamic motivation. In many cases, of course, the acting-out, particularly when it includes self-injurious behavior, is so compelling that for safety's sake it cannot be ignored. Nonetheless, it can be treated with some degree of relative indifference. Treatment of wounds should be rendered with little fanfare and as perfunctorily as is possible.

The obverse of this extinction protocol of misbehavior is to "catch them while they're being good." This includes having the treatment team make a point of providing the patient with a great deal of attention and social approval when she is behaving in an appropriate fashion. Since many of these patients show a paradoxical response to explicit praise and approval, positive social reinforcement must be tailored to their unique appetites. Lavishly praising the good behavior of a borderline patient can many times be a guaranteed way of provoking a disastrous episode of acting-out. On the other hand, a gentle and restrained demonstration of warmth and caring attention delivered to the patient contingent on mature and emotionally reasonable behavior can have dramatically positive effects.

Another variant of the operant approach successful with some higher functioning borderline patients involves the use of contingency contracting and self-monitoring. In the case of a late adolescent female borderline, contingency contracting involving written short-term treatment contractual arrangements with the treatment team was used successfully. The ingredients of the contract involved increased levels of freedom contingent upon periods of "good behavior" and the absence of acting-out behavior. This contracting was coupled with a self-monitoring strategy that involved having the patient keep a daily record of her own behavior in terms of how well or how poorly it met the requirements of the written contract. Since this patient was so sensitive to and intolerant of external control, it was important to convey to her that she was the key manager of the contracting and self-monitoring arrangement. One other operant technique that was useful with this borderline patient involved the use of "time-out" from reinforcement. Subsequent to a display of acting-out, the patient was placed in a "quiet room" where she remained until she settled down and got over her emotional outburst. Release from the time-out room was made contingent on a return to stable behavior; thus, her stable behavior was reinforced.

Just as operant principles must be creatively tailored to fit the special proclivities of the borderline patient, so too must cognitive therapy techniques be similarly adjusted. The straightforward, direct, and at times aggressive approach of Albert Ellis, the founding father of rational emotive therapy, is in most cases likely to precipitate emotional and behavioral eruptions in borderline patients. These patients cannot be told what to do or how to do it. They bristle at even mild suggestions that there might be another more adaptive way of conceptualizing and responding to a particular situation. It almost goes without saying that the first order of business and perhaps the most difficult aspect of treating these patients is establishing a positive therapeutic rapport. Ideally, the patient is to see the cognitive therapist as a benign and knowledgeable source of wisdom and counsel who is deserving of trust. Unfortunately, this ideal patient-therapist relationship is almost never achieved with this type of patient. In fact, one of the ironies presented by borderlines is that the very competence of the therapist is a threat and challenge to their chronically low self-esteem. Thus, the therapist cannot look too smart or too knowledgeable or suggest to the patient that he truly understand what motivates the patient's emotional lability and out-of-control behavior.

In the early stages of the treatment of the borderline patient, prudent cognitive therapists will, on many occasions, borrow from the repertoire of the Rogerian nondirective school of therapy. In that regard, they assume the role of listeners and observers who dispense unlimited doses of what Rogers refers to as unconditional positive regard. Sometimes, a number of months on that tack are required before a sufficient degree of trust has been established to permit the therapist to begin utilizing a cognitive approach.

Once a sufficient level of therapeutic trust has been established, it is frequently useful to have the patient embark on a course of bibliotherapy by reading Ellis and Harper's *Guide to Rational Living*,[17] along with David Burns' *Feeling Good*.[18] The 12 most common irrational beliefs identified by Ellis in rational emotive therapy are easily recognized by most borderline patients as their most cherished values. If patients perceive the bibliotherapy as part of an effort to change them, the books may quickly end up on the trash pile. A plausible rationale for the bibliotherapy is that reading books will give the patient and the therapist a common language with which to talk about the patient's problems.

With higher functioning borderline patients, group therapy based on principles of cognitive therapy can also be useful. Sometimes the borderline patient just entering treatment can benefit from exposure to higher functioning or more advanced borderline patients in a group therapy situation. One other ploy which has proven useful in cognitive behavioral treatment of the borderline patient involves identifying for the patient his or her psychological "Achilles' heel." This might include, for example, stating explicitly to a borderline patient who is in an advanced stage of treatment that she has certain more or less permanent areas of psychological sensitivity or vulnerability. One common borderline "Achilles heel" is in the area of self-esteem and self-worth. Patients may be told, for example, that because of certain life experiences they are likely to always have a high degree of vulnerability to even mild criticism and rejection. They need to be especially alert, on an almost daily basis, to their tendency to engage in distorted thinking about their own value and self-worth. Sometimes it helps to remind these patients that, by analogy, their proclivity towards cognitive and perceptual distortions of their own value and self-worth is comparable to the distorted color perception of the color-blind person. They are told that people who are color blind never completely rely on their own judgments about color and wardrobe selection. Likewise borderline patients may never be able to rely entirely on their own judgments concerning criticism, rejection, and personal self-worth. They are then instructed to depend instead on the judgments of others, particularly helpful therapists or wise friends.

Organic Mental Disorders

Cognitive behavioral therapy approaches, because of their high degree of specificity and clarity, have been found to be particularly useful in the treatment of various types of organic brain syndromes. In general, cognitive behavioral programs with this patient group have emphasized three primary goals: symptom control, social rehabilitation, and academic or vocational rehabilitation. In the area of symptom control are included such issues as toilet training, stereotypical movements, and emotional lability. For these and other forms of "symptomatic" or maladaptive behavior in the brain-impaired, the behavioral techniques of positive reinforcement of incompatible behavior, extinction, and punishment have been successfully applied.

Concerning social skills, one of the first goals in dealing with many brain-impaired patients is to teach them to "pay attention" and follow instructions reliably. In "attention skill training sessions," prompt and appropriate compliance with verbal instructions is immediately reinforced with praise and tokens. Advanced social rehabilitation with the brain-impaired involves establishing such self-care behaviors as bathing, brushing teeth, selecting clothing, dressing appropriately, and feeding. By using a combination of modeled demonstration, gradual shaping, and selective reinforcement, a remarkable degree of independent self-care can be established even in severely brain-impaired patients.

The final goal of academic and vocational rehabilitation of the brain-impaired patient is again usually achieved through the use of operant conditioning and procedures based on imitation learning. In operant based program instruction, the material to be learned is broken into its smallest components and gradually "chained" together. Along with this, immediate feedback of correct and incorrect responses and rewards for correct responses are used extensively. Microcomputers programmed to present the brain-damaged patients with cognitive and perceptual learning tasks in their area of impairment have been used successfully in rehabilitation.

Psychotic Children

Inpatient cognitive behavioral treatment of infantile autism and other pervasive developmental disorders does not differ significantly in either theory or practice from the cognitive behavioral treatment of severe adult conditions. Usually, the cognitive behavioral treatment of severe psychopathology in children begins with an effort aimed at eliminating grossly deviant behaviors, such as self-mutilation or bizarre, repetitive mannerisms. The occurrence of these highly deviant responses precludes the acquisition of more adaptive behaviors. Efforts to rid psychotic children of such highly noxious behaviors as headbanging and other forms of self-mutilation occasionally include aversive procedures. Self-injurious behavior in psychotic children is by no means a mild behavior problem. It frequently takes such severe forms as eye-gouging, biting one's own flesh to the bone, and headbanging to the point of inducing skull fracture. Often with extinction programs alone, i.e., ignoring the behavior, the initial response of the child is to increase his rate of self-destructive behavior. It is for that reason that response-contingent high intensity punishment has been used as a treatment procedure. Bucher and Lovaas[19] treated a seven-year-old schizophrenic boy who had engaged in self-injurious behavior since the age of two. During a 90-minute period of observation, the child engaged in over 3,000 self-injurious behaviors. In four treatment sessions that involved the use of 12 high intensity, contingent electroshocks, the self-injurious behavior was almost completely eliminated. The treatment protocol in this case involved having the therapist, after self-injurious behavior began, shout STOP to the child and then apply a high intensity electroshock through a grid plate on which the child was standing.

Subsequent to the elimination of grossly deviant behaviors through the use of contingent punishment or extinction procedures, most treatment programs then focus on the development of adaptive social skills. With autistic children, this typically starts with a focus on language acquisition and in some cases becomes even more basic and deals with reinforcing the child's attention to the adult therapist and the imitation of gross bodily movements. Tangible reinforcement, such as snack food or candy, are dispensed subsequent to the display of such adaptive behaviors as eye contact, social interaction, and verbalization. Self-care behaviors, including personal hygiene and dressing appropriately, and then, at more advanced levels, participating in remedial education programs become the targets of intervention.

SPECIAL ISSUES

Roles of Mental Health Professionals

In spite of the widespread popularity of cognitive behavioral therapies, clinical psychology remains the only mental health discipline that routinely includes training in this modality as a component of professional preparation. With few exceptions, clinical psychologists trained within the last decade have received both didactic and practical instruction in the theory and practice of cognitive behavior therapy. As a consequence, psychologists invariably hold leadership roles in cognitive behavior therapy clinical application, staff training, and supervision in inpatient settings. The psychologist's activities in these areas may be provided through consultations, program leadership, or direct clinical services.

Nursing and mental health worker personnel typically play the next most central role in applying cognitive behavior therapy programs in inpatient settings. While the psychologist usually designs the treatment program, it is often nursing staff and mental health workers who must implement it. This is particularly true in the case of "token economy" and other operant conditioning based forms of treatment. Nurses and mental health workers, under the supervision of a psychologist, are usually responsible for recording the patient's behavior, providing token reinforcement when appropriate, exchanging earned tokens for back-up reinforcers, and implementing time-out, extinction, and penalty procedures. Nursing and mental health workers may also be trained to implement special techniques, such as relaxation training, response prevention, social skills instruction, etc.

Social work training does not usually include a heavy emphasis on the use of cognitive behavior therapies. Thus, in most cases, social workers have a more limited role in treatment programs based on this approach. In some instances they may be involved in transmitting to patients' families information about the cognitive behavioral regimen. This work with families might also include instructing them in fundamental reinforcement principles which can be used during home visits or visits to the patient in the hospital. Social workers also become involved in the transition of the patient back into the community or employment setting. In this role they can acquire important information concerning the patient's functioning outside the hospital. This information can then lead to appropriate alterations in the inpatient treatment program. Finally, during the aftercare or post-discharge phase of treatment, the social worker may record and reinforce behaviors outside the hospital that continue to be managed via cognitive behavioral interventions.

Psychiatrists tend to have little direct role in inpatient cognitive behavioral treatment programs. One popular model has the psychiatrist managing the patient's medication, attending to physical health care issues, and providing individual psychodynamic psychotherapy, while a psychologist directs nursing care personnel in implementing a cognitive behavioral program with the same patient. Again, the role of the psychiatrist in the program is a function of training and personal interest. Certainly there is nothing inherent in psychiatry or any of the other mental health disciplines to preclude their members from acquiring the requisite skills to become bona fide cognitive behavioral therapists or consultants.

Cognitive Behavior Therapy and Psychotropic Medication

Generally speaking, the use of cognitive behavioral therapy techniques is not incompatible with the judicious use of psychotropic medication. Indeed, for a number of significant diagnostic entities, such as chronic schizophrenia in adults and attention deficit disorder in children, the treatment of first choice usually involves some combination of medication and cognitive behavior therapy. In the treatment of anxiety disorders, low doses of tricyclic antidepressants for panic attacks and a variety of anxiolytic agents such as the benzodiazepines are routinely used in combination with cognitive behavior therapy protocols. Lithium, tricyclic antidepressants, and MAO inhibitors have all been used in the pharmacological management of affective disorder patients who are simultaneously undergoing a course of cognitive behavior therapy.

However, one caution concerning the use of psychoactive drugs with cognitive behavior therapy is in order. Cognitive behavior therapies rely heavily on a learning model. An effort is made to "teach" patients new ways of thinking and behaving. Some animal and human studies have shown that various psychoactive drugs, particularly the neuroleptics and antianxiety agents, can adversely affect the acquisition and maintenance of newly learned behaviors.[20] In addition, the subject of "state dependent" learning also needs to be considered. State dependent learning refers to the fact that behaviors and skills acquired when an individual is drug free may not be retained when the patient is on medication, and conversely, behaviors acquired while under the influence of a psychoactive medication may extinguish once the medication is removed. This is a particularly significant issue in the treatment of anxiety disorders. A patient on an antianxiety drug may be able to cope with and approach a phobic situation, but this behavior may disappear entirely when the patient is unmedicated because the desired relearning did not occur sufficiently for there to be a transfer of training to the non-drug state.

Symptom Substitution

For some time the single most common and insistent criticism of the cognitive behavioral approach came from the dynamic oriented therapists and concerned the issue of "symptom substitution." The contention of the dynamicists was that the cognitive behavior therapist does little more than alter overt behavior, without affecting the underlying "psychic" causes. Their alarm was that this "superficial" approach would merely result in the emergence of new and possibly even more distressing symptoms. Suffice it to say that at this point the concern about symptom substitution has been shown to be unwarranted. Of all the psychotherapies in existence, the cognitive and behavioral schools, because of their close alliance with experimental psychology, remain among the most thoroughly researched. At this point in time there is little if any evidence that symptom substitution occurs.

Nevertheless, there are instances when patients generate new maladaptive behaviors on the heels of the elimination of old ones. One common example is in the case of the elimination of temper tantrums in children. If the primary purpose of the tantrums was to acquire parental attention and parental attention is not bestowed on the child for adaptive prosocial behaviors, then elimination of the tantrums by any means is likely to be followed by the creation of new undesirable behaviors. Cognitive behavior therapists, however, would not see this as symptom substitution in the psychodynamic sense; rather, they would regard it as evidence of additional learning, which could be circumvented with the appropriate cognitive behavioral intervention.

Simultaneous Use of Psychodynamic Therapies and Cognitive Behavioral Therapies

The factional wars between behavior therapists and psychodynamic therapists, so common in the '60s and '70s, have become far less noticeable in the present decade. Indeed, some respected authors have talked about a rapprochement between cognitive behavioral therapies and the psychodynamic school. In reality, it does seem that both approaches have something to offer one another. Psychodynamicists can benefit from familiarizing themselves with explicit behavioral methods that have been repeatedly demonstrated to be effective with a variety of clinical problems. Cognitive behavior therapists, on the other hand, can develop a greater sensitivity to the subtleties of therapeutic relationships and the less apparent aspects of patients' behavior by increasing their familiarity with psychodynamic technique. In a number of inpatient psychiatric settings, it is not uncommon for a patient to simultaneously be undergoing individual psychodynamically oriented psychotherapy and receiving a specialized cognitive behavioral regimen. When the two approaches are orchestrated and supervised by a clinician well versed in both modalities, the results can be impressive. Some patients with severe anxiety disorders show an extremely favorable response to a flooding or desensitization technique. At the same time, their response to those treatments may be enhanced by allowing and even encouraging the patient to talk about early childhood experiences. Similarly, the patient who can benefit from a psychodynamic exploration of "transference" feelings towards the therapist may also benefit from some assertiveness and social skills training to prepare for dealing with other authority figures.

Patient and Staff Acceptance

One concern frequently raised about the use of cognitive and, particularly, behavior therapies in inpatient psychiatric settings has to do with patient and staff acceptance. Will the patients perceive the treatment as overcontrolling, manipulative, or coercive? Will staff share those sentiments and have the additional concern that the cognitive behavior therapies are somehow superficial? Perhaps they don't get at the patient's "real" or underlying problems.

Experience and research with cognitive behavior therapies indicate that the level of patient satisfaction with these treatment modalities is actually quite high. Cognitive behavior therapies are perceived as equal or superior to their psychodynamic counterparts along such interpersonal dimensions as warmth, genuineness, and concern.[21] Well designed cognitive behavioral treatment programs emphasize the inclusion of the patient in the planning and implementation of therapy. When the patient formally participates in treatment planning, acceptance of treatment is greatly enhanced. The high degree of goal specificity, structure, and contingent reinforcement is of particular benefit to the disorganized patient who has difficulty "making sense" out of the less explicitly structured, traditional therapeutic milieu. When cognitive behavioral treatment programs are run on traditional "milieu therapy" inpatient unit, it is not uncommon to have patients seek to "enroll" themselves in the cognitive behavioral program because of what they perceive to be its apparent benefits.

The types of patients who stridently resist participating in cognitive behavioral programs do not appear to differ from patients who resist or fail to comply with other more traditional forms of treatment. These include severely paranoid or negativistic patients and borderline and antisocial personality disorders. Occasionally, family members resist the notion of their relative being treated with cognitive behavior therapies. These families, however, seem equally quarrelsome about other forms of therapeutic intervention.

The issue of staff acceptance of cognitive behavior therapy is somewhat more complicated. Clinicians with a zealous and unyielding commitment to psychoanalytic therapy will relentlessly oppose the use of cognitive behavior therapies. Their resistance is impervious to rational persuasion or citations of relevant empirical literature documenting the effectiveness of cognitive behavior therapy. If a higher authority requires them to "submit" their patient to a cognitive behavior regimen, their resistance sharpens and treatment is sabotaged, to the detriment of all concerned.

More commonly, the cognitive behavior therapist operating in an inpatient setting encounters staff who adopt a healthily skeptical "wait and see" attitude about the merits of cognitive behavioral interventions. The extent to which these individuals are won over to the cognitive behavior camp is invariably determined by the outcome of the treatment. Ironically, one hazard frequently encountered by cognitive behavior therapists in inpatient settings is that other staff maintain unrealistically high expectations about the efficacy of cognitive behavior strategies. This is in part the result of cognitive behavior therapy being oversold by some of its pioneers as a panacea for all varieties of mental illness. It also stems from the fact that its goal specificity leads staff to expect concrete results in the form of directly observable and measurable behavior change. By contrast, psychodynamic and traditional milieu therapies emphasize process rather than outcome, sometimes to the extent of even denigrating observable change in behavior as a valid indicator of patient improvement.

In the final analysis, the degree of acceptance of cognitive behavior therapies by both patients and staff seems to be largely a function of the "salesmanship" and expertise of the cognitive behavior therapist/consultant.

REFERENCES

1. Gruenberg EM: The social breakdown syndrome—some origins. Am J Psychiatry 1967; 123:12-20
2. Ullmann L, Krasner L: Case Studies in Behavior Modification. New York, Holt, Rinehart & Winston, 1966
3. Wolpe J: The Practice of Behavior Therapy. New York, Pergamon Press, 1969
4. Lindsley OR, Skinner BF, Solomon HC: Studies in Behavior Therapy, Status Report I. Metropolitan State Hospital, Waltham, MA, 1953
5. Lazarus A: Behavior Therapy and Beyond. New York, McGraw-Hill, 1971
6. Ellis A: Reason and Emotion in Psychotherapy. New York, Lyle Stuart, 1962
7. Bandura A: Principles of Behavior Modification. New York, Holt, Rinehart & Winston, 1969
8. Wolpe J, Lang P: A fear survey schedule for use in behavior therapy. Behavior Research and Therapy 1964; 2:27
9. Beck A, Rush A, Shaw B, Emery G: Cognitive Therapy for Depression. New York, Guilford, 1979
10. Lazarus A: Multi-Model Behavior Therapy. New York, Springer, 1976
11. Derogatis L: SCL-90 Administration and Scoring Manual. Maryland Clinical Psychometric Research, 1983
12. Weinman J, Elithorn A, Faray S: Test structure and cognitive style, In Intelligence and Learning. Edited by Friedman M, New York, Plenum Press, 1981
13. Premack D: Towards empirical behavior laws I: positive reinforcement. Psychology Review 1959; 66:219-233
14. Rachlin H: Introduction to Modern Behaviorism. San Francisco, Freeman, 1970
15. Halmi K, Powers P, Cunningham S: Treatment of anorexia nervosa with behavior modification. Arch Gen Psychiatry 1975; 32:93-96
16. Bemis K: Current approaches to the etiology and treatment of anorexia nervosa. Psychol Bull 1978; 85:593-617
17. Ellis A, Harper R: Guide to Rational Living. Englewood Cliffs, NJ, Prentice-Hall, 1961
18. Burns D: Feeling good: The Mood Therapy. New York, William Morrow, 1980
19. Bucher B, Lovaas O: Use of aversive stimulation in behavior modification, In Symposium on the Prediction of Behavior. Edited by Jones MR, Florida, University of Miami Press, 1968
20. Paul G, Tobias L, Holly B: Maintenance psychotropic drugs in the presence of active treatment programs. Arch Gen Psychiatry 1972; 27:106-115
21. Sloane B: Psychotherapy versus behavior therapy. Cambridge, MA, Harvard Univ Press, 1975

11
The Use of Medication in a Hospital Setting

John R. Lion
Joe P. Tupin

The placement of a patient within the hospital gives the clinician certain advantages he does not have on the outside. Therapy often comes to be under the scrutiny of many more people, enabling new observations to be made. Tests can be ordered and treatment rendered in the context of a safe environment. And therapeutic paradigms can be more aggressively applied. These principles hold for psychopharmacologic treatment as well.

A common reason for hospitalizing a patient pertains to the matter of drug compliance. Many psychiatric patients do not take their medication; schizophrenic patients, for example, have difficulty adhering to psychopharmacologic regimens when prescribed.[1] Within the institution, there is far less chance that a patient will miss a dose of a drug. One of the prime reasons for drug failure in the case of depression is inadequate dosing[2]; hospitalization often accomplishes the task of achieving an adequate blood level of the drug, particularly if the clinician has been reluctant to utilize a maximum dose on an outpatient basis because of side effects. Manic-depressive patients present notorious difficulties in taking mood-stabilizing drugs, particularly during the manic phases of their illnesses, and hospitalization provides for the needed drug treatment.[3] Age factors play a role here also; patients with memory difficulties or age-related disabilities may be unable to take medications according to schedule.[4] Thus, a wide array of patients manifest difficulties in appropriately handling medications, and when family or support groups fail to provide the structure conducive to compliance, in-house stay is often necessary.

In order for drug treatment to satisfactorily proceed, hospitalization is often necessary to clarify the diagnostic picture. This is particularly true in those clinical situations where observations to detect underlying affective or thought disorder components are limited.

> A young man with a history of autistic behavior and fire-setting was seen in an outpatient setting. Mental status showed no evidence of a thought disorder, but the clinician nonetheless suspected incipient schizophrenia and there was a family history of the disease. The patient was followed in weekly therapy, but his seclusiveness persisted and he did not attend school. He was finally hospitalized and at that time showed paranoid ideation and admitted to hallucinations. At this point, antipsychotic medication was begun with benefit.

The above case illustrates a common problem in outpatient practice. Patients may not reveal the extent of their symptoms, placing the clinician at a clear disadvantage. Families may also conspire in this matter of minimizing symptoms, or they may utilize denial in the observation process. In the hospital, such denial may give way to a more accurate revelation of pathology as the patient begins to trust staff and demonstrates the more insidious aspects of illness.

Effective drug treatment depends upon the recognition of target symptoms. Some of the more diffuse social symptoms of schizophrenia, such as autism or anhedonia, may be less responsive to medication than the observable behaviors of agitation and suspiciousness. Nevertheless, the treating clinician can only titrate medication effectively if he has a full grasp of the dimensions of the problem. Activities Therapy personnel may provide useful information regarding the extent of the patient's hypervigilance, irritability, or covert delusional system. But they may also furnish clues about withdrawal and seclusiveness.

> An angry and depressed borderline woman was treated with antipsychotic and antidepressant drugs during a hospitalization. Weekly team meetings assessed her progress. Although she appeared somewhat improved on the ward, the recreation therapist related that she still had little tolerance for frustration during her participation in crafts and did not allow anyone near her. She continued to be solitary and isolated during group activities off the ward and was easily wounded when criticized by others during a class exercise. The treating

clinician, taking these observations into account, increased the patient's medication with resultant improvement.

This kind of knowledge furnishes the clinician with useful guidelines to drug treatment and allows him to titrate medications upward more effectively. The behaviors are often "soft" and less likely conventional target symptoms for medication. And they may not be noticed by all ward personnel or described in routine nursing notes. Yet they are still critical to psychopharmacologic management.

In some cases of depression, hospitalization may clarify psychotic components, alerting the therapist to change medication regimens.

A middle-aged woman presented in an outpatient clinic with depression. The despondency was noted to be "classic" and many vegetative symptoms were elicited. She was placed on an antidepressant, but her mood remained low and feelings of worthlessness intensified. Finally, she overdosed at home. Within the hospital, she admitted to having had command hallucinations urging her to die. On the ward she was quite aloof, interacted in a most guarded manner, and showed a good deal of suspiciousness.

This case illustrates the worsening of an illness and its elucidation within the hospital. Whether the antidepressant medication exacerbated the depression was unclear, but she was now viewed as having a delusional depression and antipsychotic and antidepressant medication was used conjointly with success.

The depth of affective states is often difficult to assess in outpatients who show little introspection or utilize much denial. Assessment of affective components among the thought disorders may be particularly difficult.

A young man with a diagnosis of schizophrenia was noted to show some mood fluctuations. It was unclear to the therapist whether he actually had a schizoaffective illness or might have a true bipolar disorder; in any event, antipsychotic medication had limited effectiveness and he was hospitalized. On the ward, he was noted by staff to show some hypomanic episodes with grandiosity and pressured speech. Staff concurred that he should receive lithium medication. This was added to his pharmacologic regimen and had a beneficial effect.

In this case, hospitalization facilitated the use of a mood-stabilizing drug by virtue of improved observation on the part of staff who bolstered the clinician's less certain impressions. The patient, who lived apart from his family, had been seen weekly by the therapist, but extended observations of behavior and mood were lacking.

Children and adolescents with conduct disorders are commonly hospitalized for stabilization. Aggressiveness and combativeness, antisocial behavior, or drug abuse and alcoholism may prompt incarceration; in the case of younger patients, disruptive school performance and hyperactivity may lead to hospitalization. Once confined, organic or affective components of the illness may become evident, leading to possible treatment with medication.

> An adolescent with a history of temper outbursts, "hyperactivity," and school truancy was hospitalized after stealing some items at a local store. Once in the hospital, he was noted to have poor attention span and concentration, together with irritability and some hostile outbursts. There existed a history of head injury, and an EEG revealed bilateral slowing. Psychological testing for organicity showed some questionable temporal lobe pathology. Though strong characterologic issues prevailed, it was felt that the patient had an "epileptoid" component to his illness. He was begun on anticonvulsant medication to reduce his temper outbursts.

In this instance, the etiology of the patient's illness was clarified through hospitalization and the organic aspects of the disease became elucidated.

Patients who abuse alcohol and drugs may have underlying mood disorders; hospitalization in such instances enables the therapist to make the appropriate diagnosis and render pharmacologic treatment. In some instances, hospitalization clarifies not only the affective and thought disorder components of the illness, but also the toxicities of drugs utilized on an outpatient basis.

> A woman with a long history of recurrent depression was treated with lithium following an episode of hypomania. She developed mild polyuria, but her chemistries were otherwise normal. She was uninsightful and disliked taking her medication. She went on vacation, returning in a frankly hypomanic state with confusion. Her lithium level was in the toxic range despite no changes in her dosage. Because her mental status worsened, she was hospitalized. Tests revealed a high serum creatinine with a reduced creatinine clearance. With hydration, all studies returned to normal. It was felt that she had either experienced transient renal toxicity or had not adequately hydrated herself during her visit to a hot climate in the face of excessive urine output.

Side effects and toxicities can often be clarified under the controlled conditions of the hospital. In some instances, this may be accomplished simply by stopping all medications, a tactic which would be difficult on an outpatient basis. In other instances, simple observations may serve to make clear the nature of the untoward drug reaction.

> A man with a schizophrenic illness complained of intolerable motor restlessness in association with antipsychotic medication he was receiving. The outpatient therapist adjusted the dose, added an antiparkinsonian drug, and then switched to several other classes of drug without much improvement. The patient stated that he could not sit still but needed to pace all day. Because he did not take his medication due to this alleged "side effect," he was finally hospitalized and taken off all medications. Staff noted him to be very anxious, and he showed the same pacing and motor restlessness of which he had complained earlier. Antianxiety medication was next prescribed with a marked improvement, and he was eventually restarted on the antipsychotic drug without difficulty. True akathesia was never noted.

This example illustrates the value of a drug-free period. While a drug-free or "wash-out" period is often clinically desirable, it can only be undertaken if the staff can tolerate the patient's behavior. In situations where the patient has a history of violence, nursing staff may be wary of any situation in which medication is not available to control the potentially dangerous behavior and PRN orders may be necessary. But the availability of PRN medication may lead to cumulative usage in excess of what would ordinarily be prescribed for the patient. If ward personnel have experience in the management of violent patients and have access to restraint devices and seclusion rooms, drug-free periods may be feasible, provided that the milieu is conducive to the "experiment" and does not have other violent patients who detract from nursing staff's attention.

The in-hospital use of medications to handle behaviorally agitated and aggressive patients is always problematic. Appleton[5] has described the "snow phenomenon" whereby the violent patient is given increasing and repeated dosages of medication, to the point that he becomes more and more alienated from the rest of the ward. If he is then placed in seclusion, the sense of isolation is even more intensified, leading him to become more frightened and hostile. A vicious cycle ensures whereby the patient is more panicked and boisterous, and receives more medication. Wadeson and Carpenter[6] have shown that the sensory deprivation of seclusion can be strongly aversive, and serves to worsen the patient's hold over reality, fostering delusions borne of helplessness. Much more is gained by taking a patient out of seclusion and integrating him into the ward, even with the use of restraint appliances. Van Rybroek and coworkers[7] have described the use of protective aggression devices (acronym: PADS), in which leather cuffs attached to a waist belt prevent the patient from swinging back his arm to deliver a blow. In time, the cuff is removed from the nondominant hand and then altogether as part of a behavior modification scheme.

The excessive use of medication within the hospital is more an issue within clinical settings where staff/patient ratios are low and where low morale leads to an emphasis on "keeping the peace" at the expense of interaction with the patient. Suppression of motivation and alertness is always a risk in using psychotropic drugs. It is more difficult to use medications judiciously and to the point that patients can still engage in meaningful dialogue with staff. The latter is a time-dependent function. And it may mean that both staff and patients are able to tolerate some anxiety.

Hospitalization allows the clinician to treat any illness more rigorously. In the case of aggressive patients, the use of sequential parenteral dosages of a drug such as haloperidol may help produce quiescence. The rapid titration technique[8] can be used not only in the emergency room but also on the inpatient ward when agitation, hostility, and belligerence worsen. Benzodiazepine drugs[9] can likewise be administered parenterally in situations requiring rapid behavioral control. In most states, there are legal provisions and procedures which mandate how parenteral medications can be used against the patient's will.[10]

Once parenteral medication has ceased, determination of the maintenance oral dose becomes a necessity. Usually, this is some proportion of the dose required during the acute phases of the illness, but some trial and error is required, particularly in cases of acute psychosis with mania. Dosing in the hospital is a function of several parameters, which include the patient's behavior, age, and physical status. Elderly patients require frequent dosing of small amounts of medication, but some younger patients may benefit from the socially interactive process of receiving multiple doses of drugs. In theory, most antipsychotic and antidepressant medications have long half-lives and infrequent dosing is all that is needed. This spares nursing staff's valuable time.

Hospitalization also allows the clinician to treat affective disorders more vigorously.

> A 78-year-old man was given antidepressant medication by his outpatient therapist. The patient lived alone and complained of mild dizziness upon arising in the morning. His depression deepened, and the therapist eventually hospitalized him. On the ward, his cardiac status was easily monitored and a divided dose regimen of the drug

was begun without incident, significantly improving the patient's mood within a short time.

This case illustrates the concept of frequent dosing, a task often difficult on an outpatient basis. In the above case, the therapist rapidly learned about his patient's physical tolerance for the antidepressant drug. Antidepressant drugs often are the most difficult agents to use in this regard, particularly in geriatric patients who are apt to suffer from troublesome anticholinergic side effects such as constipation or urinary retention or blurred vision. But often simply removing the patient from his pathogenic environment is as useful in the management of illness as the appropriate dose.

A 40-year-old woman had a history of depression and marital difficulties. She was treated with antidepressants but failed to improve. She complained at length about her husband's negativism toward her and the children; he would not speak to her and silence prevailed in the house, making it intolerable for her to be with him in the same room. It was finally decided to hospitalize her. On the ward, she was initially withdrawn and despondent but she eventually responded to nursing staff interaction and became more active in ward activities. Her mood dramatically improved, at which time marital therapy was begun. In these sessions, her husband related his anger at her for again becoming depressed.

This case shows how hospitalization allows a therapy to proceed, though the effect of the hospitalization had more to do with the psychological and social issues than with pharmacology. But it is common experience to see patients so hopelessly enmeshed in family pathology that no drug will serve its function without some form of psychosocial intervention.

A young woman with a history of a previous psychotic illness developed the belief that her father was poisoning her. As her delusions worsened, more antipsychotic drugs were prescribed but the family pathology became intense; her mother blamed her for again becoming ill, while her father continued to dispense the medication she was prescribed. Arguments erupted at home and her condition deteriorated. She was ultimately hospitalized for a long period of time. Family sessions were held, and the patient ultimately received ECT treatments. A remission ensued.

Most clinicians working with schizophrenic patients have experienced the need to sometimes isolate the patient from the family. Precisely how family pathology negatively interacts with psychopharmacologic treatment is unclear, though workers studying the interaction of drug treatment and psychotherapy.[11,12] have commented upon the need for both parameters to be addressed in treatment strategies for maximum outcome. It is common experience, of course, to see a disturbed patient who, once removed from his environment, rapidly integrates within the hospital. This occurs with patients in adolescent turmoil as much as it does with psychotic patients and those with affective illnesses. The power of the hospital milieu in promoting psychological reintegration is considerable, and short stays within the institution may be sufficient for compensation to occur.

This improvement, in fact, may be misleading. If the clinician predicates his criteria for discharge upon the initial improvements seen in hospitalized cases, then relapse is likely. Patients need to be tested outside the hospital, for the more nurturant hospital is no substitute for the stresses of everyday life outside of the institution.

> A 35-year-old male was hospitalized with a severely agitated psychotic illness and treated immediately with antipsychotic medication. He rapidly improved and was deemed ready for discharge by the fifth day. Though almost no contact occurred between the patient and his family, he was anxious to leave the hospital and return home, and plans for outpatient therapy were made. He returned to the emergency room within 36 hours with psychotic symptomatology. A careful history was taken which revealed great conflict with his wife; she had accused him of being a failure as a husband and man and had insisted that he return to work the next morning to insure their economic survival. Her demands accounted for the patient's eagerness to prematurely leave the hospital.

This case illustrates a hasty discharge, without a test of the patient's stability by an overnight stay or leave of absence or work leave. Graduated releases from the hospital should be the rule, and the clinician should not assume that medication will confer the necessary protection for patients at risk for relapse on the outside. This is particularly true for patients with such mood disorders as a manic-depressive illness, where lithium may have to be titrated higher to more effectively enable the patient to cope with the pressures within his family and the work setting.

Another reason for delaying discharge pertains to the matter of psychopharmacologic training. Patients need to understand how to use their medications and how to deal with side effects. Those receiving lithium, for example, may benefit from attending inpatient group therapy programs which stress compliance and teach members about the concept of blood levels. Adolescent populations receiving medications may benefit from group discussions about such issues as social embarrassment and the stigma of being or having been ill. Alcoholic patients receiving Antabuse also require group instruction. Older patients receiving divided dosages of drugs can be observed to see whether they come to the nursing station to ask for their medication.

Alcoholic and drug abuse patients are often hospitalized precisely to withdraw from the drugs they are abusing. Strategies here involved slow reduction of narcotics, barbiturates, or other habit-forming substances and the use of substitute drugs. Alcoholic detoxification can usually only be carried out within a secure setting that gives the patient no access to illicit drugs. Yet it is common experience to have patients who still find the means to procure the very substances they ostensibly wish to give up. Illicit drug traffic also exists on adolescent wards, where patients may exploit benzodiazepines or deal in marijuana or cocaine. Drug traffic within a hospital is always a pernicious event, since more vulnerable patients may be susceptible to drug usage. Drug-detoxifying patients may be more demanding and put pressures on both physicians and nursing staff to prescribe "something" to alleviate discomfort. The clinician must strive for some course which renders comfort to the patient while at the same time conveying to the milieu the message that medications will not be excessively dispensed.

Often such a message is also required with other types of psychiatric patients such as borderline or histrionic individuals who loudly demand medications. The withholding of medication in the service of psychological change and introspection, albeit often painful, is of great potential benefit to the patient. But it may require that staff endure the patient's complaints and not falsely "rescue" her.

> A borderline woman articulately complained of despondency and suicidal ideation. She had been hospitalized following an overdose precipitated by a failed romance. Several nursing staff asked the doctor to prescribe antidepressants to help her, and the latter refused, indicating that the loss needed to be worked through in individual and group therapy; drugs were not the answer to her current panic and despair. In a team meeting, one nurse chastised the physician for his "coldness" in dealing with the patient, but another person pointed out to her that she identified too strongly with the patient. A discussion took place regarding the patient's manipulativeness. No medication was prescribed, and in time the patient did talk of her loss and rage, and subsequently improved.

Differences in opinion between clinician and staff may reflect a "biologic" orientation as opposed to a "psychodynamic" view of the patient's illness. Or, staff may overidentify with the patient and seek rapid pharmacologic solutions as part of the countertransference. In other instances, the tension on the ward and the critical mass of disturbed patients may directly translate into the request and utilization of more medication.[13]

One way of quantifying pharmacologic response within the hospital involves the use of rating scales for mood or thought disorders. Utilization of scales, however, requires some training on the part of staff. Some behaviors such as agitation are easily observable, while others are more complicated to evaluate. A delusion, for example, is difficult to score. Outside of research wards and institutions, few facilities use such scales. In most hospitals, changes in the patient's clinical status are viewed quite subjectively, though some more objective rating of improvement or worsening occurs during periodic assessment of the patient's individual treatment plan.

In summary, drug treatment within the hospital affords the clinician the potential of greater control, as well as the advantages of better observation and quantification.

REFERENCES

1. Van Putten T: Why do schizophrenic patients refuse to take their drugs? Arch Gen Psychiatry 1974; 31:67-72
2. Quitkin FM: The importance of dosage in prescribing antidepressants. Brit J Psychiatry 1985; 147:593-597
3. Jefferson J, Greist JH: A Primer on Lithium, Baltimore. Williams and Wilkins, 1977
4. Karasu TB, Murkofsky CA: Psychopharmacology of the elderly, in Geriatric Psychiatry. Edited by Bellack L, Karasu TB, New York, Grune and Stratton, 1976
5. Appleton WS: The snow phenomenon: tranquilizing the assaultive patient. Psychiatry 1965; 28:88-93
6. Wadeson H, Carpenter WT: Impact of the seclusion room experience. J Nerv Ment Dis 1976; 163:318-328
7. Van Rybroek GJ et al: Preventive aggression devices (PADS): ambulatory restraints as an alternative to seclusion. J Clin Psychiatry, in press
8. Donlon PT, Hopkin J, Tupin JP: Efficacy and safety of rapid neuroleptization with injectable haloperidol. Am J Psychiatry 1979; 136:273-278
9. Bick PA, Hannah, AL: Intramuscular lorazepam to restrain violent patients. Lancet 1986; 1:206
10. Applebaum PS, Gutheil TG: "Rotting with their rights on": constitutional theory and clinical reality in drug refusal by psychiatric patients. Bull Am Acad Psychiatry Law 1979; 7:308-317.
11. Lion JR: The Art of Medicating Psychiatric Patients, Baltimore, 1978
12. Group for the Advancement of Psychiatry, Report #93. Pharmacotherapy and Psychotherapy: Paradoxes, Problems, and Progress, New York, 1975
13. Sabshin M, Eisen SB: The effects of ward tension on the quality and quantity of tranquilizer utilization. Ann NY Acad Sci 1956; 67:746-757

12

Activity Therapy in Hospital Psychiatry

Diane Gibson

Activity therapy is a composite of health professions which utilizes purposeful activities in the reduction of disease symptoms and the promotion of optimal independent performance in the areas of work, care, self-care, and the constructive use of leisure time. Occupational and recreational therapy together with creative arts therapies, vocational counseling, work therapy, and horticulture typically form the activity therapies. Individual performance components, such as interpersonal relating, cognition, perception, self-concept, and motor functioning, are evaluated and treated in order to assist the patient in learning those skills and functions essential to productivity. Such creative activities as art, music, dance, and drama serve as integrating and insight-producing experiences which bring meaning and purpose to human behavior.

HISTORICAL EVOLUTION

Historically, the basic concepts of activity therapy disciplines were drawn from the moral treatment era. Early proponents of moral treatment believed that mind and body are coupled, and that anything which impinges upon one also affects the other. The work ethic was a guiding value in implementing action-oriented treatment during 19th century hospital psychiatry. Patients were expected to be "doers" in that they assumed daily work or chore responsibilities along with a balanced program of rest, recreation, and "habit training." Kindly, consistent approaches to patients were emphasized no matter how disturbed the patient.

Eleanor Clarke Slagle,[1] and Dr. William Rush Dunton,[2] early founders of occupational therapy, developed the use of planned goals and methods for promoting health through the use of activities. When he was staff psychiatrist at the Sheppard and Enoch Pratt Hospital during the 1920s, Dunton outlined principles for matching patient needs with therapeutic activities. In classifying activities regarding physical effort, attention span, repetition, and social factors, he seems remarkably modern. He wrote the first textbook on occupational therapy and assisted in developing one of the first schools for this discipline. Dunton defined occupational therapy as a treatment using instruction and employment in productive occupation. The objectives were to arouse interest, courage, and confidence; to exercise the mind and body in healthy activities; to overcome functional disability; and to reestablish a capacity for industrial and social usefulness.[3] His tenets included beliefs that:

> occupation (purposeful activity) was as necessary to life as food and drink; every human being should have both physical and mental occupations; sick minds may be healed through occupation, and all people should have enjoyable hobbies, particularly when the vocation is dull or distasteful. Lastly, every individual should have two hobbies, one outdoor and one indoor, recognizing that a greater number will create wider interests and broader intelligence.[4]

During the Second World War and the following two decades, much of the valuable original thinking regarding the inherent normalizing role of activity in hospital care was forgotten as occupational therapists assumed a reductionistic, disease-oriented model. In psychiatry, activities such as metal hammering were used to "sublimate anger" and tile trivets were employed to "build compulsive defenses." This mechanistic approach prevented the therapist from viewing the patient in a holistic way and from using activities to support remaining healthy assets in preparation for discharge to the community.

New specialties—recreation, art, dance, music, drama, horticulture and vocational counseling—emerged in the decades following the Second World War. They evolved independently but in a parallel fashion with occupational therapy, each developing its own frame of reference and methods. All of the activity therapy disciplines have grown in numbers and have developed professional status including certification, mandated education requirements, and articulated standards for treatment.

Since the 1940s, professional members of the activity therapies have become regular members of treatment teams. They contribute valuable diagnostic information gleaned from their observations of performance outside the ward and the milieu. For example, occasionally a borderline or narcissistic patient may demonstrate attention-seeking and regressive behavior while "at home" on the ward while simultaneously functioning in a responsible manner in the patient government or work therapy assignment. Setting clear expectations for behavior and asking the patient to take responsibility in a work-oriented setting assist the patient in functioning, at least temporarily, at a high level of performance. Such information is valuable to the team as a measure of improvement.

BENEFITS OF HOSPITALIZATION

The impact of the massive move toward deinstitutionalization and the significant cutbacks in length of stay brought about by cost-conscious third-party payers may serve to prohibit long-term hospitalization with its many positive benefits, especially for the patient who has failed to respond to other forms of treatment. In the author's opinion, long-term hospitalization continues to be the only form of treatment which can assure the highly structured and carefully supervised environment needed by the severely disorganized schizophrenic or the erratically self-destructive borderline personality.

Hospital admission[5] is indicated when skilled observation is needed for diagnostic clarification; when the patient, his family, or society need protection from suicidal or homicidal behavior; when the patient is too disorganized to function in the community; when specialized services such as medical, nursing, or rehabilitative treatment are required. The psychiatric hospital may provide the only effective institution in dealing with difficult and recalcitrant problems because of its concentration of skilled professionals, including psychiatrists, psychologists, social workers, nurses, and members of activity therapy disciplines.

Many mental health professionals have only vague understanding of the purpose and nature of activities used to treat hospitalized patients. Perhaps this is in part due to the difficulty occupational therapists and other activity therapy staff have in clearly defining their own role and in clarifying that role to treatment teams. As a result, some practitioners view activity therapy as diversional engagement, thus missing the important role of activity in psychiatric rehabilitation.

On the other hand, many contemporary activity therapy staff clearly articulate their function and have become laudable members of clinical teams. Insurance companies have recognized the role of activity therapy as a treatment modality for the last 15 years. Commercial insurers, such as Blue Cross, and federal payors, such as Medicare, fully fund activities provided by certified and/or licensed staff in activity therapy. For example, insurance companies will cover goal-oriented activities when they specifically involve treatment objectives oriented toward diminishing symptomatology and training for living outside the hospital. Activities of daily living, social skills, training, and prevocational training are examples of fee-for-service treatments. In hospitals where no fee for service exists, most insurance companies pay for a daily rate which includes activity therapy just as it includes nursing and board and room.

Insurance does not typically cover outpatient activity therapy at this time, unless activity group therapy is co-led and supervised by another professional who receives coverage. For this reason, almost all psychosocial rehabilitation conducted by members of activity therapy disciplines takes place within hospitals. Occasionally when vocational counseling, art therapy, dance therapy, and recreational and occupational therapy are *only* available within the hospital, these services may act as a drawing card for some referrals. For example, a chronic patient who has never held a job and is unaware of his aptitudes may be referred to a hospital offering vocational counseling rather than to a psychiatric unit in a general hospital.

ASSESSMENT AND TREATMENT PLANNING

Certain etiological concepts are important in understanding the role of activity therapy in treating the mentally ill. Mental illness develops when an individual is no longer able to deal effectively with life stresses. Commonly used defenses are not sufficient to cope with overwhelming stresses, whether the origin be primarily intrapsychic, genetic, organic, or environmental. Most persons who are ill enough to be hospitalized also have chronic interpersonal problems, such as loneliness and isolation, poor social skills, sexual concerns, conflicts with authority, anger, and dependency. The patient's symptoms represent his effort to return to a more stable level of adjustment. They may cause or accompany a breakdown in previously learned functional capacities in work, leisure, and self-care, or they may have precluded the initial learning of functional skills.

Regardless of whether the patient needs habilitation or rehabilitation, an assessment of current performance must precede treatment to facilitate design of an activity therapy treatment program to address his or her individual needs. The activity therapy assessment is presented at the team's diagnostic session and is integrated into the master treatment plan along with assessments of other disciplines. It is essential that the patient be included as much as possible so that he or she will become invested in the treatment program. A typical assessment involves both a semi-structured interview and observation of performance skills. The interviewer gathers data involving the patient's work, education, leisure, and self-care history. Interests, goals, problems, and level of self-esteem are reviewed in an effort to understand strengths and limitations that may enhance or diminish the patient's ability to fulfill such life roles as worker, retiree, parent, or student. Basic cognitive and social skills are evaluated during individual and group tasks while gross motor skills are assessed in group games (see Table 1 for listing of common assessment instruments). The activity therapy assessment includes not only the patient's strengths and deficits but also objectives stated in behavioral terms and a recommended action plan and time frame. Long-term objectives are designed to promote the team's overall objectives. For example, a schizophrenic patient may lack elementary social skills. The activity therapy objective might read, "Patient will initiate conversation with peers at least three times during the next week." The action plan might involve attending communication skills twice weekly.

Specific performance areas which are amenable to activity therapy treatment and which can be evaluated during the assessment period are:

- *Work skills*: Skills essential to securing and maintaining a job, for example, punctuality, dependability, coordination, problem-solving, task completion, attention to detail, frustration tolerance, awareness of vocational skills and opportunities for placement, comfort with job interviews and with authority.
- *Self-Care skills*: Skills essential to independent functioning in everyday activities, for example, self-grooming and feeding, use of public transportation, money management, budgeting and cooking, and use of community resources.

**Table 1
Test Instruments**

Visual perceptual motor
    Schroeder Block Campbell Adult Psychiatric Sensory Integration Evaluation (SBC)
    Southern California Sensory Integration (SCSI)

Activities of daily living
    Kolman Evaluation of Living Skills (KELS)
    Routine Task Inventory (RTI)

Functional performance
    Comprehensive Occupational Therapy Evaluation (COTE)
    Bay Area Functional Evaluation (Ba FPE)

Vocational
    Strong Campbell Interest Inventory (SCII)
    General Aptitude Test Battery (GATB)
    Career Assessment Inventory (CAI)
    Career Decision-Making System (CDMS)
    Myers Briggs Type Indicator (MBTI)

- *Leisure skills*: Skills essential to constructive use of leisure time, for example, knowledge and skills necessary to engage in sports, games, and hobbies.
- *Cognitive skills*: The level, quality and/or degree of comprehension, communication, concentration, problem-solving, time management, conceptualization, integration of learning, judgment, and time-place-person orientation.
- *Motor skills*: The level, quality, and/or degree of motion, gross muscle strength, muscle tone, endurance, fine motor skills, and functional use.
- *Perceptual motor skills*: Presence and level of function in spatial discrimination, laterality, eye-hand coordination, figure-ground discrimination, and depth perception.
- *Psychological skills*: The level, quality, and/or degree of self-identity, self-concept, and coping skills[6]: (a) *self-identity* and *self-concept*—the ability to perceive self-needs and expectations from those of others; identify areas of self-competency and limitations; accept responsibility for self; perceive sexuality of self; have self-respect; have appropriate body image; view self as being able to influence events; (b) *coping skills*—includes the ability to sublimate drives, find sources of need gratification, tolerate frustration and anxiety, experience gratification, and control impulses.
- *Social/interpersonal skills*: The level, quality, and/or degree of dyadic and group interaction skills:[6] (a) *dyadic interaction skills*—abilities in relationships to peers, subordinates, and authority figures; demonstrating trust, respect, and warmth; perceiving and responding to needs and feelings of others; engaging in and sustaining interdependent relationships; communicating feelings; (b) *group interaction skills*—abilities in performing tasks in the presence of others; sharing tasks with others; cooperating and competing with others; fulfilling a variety of group membership roles.

A case study is included at this point to exemplify activity therapy assessment and treatment planning as well as how these components fit into the master treatment plan.

Case Study I: Assessment and Treatment Plan for an Anorectic Patient

Summary of Physician's Admission Note. This is the fourth hospitalization for this 21-year-old single, white female (Ms. E.). She has a history of anorectic symptoms, including an intense fear of becoming obese that does not diminish as weight loss progresses. Ms. E. has a profound disturbance of body image. She weighs 68 pounds and has experienced weight loss of greater than 25% of her original body weight. She has refused to maintain her weight over a minimal normal weight for age and height. With her restricted pattern of eating, she has been eating approximately 300 calories per day. Bulimic symptoms include self-induced vomiting up to two times daily along with the use of cathartics at an average of 45 Correctols daily. Although there is no history of bingeing, she has used up to 75 Correctols in the past and denies use of diet pills and diuretics.

Ms. E. has been preoccupied with her weight since the age of 13, when she weighed 180 pounds. During the next six years, she lost and gained as much as 60 pounds. At age 19, she began a steady weight loss despite a three-week medical hospitalization in a general hospital. She undertook outpatient treatment with a social worker who refused to treat her when her weight dropped below 90 pounds.

Her father died unexpectedly from a heart attack when she was 20, after which she gradually reduced her weight to 68 pounds. During the following year, Ms. E. was hospitalized twice at a general medical hospital because of dehydration and gastroenteritis as a result of her eating disorder, which again included restriction of caloric intake, vomiting, and catharsis. During the last hospitalization, her potassium and sodium levels were dangerously low. When her medical condition stabilized, she was referred to the present hospital for inpatient treatment of her psychiatric disorder.

Currently, Ms. E. lives with the mother and sister. No significant psychiatric history exists in the family. Her sister, 24, is obese, weighing approximately 300 pounds. Her mother is also overweight and has attended various diet workshops in the past. Apparently, she is very closely tied to her own parents. Ms. E. herself has never lived away from home. It is notable that she was an A student in high school and graduated as a member of the National Honor Society. Despite these achievements, she did not consider entering college, stating that she had always wanted to be a secretary. She worked for approximately one and a half years in various departments of the Social Security Department. She had to quit work as a result of her eating disorder and has lived at home since then. Ms. E. has dated on a superficial basis and notes that the longest time she has gone out with a male has been one month. She has not had sexual relationships with males.

Developmentally, Ms. E. was a product of a normal prenatal period. She was delivered vaginally without complications and weighed seven pounds, 13 ounces. Her mother relates there was no delay in achievement of developmental milestones. However, her recollection may be somewhat amiss, as she recalls that the patient was talking at the age of one year. Her mother quit work seven months after the patient was born and has worked as a housewife since that time.

Summary of Activity Therapy Assessment. Ms. E. was cooperative and spontaneous throughout the evaluation procedures. She attended two out of the three evaluation sessions after being on hall restrictions for two and a half weeks. She spoke easily, although she sat in a fetal position holding her knees tightly with her arms, as if to cover herself.

Ms. E. values both creative, altruistic self-development and social activities. However, in the past three to six months, she has discontinued all of her activities except socializing with friends. She indicated that she was unable to structure her time in order to pursue needed and valued activities and did not know how to use community resources for this purpose. Her self-attitude survey revealed that while she spends time with friends, she feels taken advantage of and gives in to others in order to be part of the group. She reported that she would go out of her way to do extra things for people, but that her friends abused this quality in her. She reported having difficulty asserting herself with them.

A vocational assessment was completed. She spoke of being well thought of at her secretarial job, and although she was glad about that, she did not feel any sense of personal accomplishment concerning the tasks of her job. She was considering going to college to become a teacher.

An assessment of the patient's independent living skills revealed that she is competent in areas of money management and general household skills but that she has never lived independently of her family. She lives with her parents, manages her own finances, and is afraid to live on her own in an apartment.

For purposes of illustration, only the physician and activity therapy assessments have been included here. After ten days, all discipline assessments were reviewed and incorporated into the master treatment plan as follows:

Master Treatment Plan Summary

Problem	Objectives	Action Plans
A. *Physical*		
Malnourishment	Gain approximately 46	*Nursing:*
Electrolyte imbalance	pounds by discharge	Refeeding program
Secondary amenorrhea		Feelings group
B. *Emotional/Behavioral*		
Anorexia/bulimia	Recognize illness	*Psychiatry:*
Depression	Examine control issues	Individual psychotherapy
Low self-esteem	Seek help in assessing	Group psychotherapy
Perfection	physical states	*Activity Therapy:*
Cannot discuss feelings and values	Develop realistic body image	Assertiveness training Dance therapy
Lack of belief in efficacy of skills	Identify feelings and values Develop greater confidence in skills	Patient publications Patient government

Master Treatment Plan Summary

Problem	Objectives	Action Plans
C. *Social/Interpersonal* 　Lacks autonomy 　Overly dependent on family	Develop independent behavior Develop family understanding of controlling interactions with patient	*Social Work:* 　Family therapy
D. *Vocational/Avocational* 　Lack of leisure interests 　Vocational uncertainty	Identify leisure values and projects with emphasis on pleasure, not achievement Explore career options	*Activity Therapy:* 　Leisure counseling 　Recreation with crafts 　Vocational counseling 　Work therapy in journal office

Course in Hospital. During the early phase of treatment, Ms. E. was ward restricted in order to control her refeeding regimen and weight gain. After three weeks, she was referred to assertiveness training to develop self-esteem and directness in communication, and to leisure counseling to identify and structure leisure interests and free time. After several sessions in these group activities, Ms. E. began to initiate conversation with peers, although she needed considerable reassurance from staff. She was able to state that peer pressure for her to focus on nonweight-related issues, such as interests and feelings, felt "threatening" and "unsupportive."

At times, Ms. E. was resistant to the eating disordered program. She used the men's bathroom to avoid being observed taking laxatives or vomiting. When confronted, she became angry and placed a three-day notice to leave, which she later withdrew.

Ms. E.'s perfectionism, competitiveness, and low self-esteem were addressed in assignments to horticulture and patient publications. In these activities, she was able to complete successful projects and encouraged to acknowledge her accomplishments. Her need to be perfect and her low self-esteem were evidenced in her disinclination to experiment and to take risks. Her depression was masked by a superficially cheerful demeanor; however, when pressed regarding behavior and feelings, she became tearful quickly.

Since Ms. E. believed she made a serious mistake in terminating employment, she was referred to vocational counseling to explore educational and vocational options. She attended a career exploration group and began regular participation in work therapy. In the journal office, she frequently asked for feedback on her personal appearance and work performance. The work therapy position, assistant to the hospital's journal editor, was selected based on her interest in writing, her skills in organizational content, and her need to improve self-esteem. Her response to the responsibility and the limited setting of her work were good, and she gradually became able to accept and integrate feedback.

Within the dance therapy and art therapy groups, focused on identifying and accepting feelings, she spontaneously began to interact with other members of the group and to eliminate her tendency to cry.

Assuming continuously greater initiative, Ms. E. was elected ward chairman of PAC (patient government). In that capacity she set high standards for her own performance, yet was able to negotiate and facilitate appropriate work of other patients. As she neared discharge, she and the vocational counselor agreed on her considered decision to matriculate in a medical technology course; although these plans were postponed on the advice of the treatment team, Ms. E. was able to volunteer in a similar role at a local hospital during the summer while she waited to enter school in the fall.

The psychotherapist noted at discharge (after three months' treatment), "Ms. E.'s condition was much improved, her weight having reached the desired range. She returned home to live with her mother until she could complete her training and secure a job. Her self-esteem had improved significantly, and she had undertaken responsible activities. She was no longer a danger to herself, and her cognitive distortions consistent with her eating disorder were diminished. The patient still had difficulty in the area of trust, which would be a continued focus in outpatient work."

TREATMENT ASSUMPTIONS

The following guidelines are essential to contemporary activity therapy and tend to differentiate this modality from the somatic and verbal treatments offered by psychiatrists, psychologists, social workers, and nurses:

1. Health is defined as having achieved mastery in work, leisure and self-care, as well as a sense of self-acceptance and satisfaction interpersonally and intrapersonally.
2. Purposeful activities may be individually tailored to assist the individual patient in learning skills that may have been retarded or neglected due to illness.
3. Activities include a broad range of human involvement. They may be goal oriented or nondirected, work or leisure oriented, or symptom-reducing and/or skill-developing in nature. Examples include creative, expressive, and symbolic activities; sports, games, and crafts; discussions and work or organizational tasks.
4. The use of activities focuses upon "doing" rather than "receiving" in the sense that emphasis is given to participation, involvement, and/or productivity. The group in which the activity may take place and

the interaction between the activity therapist and the patient are matched and shaped to meet the developmental needs, level and interests of the patient.
5. Activities reflect and relate to real-life situations and conditions as much as possible in order to prepare the patient for successful reinvolvement with his/her anticipated role and environment. The total treatment schedule represents a balance in work, rest, leisure, self-care, and sleep.
6. Activities incorporate the patient's or patient group's responsibility to make decisions for themselves. Growth toward independence and self-determination is an important aspect of rehabilitation. The use of activities is designed to foster growth in mastery and competence, curiosity and self-awareness, and creativity.
7. Activities provide "here-and-now" social and task situations in which patients give and receive regular feedback and positive reinforcement.

THERAPEUTIC VALUE OF ACTIVITY

Activity therapy disciplines place the process of *doing* center stage in assisting patients to learn necessary adaptive skills. Fidler[7] has stated:

> If health professionals are to assume a major responsibility for designing environments and experiences for the prevention of illness, for the maintenance and restoration of health, they need to achieve a more sophisticated understanding of *doing*. The word *doing* is selected to convey the sense of performing, producing, or causing. It is purposeful action in contrast to random activity that the action is directed toward the intrapersonal (testing a skill), the interpersonal (clarifying a relationship), or the nonhuman (creating an end product). Doing is viewed as enabling the development and integration of the sensory, motor, cognitive, and psychological systems; serving as a socializing agent; and verifying one's efficacy as a competent, contributing member of one's society.

Activities enable patients to try out and practice their capacity for experiencing, responding, managing, and controlling, thus creating a reservoir from which to draw in coping with problems of everyday life. "People can become competent and confident through what they do. Doing enables them to become more fully human as they develop their potential and earn their membership in the culture through their contributions."[8]

Competence and its by-product, self-esteem, evolve from direct and repeated real encounters with task experiences. Task groups are designed to provide the *doing* which results in validation of efficacy of action via verbal and nonverbal feedback from patient peers and staff. The intrinsic gratification of accomplishment and even the sheer pleasure involved in moving or creating are further subtle aspects of the human experience which contribute to self-esteem. Patients say, "It feels good to dance," or, "I'm pleased I could draw the flower the way I see it." The inherent human drive toward mastery is powerful; it explains the joy and gratification of being a cause, of having an effect, and of accomplishing something from within one's own resources. Motivation of this kind lies behind the desire of the resident psychiatrist to learn psychotherapy techniques as well as his patients' desire to learn how to use the potter's wheel.

Despite their need for purposeful activity, many patients are resistant to becoming involved in action-oriented experiences. Why? Early negative feedback from others and lack of success in manipulating nonhuman objects have left these patients with a sense that "to do is to verify one's incompetence." Hence, rationalizations such as "activities are dumb and boring" are used to defend against potential failure. Starting from this position, it is doubly important that the therapist skillfully match the activity with the patient's functioning level, interests, and goals so that success will be experienced in the activity. Furthermore, the activity must be recognized as socially and culturally relevant to the values and needs of the individual patient. Cultural relevance was exemplified by the case of a depressed woman who refused to discuss her feelings and problems with her psychotherapist as she improved, yet regularly attended a cooking group in which she demonstrated pleasure in cooking and serving other patients. The psychiatrist hesitated in discharging her until she understood her own feelings and the problems which had brought her into the hospital. Her husband, a blue collar worker, explained that he and his wife were happy that she was now well and could return home to cook for the family. Their definition of health included functional work skills, not verbal skills or insight into problems, which are middle-class values.

ROLE OF ACTIVITY THERAPY STAFF

The role of an occupational, recreation, or creative art therapist varies greatly depending on the diagnosis and age of the patient and the content and purpose of the activity. Although the classic therapeutic relationship focuses on feelings and on the analysis of unconscious elements in relationships, the relationship of an occupational therapist may act as teacher, supervisor, coach, or crafts person, as he or she teaches and facilitates prevocational habits, recreational pursuits, and self-maintenance tasks. These aspects of role are unique to activity therapy in that they flow from the "doing" or experiential content of this treatment.

Given a therapist's prime function of engaging patients in productive, goal-oriented activity, the therapist must know how "to do" the activity, whether it encompasses crafts, art, music, or social skills; she or he also must believe that the learning of the activity and its processes will help the patient. To this end, the therapist must also be a source of hope and affirmation to the patient. There is an apprentice-like association which allows the patient to acquire requisite emotional and informational resources.[8]

In most group activities, but particularly in those involving play or spontaneous, interactional activities, the therapist becomes a truly participating member of the group, thus helping create the spirit and meaning of the group occupation. The therapist must lead sessions sensitively in a manner which offers patients tangible benefits. He or she must be self-revealing, allowing patients to observe and role model healthy behavior. The therapist focuses primarily on here-and-now interactions in groups, giving special attention to providing severely ill patients with supportive, pleasant, and constructive experiences.

Patients experience hospitalization as failure and defeat — affects which further compound the stress, disorganization, and demoralization they have already experienced.[9] Hospitalization further compounds the sense of isolation and estrangement from family and friends, despite the patient's removal from a possible noxious environment. These factors legitimize the patient's surrender to dependency and regression. The role of the therapist is a delicate one, in that she or he must remain empathic and supportive to the patient while guarding against tendencies to promote dependent regression within the hospital. Clear expectations of responsibility, such as attendance at hall meetings, activities, and work therapy, assist the patient in assuming an adult role. Frequently, patients are capable of organizing and planning functions in activities when they are allowed to "own" responsibility for decision-making and leadership. Psychotherapists are occasionally surprised to find that the same patients who hallucinate or refuse to accommodate to rules on the hall are capable of chairing weekend planning committees requiring that they orient, guide, and coach other patients. The author recalls an ironic incident in which a patient chairman eloped from his hall but returned just in time to lead the movie club because, "I was the only one who could operate the projector."

Conversely, staff working in activities therapy must be careful not to place demands on patients that are beyond their capacity. Middle-class mental health professionals place high value on personal growth, self-knowledge, and self-actualization, and they feel successful when their patients are able to attain a measure of these lofty goals. However, the role of the hospital therapist is to provide basic safety and security and to provide the building blocks to gain and retain skills in a protected environment. Further insight-oriented therapy and skill refinement can be continued after discharge.

GROUPS IN ACTIVITY THERAPY

In most activity therapy departments, services are typically delivered in group settings. This practice is sound for both economic and clinical reasons. Many psychiatric patients suffer from interpersonal isolation which may be relieved by participation in various hospital groups. Gradual social learning in a setting of interpersonal comfort allows patients to develop friendships, sometimes for the first time in their lives. Occasionally, patients comment that learning how to make a friend, how to trust and share, is a significant step back into "the real world."

Gould and Glick[10] have stated that different kinds of patients benefit from different group approaches. In their study borderline and neurotically depressed patients stated that they highly valued group therapy, which emphasized interpersonal interaction and the challenge of asking them to assume responsibility for their own treatment. Traditional nondirective group therapy, designed for neurotic outpatients, is not effective and can even be countertherapeutic for inpatients.[9] Inpatients require clearer structure in the form of orientation, instructions, here-and-now emphasis, and a focused agenda; hence, major modification in the classic format is required.[11]

Although members of activity therapy disciplines do not typically lead verbal group psychotherapy sessions, they do apply group dynamics principles to their groups and are sensitive to group process issues. Interpersonal skills, communication, and assertiveness training groups are focused on skill acquisition and therefore are notable in their task orientation. Groups which are led strictly on a verbal basis are usually geared to high level patients who are intellectually intact and moderately well-organized.

Schizophrenic patients prefer groups which are supportive, highly structured, and place few demands on them. They need to perceive themselves as able to perform the group task, usually of a concrete, simple nature—one at which they can succeed. They do not rate group therapy as highly as borderline patients. In one study, schizophrenic patients rated group therapy third of nine therapeutic approaches. Reality-focused groups which offer opportunities for sealing over rather than opening up emotional issues are more successful.[9]

Groups for low level schizophrenics provide support and structure to help orient patients to their temporal and spatial surroundings, to increase attention span, to facilitate socialization with staff and other patients, and to enable them to take part in the hall program. Tasks are designed to allow regressed patients mastery of elementary social, physical, or work skills and thus provide them with a sense of success and safety. Tasks may include simple games, physical exercises, social skills training, and basic prevocational jobs. For example, a small group of chronic schizophrenic patients might cook and eat a spaghetti dinner together, or they might collate and staple the hospital newspaper as part of the program which teaches basic work skills.

Occupational therapists have been trained to analyze activities and tasks in order to provide appropriate behavioral expectations for patients with varying degrees of ego integration. This skill makes them particularly useful in designing, leading, or consulting to therapy groups for disturbed and chronic patients. Protocols are useful in helping staff conceptualize and design treatment. Some hospital departments require them prior to initiation of a new group. A sample group protocol can be found in Table 2.

Table 2
Assertiveness Training Protocol

I. *Format*
  Time: TUESDAY/THURSDAY 1–2
  Place: Room 12
  Size: 8–10 Patients
  Leaders: OTR

II. *Purpose*
  Assertive Training is based on the assumption that effective communication is a learned behavior. Using a behaviorial frame of reference, assertive training focuses on common everyday situations (e.g., being shortchanged, dealing with "put-downs," making and refusing requests). It assists patients in examining interpersonal rights (e.g., right to say no, right to change your mind, the right to privacy), and the consequences of behavior. It provides an opportunity for exploration and practice of alternative methods of coping effectively with conflicts of everyday living in order to decrease anxiety and improve self-concept.

III. *Goals/Behavioral Objectives*
  A. Increase self-esteem

   Patient will: demonstrate the ability to make own decisions; be aware of own interpersonal rights; convincingly state opinions and disagree without aggression.

  B. Decrease anxiety

   Patient will demonstrate: improved eye contact, absence of nonproductive behaviors (rocking, playing with hands, etc.), an audible tone of voice, comfortably erect posture, emphatic gestures, meaningful facial expression; spontaneity and flexibility in expression of self.

(continued)

Table 2
Continued

C. Develop verbal communication ability

Patient will be comfortable carrying on conversations, expressing feelings and opinions without undue anxiety.

D. Develop appropriately assertive behavior

Patient will be able to stand up for his/her interpersonal rights; will act in own best interest without infringing on the rights of others.

IV. *Criteria for Patient Referral*
   A. The patient should demonstrate a willingness to participate and to accept constructive feedback. (The use of role-play as a primary treatment modality indicate the importance of this criterion.)
   B. Patients referred to this group should be able to participate in the cooperative group level:[6]
      1. can attend to the task for 60 minutes without a break;
      2. can think through cause and effect relationships;
      3. can establish own goals;
      4. can conceive end result;
      5. can think through alternatives via covert imagery;
      6. can follow three or more written or verbal directions.
   C. Patient may be verbally limited and inhibited, may internalize anger while showing potential to become more verbally expressive.
   D. Inappropriate referrals
      1. Severely regressed, totally nonverbal, or extremely anxious patients.
      2. Severely aggressive, i.e., physically combative and verbally abusive patients.
      3. Patients who are actively psychotic and/or paranoid.

V. *Methodology and Leadership*
   A. The group will operate by means of conversation and rehearsed (role-play) situations with limited use of audiovisual equipment, environmental props (e.g., chairs, hat, book), and occasional outings into the community (e.g., restaurants, stores) to practice assertive behavior.
   B. Leader will:
      1. be a role model for assertive behavior;
      2. consistently communicate the group's purpose and behavioral objectives to the group members;
      3. offer and promote behavioral feedback;
      4. initially choose situations for rehearsal, gradually increasing their difficulty;
      5. intervene, giving feedback and using role modeling or role reversal, when necessary;
      6. eventually expect group members to supply situations for rehearsal;
      7. encourage increasingly more independent resolutions.

VI. *Evaluation*
   Evaluation will be determined using the assertive training evaluation form in Table 3.

From the Sheppard and Enoch Pratt Hospital activity therapy department

Table 3
Assertive Training Evaluation

Key:
1. Seldom
2. Occasionally
3. Frequently
4. Consistently

Patient's Name _____ Case _____ Hall _____ Date _____

A. T. Staff _____

	1	2	3	4

A. *SELF-ESTEEM*
   1. Able to make own decisions _____
   2. Aware of interpersonal rights _____
   3. Convincingly states opinions _____
   4. Disagrees without aggression _____

B. *ANXIETY*
   1. Maintains eye contact _____
   2. Absence of nonproductive behaviors, e.g., rocking, playing with hands _____
   3. Audible tone of voice _____
   4. Comfortably erect posture _____
   5. Emphatic gestures _____
   6. Meaningful facial expressions _____
   7. Spontaneity in expression of self _____
   8. Flexibility in expression of self _____

C. *VERBAL COMMUNICATION*
   1. Comfortable carrying on conversations _____
   2. Comfortable expressing feelings, opinions without undue anxiety _____

D. *ASSERTIVE*
   1. Able to stand up for interpersonal rights _____
   2. Acts in own best interest without infringing on rights of others _____

COMMENTS:

From the Sheppard and Enoch Pratt Hospital Activity Therapy Department.

MODALITIES OF ACTIVITY THERAPY

Creative Art Therapies

The creative art therapies, which include art, dance, music, and drama, have therapeutic factors and theory in common. They use nonverbal media to foster expression and stimulate communication. Psychodynamic principles are essential to the understanding of patient etiology, and symbolic processes are viewed as important in facilitating patient awareness of unconscious material. The creative process itself involves a healing element. Creative art therapies may be implemented on an individual basis for the regressed or difficult patient or, more commonly, on a group basis. When the uncovering of unconscious issues is not viewed as appropriate, as is sometimes the case in short-term educational treatment or long-term behavior modification, the creative art therapies may be contraindicated. Art therapy may not be recommended at a time when the uncovering process may be too threatening and anxiety-producing. However, art, dance, or music may be structured toward skill acquisition (such as learning how to paint) rather than the uncovering of psychodynamic processes, depending on the frame of reference.

Art therapists work with a variety of materials including finger paint, oil paint, tempera, and clay in unstructured, spontaneous sessions and with pastels, felt-tip markers and crayons in structured sessions. Typically, the patient group draws or paints during the first half of the session and discusses the drawings during the second half. Art therapy goals encompass uncovering feelings, providing a cathartic experience, strengthening ego defenses, reducing guilt, developing impulse control, and increasing tolerance for social and group experience.[12]

Music therapy uses the elements of music, such as rhythm, melody, pitch, and harmony, in providing a nonverbal therapeutic modality. By employing a patient's skill in music and the communicative nature of rhythm, lyrics, and counterpoint, the music therapist can enhance the potential for behavioral change and for insight. Training in human development, psychodynamics, group process, and music is essential.

Dance/movement therapy is the psychotherapeutic use of dance/movement to further the physical and emotional integration of the individual. Dance/movement therapy assumes that mind and body are an integrated whole, each affecting the other. Mental conflicts and thought patterns are directly reflected in the body's postures, gestures, and movement. When dance/movement is used for therapeutic intervention, the resulting self-expression and psychophysical changes can reflect a healthier mental function. As the movement repertoire expands, so does the behavioral repertoire,

Activity Therapy in Hospital Psychiatry

thus enabling individuals to meet their needs more effectively and to facilitate appropriate adjustment to the demands of the environment.[14]

The dance therapist helps patients use movement interaction to examine, clarify, and organize their behavior and its symbolic movement. Patients learn to identify and cope with feelings and problems through movement. For example, motor responses to anger, such as sublimation or controlled aggressive discharge, can be taught with the additional benefit of verbalizing feelings rather than acting them out in an unproductive manner.

Drama therapy intentionally uses creative drama to further psychotherapeutic goals. It is not the same as psychodrama, which involves structured action methods, such as sociometry, enactment, and social systems analysis, to alter cognitive patterns. Drama therapy includes any therapeutic use of role-playing employing improvisational theater for purposes of emotional insight and personal growth. Improvisation and free expression form the core of the role-play, in which the patient assumes the identity of another person. When a vague situation is all that has been identified, the actor-patient must use his/her own resources to create a role identity. Both conscious and unconscious aspects are revealed as one draws on memories, habits, and feelings. The drama therapist helps the patient examine patterns of behavior through these role-plays and in doing so assists the patient in understanding their origins. Experimentation with new, more satisfying behavior is encouraged by a supportive group. Props, costumes, mime, and scripts may all be used to enhance the role-playing process.

Occupational therapy

In psychiatry, occupational therapy[13] is the use of goal-oriented, purposeful activity to maximize independence, prevent disability, and maintain health with individuals who are limited by psychosocial dysfunction. The emphasis is on health and on helping the patient attain skills necessary to function adequately and appropriately in the community after discharge from the hospital. Specific occupational therapy services include:

1. teaching daily living skills, such as grooming, food preparation, budgeting, transportation, and apartment living;
2. teaching prevocational skills, such as following instructions, relating to authority, developing memory and attention span, and interacting with a work group;
3. teaching social and communication skills, such as directness in communication, eye contact, nonverbal behavior, initiating and carrying on conversation, and social empathy;

4. developing perceptual motor skills, such as laterality, spatial discrimination, depth perception, figure-ground discrimination, and eye-hand coordination.

The occupational therapist may lead groups concerned with communication skills, prevocational training, activities of daily living, community outings, or discharge planning. These are generally taught in a setting which simulates a real situation outside the hospital as closely as possible. For example, in a communication skills group for low-level patients who have difficulty interacting with others, the occupational therapist may lead an exercise in which each patient practices eye contact and gestures while telling the group a brief story about a trip he took. The leader and group review the objectives of the session and give positive feedback to the patient. Patients are expected to practice these skills outside the group and may even be given "homework" between sessions. Crafts, such as ceramics, leatherwork, and sewing, are taught not as diversional activities but as pleasurable experiences which involve objectives relating to cognitive, socio-leisure, or skills improvement.

Recreation Therapy

Play, leisure, and recreation are vital elements in normal growth and development, in social and family relationships, and in promoting the overall quality of life. Recreation therapists facilitate the development, maintenance, and expression of appropriate leisure lifestyle for individuals with psychiatric, physical, or social limitations.

Play for children is critical to the development of adult behaviors. In play, children learn to deal with rules, symbols, and competitive and cooperative relationships. They learn how to take risks and explore their environment in ways which eventually lead to complex social interaction and role assumption. Just as the environment needs to be conducive for children to play by providing interesting objects, people, and events, the environment for adults should offer stimulating recreational sports, games, dance, and social happenings. Sports allow patients to experience and resolve issues of competition and collaboration while learning appropriate role behaviors. Furthermore, recreational activities generate feelings of communality and common purpose, which are distinct values in overcoming the alienation and aloneness experienced by many patients suffering from mental illness. Active physical exercise and sports are frequently recommended for the anxious young adult or the compulsive, driven executive, both of whom need outlets for psychomotor tension and constructive means for relaxation. Usually physical exercise is coupled with stress management education as well as leisure planning and community outings to assist the patient in learning more adaptive patterns of behavior.

Recreation therapy goals include:

1. patient identification and development of socio-leisure interests and skills;
2. amelioration of patient pathology and existing disability;
3. patient understanding of the significance of leisure and balance with work;
4. patient awareness of and participation in community leisure resources;
5. reduction of isolation, loneliness, and boredom of hospital by provision of pleasurable social/recreational activities.

Recreation therapists are skilled in leading and understanding the theory and value of games, sports, and community events; hence, groups they lead may include leisure counseling, leisure planning, relaxation training, and stress management, as well as swimming, weight training, and various sports.

Vocational Planning/Work Therapy

Vocational development is a lifelong process involving choices at various stages of life. These choices involve the interplay of individual determinants, such as abilities, interests, and aptitudes, and environmental demands.[14] Work behavior or work habits evolve from a long developmental process. At any point along the vocational developmental continuum, growth may be interrupted, delayed, or misdirected. Individuals in need of further development in the areas of career decision-making skills and development of optimal work behavior can be assisted through vocational and/or work counseling, guidance, and planning, as well as thorough experiential learning opportunities provided in work therapy. Vocational counseling and work therapy programs are developed for each patient according to his/her individual needs. These programs relate to and reflect real-life situations in order to adequately prepare each individual for reentry into the worker role.

Both mental health staff and patients view the capacity to work as a sign of getting well and an indication of readiness for discharge. Work in the hospital may range from simple prevocational chores such as stapling or collating to regular, supervised work in the kitchen, library, or grounds. Simple work modules including regular household chores and clerical tasks may be implemented within unit-based activity programs. Community volunteerism can be used as a final step in trying out work skills and behaviors.

Associated work support groups may assist the patient in job interviewing, resumé writing, or newspaper ad scanning.

Federal regulations stipulate that patients may work not more than one hour per day, five days per week, for a total of 90 days in a work therapy setting. These regulations were designed to prevent psychiatric hospitals from exploiting unpaid patient labor, a condition that was known to exist in state hospitals. Such regulations seriously hinder the hospital in fully using the treatment potential of work therapy. Some hospitals have circumvented the problem by paying patients for work on a subminimal scale, a legitimate practice if substandard work performance can be demonstrated. In such cases, the hospital must be granted an exception to federal regulations by the Labor Department. Within the last few years, the short-term nature of most hospital treatment, as well as the increased administrative load necessitated by work payments, have all but eliminated extensive work therapy programs.

Vocational testing and counseling are available in some hospitals or from state divisions of vocational rehabilitation to assist the patient in assessing his vocational interests and skills and to support his attempts to locate a job after discharge. Emphasis is placed on developing the patient's ability to find and secure the job himself/herself; job finding is not the vocational counselor's role.

Vocational planning and work therapy goals include:

1. developing and maintaining basic work habits (punctuality, attendance) and basic work skills (interpersonal, supervision, following direction);
2. developing a sense of accomplishment, risk-taking behavior, self-esteem, self-confidence, and acceptance of constructive criticism;
3. examining underlying reasons for problems, such as poor attendance, lateness, an inability to attend to a given task, lack of personal motivation, poor sense of responsibility, and/or lack of self-discipline, and emphasizing both internal and external ways to motivate oneself;
4. exploring alternative social responses to such problems as lack of social assertiveness, minimal interaction with supervisor and co-workers, and a lack of awareness of others' needs and feelings;
5. developing productivity and an interest in work activity;
6. assisting the patient in identifying where work adjustment difficulties lie and encouraging the patient to modify unacceptable behavior;
7. developing and maintaining work behaviors appropriate for gainful employment and volunteer work;

8. developing more positive work attitudes (for example, regard for supervision, realistic expectations);
9. expressing interests and recognizing abilities resulting in a realistic overview of own skills and work behaviors;
10. assessing, counseling, and referring for vocational programs, job placement, training, volunteer work, school.

The following case studies demonstrate the usefulness of activity therapy services in treating a hospitalized borderline patient and a chronic schizophrenic patient.

Case Study II: Long-Term Treatment of a Borderline Personality

Ms. B., a young, separated female with two children, was admitted to a long-term unit for comprehensive care after an unsuccessful hospitalization in a short-term unit and a near fatal suicide. She had made many suicidal gestures in high school, particularly following rejections from men, which left her feeling unimportant and despairing.

Ms. B. had married after her third year in college, but her marriage was stormy and marked by angry outbursts toward her husband. Her husband left her during her second pregnancy, after which she became unable to function on her own or care for her children. She focused solely on others' expectations and could not describe her own experiences, a problem which was seemingly related to her fragmentation and chaotic internal state. Although she did not appear psychotic, her sense of self and differentiation were tenuous, and her relationships were filled with confusion, frustration, and disappointment. Her desperate lack of feeling needed or valued by anyone ended in suicidal gestures and attempts. She was diagnosed borderline personality. She was referred to activity therapy, social work, and psychological testing. She received individual psychotherapy three times per week. No psychotropic medication was ordered.

The activity therapy assessment revealed the following information: Ms. B. had difficulty in providing the appropriate degree of structure in her life, perhaps due to the level of internal disorganization. She did not have sufficient energy and insight available to control or even to recognize her own feelings. She lacked independent living skills, particularly in money management and apartment living. Although her cognitive and physical skills appeared intact, she lacked clarity regarding her own values and demonstrated trouble in organizing and communicating her thoughts and feelings. Socially, she seemed guarded with passive-aggressive trends. Ms. B. did not finish college and had a sporadic work history, although she held a job as a coach with the department of recreation. She stated her goals for hospitalization were to gain self-esteem, assertiveness, and daily living skills, and to become a more productive person.

The above problems were restated in objectives with the following recommendations: dance therapy to address awareness and organization of feelings and thoughts; daily living skills to address money management and apartment living; values clarification to address individuation; work therapy to assist in understanding and complying with work constraints; and patient government to deal with issues of responsibility and communication skills.

During the initial dance therapy session, Ms. B. expressed anger repeatedly by refusing to attend on certain days until hall staff met her sign-out demands. Issues of powerlessness and the need to control gradually diminished as Ms. B. continued to be accepted as a group member despite her defenses of displacement and projection.

Ms. B. began a values clarification group with apprehension, yet curiosity. She was not able to identify any positive features in herself, and she discovered major discrepancies between her values and her practices. She found identification of values difficult because she perceived this learning would lead to the demand that she assume adult responsibility.

Attendance at money management sessions was typified by her ability to understand concepts easily; yet she was filled with ambivalence regarding any information or expectation that might lead to independence. Given extensive support and structure, she did manage to set up a monthly budget designed along potential post-discharge needs. As she participated in apartment living counseling sessions, her anxiety regarding pending separation from the hospital and resentment toward her husband surfaced. She eventually arranged for transitional housing, although she continually denied need for support systems and showed difficulty in self-structuring in leisure and work.

Toward the end of her first year of hospitalization, Ms. B. began work therapy in the hospital school, toward which she felt extreme anxiety, given her high expectations and ambivalence about independence and responsibility assumed in the work role. Her anxiety gradually decreased as she was allowed to be dependent on her supervisor for direction and support. Her performance remained high, and her attendance was regular.

Her psychotherapist noted, "One-to-one supervision is necessary to accomplish even the most basic tasks; otherwise, the patient becomes extremely ambivalent, oppositional, and disorganized in her ability to concentrate on the task at hand. A significant change is her capacity and willingness to work with someone else on those tasks which are so frightening to her; they ultimately mean more than the loss of a dependent stance which she needs to overcome if she is to gain something useful."

In contrast to her difficulty in approaching personal feelings and issues, Ms. B. assumed the chairmanship of the Patient Activities Committee (patient government) which she handled with diplomacy and clear, careful thinking. In this role, she slowly integrated her many areas of growth — assumption of work responsibility for planning patient-run activities, dealing directly and effectively with others, and revealing feelings openly without resorting regularly to angry or controlling responses.

After 18 months of hospitalization, Ms. B. was discharged to a transitional home for women and a part-time job. She was able to regularly visit her children and proceed through a difficult divorce. One year later, she continues to see her psychotherapist once per week and her vocational counselor as needed.

Case Study III: Long-Term Treatment of a Chronic Schizophrenic

Mr. C., a white male, had been admitted to psychiatric hospitals many times. He was single and unemployed. Diagnosed chronic undifferentiated schizophrenia, he usually appeared disheveled, bewildered, and severely disorganized. He admitted to vague paranoid delusions and auditory hallucinations. Insight and judgment were poor.

He had a history of slow, gradual improvement during each hospitalization which was followed by day treatment and living in a halfway house. During each of several short-term hospitalizations, he was cautiously prepared for discharge, and although he had difficulty in separating from the hospital, he was cooperative and agreeable. Attendance at day care centers was erratic, since he could not mobilize himself to get out of bed in the morning. Mr. C.'s ability to take his medication was limited.

Community readjustment was marred by stresses upon Mr. C. which ended in symptoms and disorganization, leading to police involvement, minor arrest charges, and then rehospitalization. For example, during the Christmas holidays preceding the hospitalization in question, Mr. C. made plans to return to his hometown in a distant state. He missed one bus and took a late bus which got him into his home city in the middle of the night. Since he did not notify family members of his change in arrival time, they were concerned about his whereabouts. After staying in the bus station all night, he wandered around town the next day while trying to figure out how to contact his relatives. Finally, they were located and he spent several days with them; then he returned to his halfway house only to find his therapist on vacation and unavailable for support. With a growing sense of apprehension, he pulled a fire alarm and waited at the alarm until the fire engines came. He was picked up, charged, taken to jail, and then referred to the hospital under court order.

Mr. C. was admitted to a short-term unit in a private psychiatric hospital. The activity therapy initial summary indicated the same grossly psychotic thinking and behaviors described above as well as significant deficits in task, communication, self-image, leisure, and independent living skills. During a task evaluation, he was unable to follow any of four verbal directions; however, his end product approximated the correct form, suggesting that he was able to understand the general concepts but unable to remember specific details. A fine motor tremor was noted. Leisure interests were chronically limited, his only activity having been bowling, which was undertaken in the structured program of the hospital. He stated he valued friends but had not been able to develop and maintain friendships due to his ongoing illness. His self-esteem was impaired, and he lacked the confidence and skills to explore new activities. Concerning independent living skills, the patient was unable to live independently and needed significant help to carry out and maintain self-care. Disorganization and poor self-control interfered with his ability to learn as well as maintain a simple budget.

Mr. C. remained on the short-term unit for several weeks until he was transferred to a long-term unit. He began work therapy in the print shop, where he successfully handled simple tasks. In individual money management sessions, he learned simple procedures for monitoring and spending his money. During the next few months, he gradually increased his involvement in structured activities, such as bowling and the prevocational work group. He felt afraid to venture far from his hall due to his fear of the unfamiliar and his difficulty in asking others for assistance and clarification.

After six months of hospitalization on the long-term unit, Mr. C. was transferred to a token economy unit designed especially for chronic schizophrenic patients. The problem list included tremors, incoherence and paranoid delusions under stress, withdrawal, inconsistent hygiene, moodiness, and poor social judgment.

The activity therapy program involved physical exercise, prevocational work, individual perceptual motor training, meal planning and cooking, and a community outing once per week. Attendance at the activities was rewarded with tokens. The activity therapy program was part of a highly structured milieu in which expectations were made very clear and positive feedback was given regularly. After six months on the token economy unit, Mr. C. was discharged to a halfway house and a transitional day program, where he has remained for four months.

We do not expect that this patient will ever be "cured" of his illness or that he will be able to live independently. However, with sufficient structure, medication, and appropriate support systems in the community, he may be able to remain out of the hospital for years at a time, or, if he does need to return to the hospital, perhaps the episode can be handled on a short-term basis.

FUTURE TRENDS

Knowledge Base

Activity therapy disciplines need to generate research data to support the value and effectiveness of activity in psychiatry. Outcome studies which delineate how activity promotes functional improvements in psychiatric populations are needed. Occupational therapists must then offer new, clear definitions of practice and provide continuing education in this vein. The gap between basic research and valid implementation is large and may typically involve premature application of studies which have not been replicated or cannot be generalized.

Hemphill[15] has stressed the need for standardized evaluation methodology in psychiatric occupational therapy. Serious discrepancies exist between what is taught in the universities and the clinics. Standardized interview formats are currently being formulated in relation to occupational behavior theory, and these should be available by the late 1980s.

Managers of activity therapy departments can encourage these development efforts by supporting a system in which research is facilitated—one which emphasizes documentation standards, evaluation processes, reporting methods, quality assurance, chart audits, integration of information from credentialing bodies, and productivity standards.[16]

Economic Issues and Trends

Cost containment has become a serious issue, one which is affecting private and public hospitals alike as soaring health care costs have been brought under regulatory control by federal prospective payment systems and insurance companies. These agencies and consumers alike have assumed control in asking, "What do I get for my buck?" or "How do I know this treatment is effective?"

As national health care conglomerates assume control of increasing numbers of psychiatric facilities, local activity therapists will no longer be able to continue their historical autonomy in defining treatment practices and length of stay. Cost-effective outcomes utilizing the lowest priced treatment will eventually replace ambiguously defined and higher priced services. In the past, insurance carriers have been fairly liberal in payment policies. Today they employ increasing scrutiny in determining length of stay and defining active treatment.

Cost containment issues will play a vital role in manpower supply and demand for various levels of staff—professionals, assistants, and aides; it behooves the departmental manager to think prospectively and creatively in adapting to environmental constraints. Cost containment will also affect treatment scheduling, inasmuch as short-term hospitalization brings various professionals into competition for the patient during the day. Evening and weekend activity scheduling may be both clinically and administratively indicated.

Population Trends

The proportion of the elderly has steadily grown since 1900, and it is estimated that by the year 2030 there will be more than 30 million persons over age 65.[17] Occupational therapists and members of other activity therapy disciplines will need specialized training to provide effective treatment for increasing numbers of the psychiatrically impaired elderly. Emphasis on this population will increase the use of home health care and psychiatric consultations in nursing homes. Helping the aged to understand their adaptive capacities in executing activities of daily living is an ideal function for occupational therapy.

The deinstitutionalization movement will continue to extend the range of service delivery systems for chronic patients. The decline in state mental hospitals has been offset by an increase in outpatient programs in both private and public settings. Community facilities include day treatment centers, halfway houses, group homes, and foster homes. Patients have a difficult time consolidating behaviors learned during short hospitalizations when outpatient programs are not available for transfer and generalization. In addition, some hospitals are debating whether hospitalization should be used to reduce symptoms and acute signs of illness or whether it should be used to develop community survival skills. Activity therapy disciplines are well qualified to treat chronic patients, since these professions are skilled in teaching concrete community living skills and can adapt activities to meet the individual needs of patients.

REFERENCES

1. Slagle EC: Training aids for mental patients. Arch Occup Ther 1922; 1:11–17
2. Dunton WR: Prescribing Occupational Therapy. Springfield, IL, Charles C Thomas, 1928
3. Dunton WR: Occupational therapy, in Barr's Modern Medical Therapy in General Practice, 1. Edited by Barr DP, Baltimore, Williams & Wilkins, 1940
4. Dunton WR: Reconstruction Therapy. Philadelphia, W.B. Saunders, 1919
5. Group for Advancement of Psychiatry Report No 72: Crisis in psychiatric hospitalization. Vol 7, 1969

6. Mosey A: Three Frames of Reference for Mental Health. Thorofare, New Jersey, Charles B Slack, 1982
7. Fidler G, Fidler J: Doing and becoming: purposeful action and self-actualization. Am J Occup Ther 1978; 32:305-310
8. Barris R, Kielhofner G, Watts J: Psychosocial Occupational Therapy, 2nd ed. Baltimore, Waverly Press, 1983
9. Yalom I: Inpatient Group Psychotherapy. New York, Basic Books, 1983
10. Gould E, Glick I: Patient-staff judgments of treatment program helpfulness on a psychiatric ward. Br J Med Psychol 1976; 49:23-33
11. May P: When, what, and why? Psychopharmacology and other treatments in schizophrenia. Compr Psychiatry 1976; 17:683-693
12. Karasu TB: The Psychosocial Therapies, Part II. Washington, American Psychiatric Association, 1984
13. Reed R, Sanderson S: Concepts in Occupational Therapy, 2nd ed. Baltimore, Waverly Press, 1983
14. Activity Therapy Program Description. Sheppard and Enoch Pratt Hospital, Towson, MD, 1986
15. Hemphill BJ: Mental health evaluations used in occupational therapy. Am J Occup Ther 1980; 35:721-726
16. Scott AH: Occupational therapy: The profession as a system. Mental Health SCOPE: Strategies, Concepts, and Opportunities for Program Development and Evaluation. Rockville, MD, American Occupational Therapy Association, 1986
17. Fine S: Trends in mental health. Mental Health SCOPE: Strategies, Concepts, and Opportunities for Program Development and Evaluations. Rockville, MD, American Occupational Therapy Association, 1986

13
The Role of the Psychiatric Nurse

Ann Marie T. Brooks

HISTORY

The history of psychiatric nursing has been marked by its consistent contributions to patient care. The establishment of psychiatric nursing as a specialty came about in the 1880s with the founding of a school at McLean Hospital in Boston.[1] This program prepared nurses to care for the mentally ill. The establishment of a specific psychiatric nursing curriculum was seen as the first step in setting forth the professional role of the psychiatric nurse. The first graduate psychiatric nurse in the United States, Linda Richards, served as a spokeswoman for the specialty[2] and was active in creating schools of nursing in state hospitals.

Primary responsibilities of the psychiatric nurse for the next 50 years included such tasks as administering sedative drugs (whiskey, chloroform, and paraldehyde) and preparing patients for hydrotherapeutic measures (hot and cold douches, showers, and continuous baths). The evolution from a custodial to a therapeutic role was slow. Active involvement in psychodynamic interventions was not considered a part of the nurse's role. Development and use of such somatic treatments as insulin therapy, cold wet sheet pack, and electric shock therapy in the 1930s aided role development because nurses needed specific professional training to carry out these activities. Observing and reporting to the physician the reactions of the patient were the essential responsibilities of the nurse. The nurse was viewed primarily as a caretaker and was expected to undertake only those interventions ordered or sanctioned by the physician. Since care was viewed as a long-term process, the nurse served as an important link in the continuity of treatment and as an assistant to the physician. There was little expectation of involvement by patient or family in planning the direction of care. The psychiatric nurse was expected to assist the patient and family in assimilating the symptoms of illness and exhibiting patience and understanding in coping with the requirements of treatment.

During this time nurses began to recognize that different psychiatric nursing interventions were needed if they were to expand and enhance the practice of this specialty within the discipline of nursing. Through its funding of psychiatric nursing education, the National Mental Health Act of 1946[3] directly contributed to the development of psychiatric nursing as a specialty. Support from this legislation resulted in the establishment of graduate programs in psychiatric nursing. These programs produced nurse graduates who entered direct practice, as well as qualified teachers of psychiatric nursing. Funding earmarked for the integration of mental health concepts also influenced nursing practice, as qualified nurses were hired to teach in a nursing program.

An important change in nursing came about with a shift to seeing each patient as an individual. In the '50s, illness was seen as generic and labeling was common. Thus, a nurse was ordered to minister to a "schizophrenic" or a "depressive" rather than to a patient with schizophrenia or depression who required a specific and unique treatment plan. The publication in 1952 of Peplau's book, *Interpersonal Relations in Nursing*,[4] was a turning point. The author recognized nursing as a significant therapeutic process and pointed out that the establishment of a nurse-patient relationship was critical to the healing process. She provided a systematic framework for psychiatric nursing practice and stated that "the nurse is an active participant in all aspects of patient care." Peplau considered continual evaluation and refinement of the nurse-patient relationship to be a critical component of successful inpatient care. How patients responded to nursing interventions was identified as a key ingredient of effective delivery of nursing care.

Tudor[5] also stressed the skills and processes associated with patient care. For example, Tudor asserted that psychiatric nurses exerted their influence on patient care in three ways: facilitating the patient's communication; facilitating socialization; and fulfilling the patient's needs. These experts and others took part in a major effort to examine the interaction between patient and nurse and to identify essential skills; the nurse was no longer seen as a servant to the physician but rather as an autonomous clinician.

One approach utilized by nurses at the Menninger Clinic gained widespread acceptance in the 1950s. In this process, known as "attitude therapy,"[6] the nurse and all other staff utilized a variety of prescribed attitudes to assist inpatients in regaining mental health and learning adaptive patterns of behavior. These attitudes included: active friendliness, indulgence, passive friendliness, watchfulness, matter-of-factness, and kind firmness. These attitudes were usually agreed upon by the treatment team and the physician. A nurse, for example, would be instructed to interact with the patient in an actively friendly manner, following a basic principle of giving the patient attention before it is requested. The expectation was that the patient would learn to imitate the style of behavior and become more animated and interested in life. This "recipe" style of interaction fostered standardized types of nurse behaviors, in contrast to modern-day spontaneous behaviors between patients and staff.

During the 1960s, the concept of the therapeutic community gained acceptance. In addition, psychopharmacology became an important part of psychiatric practice, resulting in new responsibilities for nurses. More actively involved in the dispensing of medications with complex effects, nurses assumed added responsibilities in determining some aspects of the pharmacologic needs of patients. Thus, nurses were asked to make clinical judgments in dispensing medications, teaching patients about them, and monitoring the effects. Medication also significantly influenced the discharge process and the role of the nurse in this process. With medications, patients were able to live outside the hospital; consequently, helping persons to return to society became a nursing agenda.

In the early 1960s, publication of *Toward Quality in Nursing*[7] and subsequent landmark mental health legislation provided funding initiatives for nursing education. The report recognized the contribution of nurses as primary caregivers and augmented funding for role development. Stipends and traineeships enabled many nurses to obtain baccalaureate and graduate degrees in psychiatric nursing. The first nurse to obtain a Doctorate of Nursing Science was in psychiatric nursing at Boston University; this accomplishment was seen as part of a movement toward doctoral education for nurses in clinical practice.

CONTEMPORARY PERSPECTIVE

Modern psychiatric nursing practice has been affected by societal changes. The women's movement in the 1960s and '70s brought about significant gains for women. Increased opportunities in education and in the workplace augmented career choices. Nursing, as a traditional female occupation, was viewed by feminists and others in society as providing inadequate opportunities for women; consequently, potential recruits were not encouraged to pursue nursing as a career. In the intervening years, career-oriented women have been drawn away from nursing to other professions and higher-paying jobs. At the same time nursing has shed the image of a weak, female occupation under the control of medicine.

The inability of the nursing profession to successfully resolve the entry-into-practice dilemma continues to adversely affect nursing practice. Since 1965,[8] when the first position paper by the American Nurses' Association proposed that baccalaureate nursing education become the recognized entry level for the professional nurse, the controversy over professional vs. technical has raged without successful resolution. At the present time, there are three educational routes to becoming a professional nurse: baccalaureate, associate degree, and diploma. The lack of agreed-upon, clear-cut levels of nursing education and uniform pathways for entry into practice has divided nurses within the profession and hampered educational development. Nevertheless, most professional nursing organizations have made public commitments to the baccalaureate level of preparation, and the American Nurses' Association, through state nurses' associations, has continued to struggle with implementation of its plan in a timely fashion.

In most psychiatric settings, whether private or public, nurses are selected on the basis more of their abilities and experience than of their educational preparation. It is the exception rather than the rule to find that psychiatric nurses are financially compensated for their educational preparation, clinical knowledge and skills rather than their years of nursing experience. However, the baccalaureate degree is still preferred by hospitals in employing nurses.

Recruitment and retention within nursing are major issues affecting practice.[9] While the acute shortage of nurses that occurred in the late 1970s and early '80s had seemed to subside, a decreased pool of applicants to nursing programs, lack of satisfaction with the nursing role, and an increased demand for nurses point to a continuing problem. Recruitment has suffered a dramatic decline in the past decade. While the difficulty can be simply attributed to decreased supply and increased demand, it is important to examine the factors contributing to this situation.

A major factor is the decrease in the number of individuals entering the profession. With numerous options now available to high school graduates, some of the bright and energetic women who traditionally would have chosen nursing as their profession have headed elsewhere. The stigma of mental illness and lack of understanding about the role of mental health professionals and specifically of psychiatric nurses have led to a basic negativity about becoming a psychiatric nurse. Apparently limited opportunities for the nurse within the psychiatric hospital are also a factor, especially since lack of exposure to inpatient settings prevents students from seeing the possibilities available to them. Rarely do nursing instructors encourage students to enter this specialty immediately following graduation. More commonly they advise new graduates to "get a year of medical-surgical experience under your belts" before entering psychiatric nursing. This in itself serves as a barrier for recruitment and retention. The appeal of "high tech" and the emphasis on quantifiable skills have added to recruiting difficulties, as well as decreased federal support for students at both the baccalaureate and graduate levels.

THE ROLE OF PSYCHIATRIC NURSING IN 1980s

As we have seen, over the past century the role of the nurse in psychiatric care delivery has evolved from passive participant to active team member. In 1976 the Division on Psychiatric and Mental Health Nursing of the American Nurses' Association formulated Standards of Practice for this specialty,[10] noting that "psychiatric nursing is a specialized area of nursing practice employing theories of human behavior as its scientific aspect and purposeful use of self as its art." This definition provides the overall framework for role implementation within psychiatric nursing practice. The standards require that the nurse possess a sound theoretical knowledge base, ability to use the nursing process, skill in effectively collaborating with other disciplines to plan and evaluate treatment, ability to establish a relationship with the patient, and skill in provision of independent nursing interventions. A major revision of these standards, published in 1982,[11] stresses incorporation of an expanded knowledge base in the role of the nurse in psychiatric care delivery. The standards differentiate between a generalist level of practice for the baccalaureate nurse graduate and a specialist level of psychiatric nursing practice for graduate level training. In 1985,[12] standards for child and adolescent psychiatric nursing were established and implemented. Publication of these subspecialty standards was considered a major breakthrough because it publicly recognized the important and distinctive contribution of psychiatric nurses in the treatment of children and adolescents.

The matter of standards has a direct bearing on inpatient management. Standards have shaped the education of nurses and affected both their degree of sophistication and their ability to handle complex diagnostic and therapeutic issues as they arise on the units. For instance, a standard emphasizing health education has a significant effect on the method used by nurses to carry out and document activities related to teaching patients about their illness. It may involve sitting down with the patient and family and reviewing the types of medications the patient will receive following discharge or convening a formal group to discuss a plan for compliance to a medication regimen.

Psychiatric nursing at the generalist level is carried out primarily in inpatient settings. Here the major variables affecting the role of the nurse are: types of patients, philosophy and mission of the facility, types of treatment programs, goals of active treatment, and staffing levels.

Basic activities for the nurse in an inpatient setting include:

1. Establishment of nurse/patient relationship;
2. Active participation in the therapeutic milieu;
3. Implementation of physicians' orders and ongoing collaboration and consultation with the physician/therapist regarding planned treatment;
4. Active psychiatric interventions in response to various behavioral patterns related to presenting illness;
5. Application of a problem-solving approach (nursing process) in carrying out nursing care in coordination with other nursing staff;
6. Provision of nursing care activities in response to medical problems and needs;
7. Distribution of medication, including education related to medications, their effects and implications for functioning;
8. Documentation of all relevant information related to provision of safe, effective nursing care;
9. Supervision and delegation of tasks to other levels of nursing personnel as necessary;
10. Participation in self-evaluation, peer review, and quality assurance activities;
11. Adherence to established nursing standards, practices, and procedures; and
12. Participation in discharge planning.

The professional nurse is responsible and accountable for the quality of nursing care delivery on the unit. She is recognized as a legally accountable agent who directly implements physicians' orders and monitors the implementation of active treatment on a 24-hour, seven-day-a-week basis. Other nursing personnel work with the professional nurse in supportive roles and report to her for supervision, monitoring, and assignment of their activities.

The nurse's independent, interdependent, and dependent functions demand open communication, coordination, and decision-making with all other health professionals involved in care. While the physician is accountable for the direction of active treatment, the nurse is responsible for carrying out the orders and coordination of treatment.

MILIEU MANAGEMENT

The nurse plays an important role in the therapeutic milieu (see Chapter 8). She uses various formal and informal activities to promote patient interactions and encourages patients to take advantage of all the learning opportunities available. The nurse is also expected to provide care, support, and feedback, and to implement specific interventions related to the treatment plan as part of the milieu process.

Maintaining a safe and clean environment for patients within the milieu is a challenging but necessary component of the nurse's role. The nurse may directly intervene with a patient or group of patients to maintain a calm, safe environment. At times, the nurse may need to decide to change the activities of the milieu because of presenting patient behaviors. Examples of such clinical decisions are restriction of patients to the unit, canceling an outing, and calling a special community meeting. Instituting a level of observation requiring additional patient monitoring is another technique commonly used by the nurse to ensure safety. These clinical judgments are made in collaboration with the physician/therapist.

Nurses participate in the milieu and assume various leadership roles in community or unit meetings. They may initiate or coordinate structured activities while monitoring the total environment. The head or charge nurse works in close collaboration with other staff to provide ongoing assessment and feedback to the physician and other treatment team members regarding the effectiveness of the therapeutic environment. Structured activities are often used by the nurse to facilitate a patient's entry into the hospital system and assumption of the patient role. These activities are creatively designed to meet the needs of the population being served. Activities within the milieu can also enhance the development of positive alliances and networks for effective communication among patients and staff. The nurse also contributes to the functioning of the milieu by evaluating whether the atmosphere, communication patterns, rules and policies of the milieu are effective and conducive to growth, as well as humanistic and supportive of active treatment.

The role of the nurse in the milieu is shaped both by the person's knowledge and skill and by the philosophy, type of treatment program, length of stay, and characteristics of the patient population. In a short-term treatment setting, it is critical that the nurse facilitate patients' quick and effective entry into the environment. The nurse plays a pivotal role in helping patients understand the rules and responsibilities. This initial orientation can set the tone for patients' constructive use of their hospital stays.

Treatment program responsibilities take up the majority of nurses' time. The complexity and variety of tasks and responsibilities require constant updating, effective time management, and consultation with others. Treating the medical and emotional needs of patients is more than merely handing out medications and monitoring participation in the milieu or adherence to program rules and regulations. In current psychiatric practice, the nurse must possess an in-depth knowledge of psychopharmacologic agents and be able to discuss with patients their medications, intended results, and ways to evaluate effects. The nurse needs to be familiar with the normal dose range of various drugs to work effectively with the physician and other members of the treatment team in documenting and monitoring therapeutic effectiveness. Also, patients who have been on long-standing medication regimens can become skeptical if changes are made without adequate communication or justification for the need for this action.

Refusal of medication by a patient can become a major nursing problem, slowing recovery and indicating that the patient may stop medication upon discharge. Since such noncompliance is a major determinant in readmission, the nurse must not only teach patients about medication regimens but also evaluate their grasp of this knowledge prior to leaving the hospital. The actual time devoted to distribution of medication may be brief, but the process and the setting in which it takes place are important. The nurse should give out medication in an environment which promotes independence, knowledge, and understanding of the medication regimen and allows time and opportunity for questions and communication of concerns. In many settings, medications are distributed before or after community meetings or other scheduled activities. This helps to ensure the availability of patients. Unfortunately, the nurse is often hurried because of the number of patients and other competing activities and consequently is not able to converse with patients about medication issues.

During hospitalization, patients may discuss their medications with other patients and staff. These interactions can influence their cooperation with their medication regimen either positively or negatively. It is important that common concerns and myths regarding the expected and side effects of medications be addressed in an ongoing, open fashion in order to promote understanding and respect for this necessary component of active psychiatric treatment.

Responding to complex medical and psychiatric problems is part of the nurse's role. Changes in reimbursement systems and insurance coverage have resulted in admission or transfer of patients with medically unstable conditions to settings neither staffed nor equipped to routinely handle such cases. While backup with an acute care facility is a standard, psychiatric patients are usually not welcome in acute care settings because of staff attitudes. As a result, a patient recovering from a self-inflicted gunshot wound or a broken leg sustained from jumping out a window may be transferred when barely stabilized. An eating disorder patient who is diabetic or a substance abuse patient with multiple sclerosis needs aggressive monitoring and evaluation of care on a 24-hour, seven-day-a-week basis, increasing demands on nursing staff.

The physical environment of a facility plays an important role in psychiatric treatment, since it is a catalyst for the therapeutic process and affects nurses' ability to deliver safe and effective care.[13] The overall quality of day-to-day living and working in a psychiatric environment is dependent on an atmosphere which is both conducive to socialization and responsive to presenting patient needs. Expectations for use of the physical environment may differ in various types of inpatient settings (public, private, acute care hospitals), but the identified overall goal should be to provide adequate space to fit program and population needs. Combining various types of patient populations for the sake of program flexibility and financial viability can pose particular challenges because of differences in maturational levels and physical capabilities.

Physical layout should allow staff to safely monitor patient interactions and activities. Barrier-free design facilitates observation of patients. While cleanliness is a basic assumption, other factors can either promote or interfere with program objectives. For instance, if an adolescent unit contains furniture that is damaged or uncomfortable and does not fit the population or promote a comfortable, home-like atmosphere, patients may deliberately destroy the interior furnishings to release excess energy and aggression. In new facilities more attention is being devoted to planning for patient movement and access. At the Menninger Clinic in Topeka, a newly built hospital has patient units with an exercise room adjacent to the living area. This allows patients ample access to recreational activities involving physical release of energy while still in close proximity to the staff.

Seclusion rooms and locked doors are still routinely used in psychiatric hospitals. Even though state and federal legislation requires use of least restrictive measures, the need to contain patients for their own safety and the safety of others persists. The nurse plays a pivotal role in using the physical environment and restrictive measures in preventing patient self-harm or harm to others. Newer facilities or those recently renovated have more normal-appearing seclusion rooms; although these are still resistant to damage they communicate expectations different from those of the traditional, incarceration-like room.

It is common to find a combination of open and closed units within any operating facility. It is unusual to find large psychiatric facilities that are totally unlocked and permit patients free access to other areas of the hospital and the outside. The trend in smaller, newly opened psychiatric facilities is toward an open system model.

Within the structure of the milieu setting, various professionals are expected to work together collaboratively. Disciplines such as psychiatry, psychology, social work, and activity therapy are expected to come together with nursing to provide active treatment. Because of the intensity and ongoing provision of services by nurses, other professionals, most often psychiatrists, are somewhat dependent upon nurses to provide information necessary for planning and monitoring of treatment. For example, the physician may rely on the nurse and other nursing team members for specific information related to patient functioning during the 24-hour cycle, including reaction to treatments and medications, interactions with patients and staff, and sleeping patterns. Effective role functioning for each discipline requires strong communication networks and collaboration based on mutual understanding, respect, and commitment to common treatment approaches and modalities. Part of the nurse's role is to demonstrate and teach the physician and other caregivers what nurses do that makes a difference to patient treatment and outcomes. It is also important for other disciplines to share their unique contributions as part of ongoing team-building and enrichment of patient care.

Disagreements about specific treatment interventions or overall care are not necessarily a sign of poor team functioning. Because of the diversity of educational preparation and experiences within the cadre of professionals providing care, it is unrealistic to believe that consensus is an automatic outcome of a team assignment. However, when disagreements in approach result in serious communication breakdown and affect patient care through splitting of staff on goal-setting and inconsistent approaches in care delivery, it is necessary for the team members to address these problems directly. If the problems emanate from disagreements surrounding treatment orientations, the leadership (physician, nurse, and appropriate others) may need to step in to assist the staff in successful problem resolution.

Practice models for physician staffing also affect the role of the nurse and functioning of other treatment team members. In a closed model, the availability of the physician is greatly enhanced. The physician has time to interact with patients and staff and is considered a member of the team. The communication between the physician and staff is strong and patient-focused. On the other hand, with an open staff model, establishing coordination of care and communication may be difficult. A great deal of energy on the part of the physician and staff is needed to assess, plan and evaluate treatment, but the physician with privileges at several hospitals and a large private practice has time for only limited communication with the inpatient staff. If the primary communication method is the medical record, the richness of interaction between direct care providers and physician is lost.

Traditionally, nursing staff are involved in many inpatient therapeutic interventions that occur in the absence of physicians. Leadership of various groups, handling medical and psychiatric emergencies, communicating with families, and ongoing coordination of care fall to the nurse. In addition, the nurse serves as a bridge for communication between patient and physician and can be called on to interpret a treatment team decision or a change in medication to the patient and family. For example, the nurse may be left to explain to the family why a weekend pass was canceled by the physician. Although not personally involved in the decision-making process, she is expected to communicate to the family empathy and understanding, as well as the rationale for the decision.

The nurse is most often responsible for handling psychiatric emergencies. Violence and assaultive behavior have received more attention as the number of assaults toward staff has increased. Nevertheless, many incidents are not reported. According to Lion and Reid,[14] this underreporting is due to staff's belief that assault is related to performance failure, acceptance by staff of assault as part of the role, and the avoidance of tedious form completion and reporting. In addition, nursing staff have not felt supported by the recapitulation and review that follow an incident. The physician, other nursing staff, and other members of the treatment team often criticize the process and outcome.

A major problem for nursing staff working with potentially assaultive patients is that these patients still require treatment during the acute or prolonged period of unpredictability. Options for treatment may be limited, and the lack of alternatives is at times both frustrating and demoralizing for nurses and other staff. Restrictive measures, such as leather restraints, may adequately limit patient movement for a specific period of time, but are only seen as temporary measures and do not necessarily promote effective communication. If a severe assault on staff occurs, there may be a general tendency to maintain the patient in restraints or seclusion until the staff feel very secure that this behavior has subsided. Clear expectations about the limits of behavior and the consequences for breaking limits contribute to an atmosphere of security for both patients and staff. In recent years, psychiatric nurses have begun to take a leadership role in addressing these problems and are attempting to document through research the effect of patient assault on nursing staff.

CLINICAL ROLE OF THE NURSE

The basic aim of the nursing process is to regard the patient as a partner in the process of treatment rather than as a recipient of a plan or solution. The steps within this process include: assessment, planning, implementation, and evaluation. Continual modification and enrichment of nursing care are aided by the activities within this process.

Assessment is designed to provide an opportunity to carefully evaluate the patient in a holistic manner.[15] A usual part of this process is the completion of a formal nursing assessment within the first 24–48 hours of hospitalization. This step involves examination of the patient's physical and emotional needs based on presenting patient data. Social and cultural background and other important information pertinent to patient care are sought by the nurse as baseline data to guide initial treatment planning and to provide a safe environment. Subjective data, obtained by inquiry into patient's perceptions of the immediate presenting problems and goals for hospitalization, are an important part of the assessment. Sample questions can range from "Have you thought about harming yourself?" to "What are your usual patterns of sleep?" Special nursing needs based on presenting medical and/or psychiatric conditions are also identified.

As with all psychiatric patients, the suicide potential of the patient must be assessed. Past history and usual coping strategies are useful but do not provide a complete clinical picture. The questions that are asked by the nurse are direct, and this information is then used by the physician in collaboration with other experts to make decisions about the type of monitoring needed. All information gathered by the nurse and nursing staff as part of the assessment process serves to strengthen the understanding of behavioral needs. It also gives the nurse indications regarding the patient's perception of his/her situational resources, which can then be used as part of treatment. Assessment is continuous throughout the patient's course of hospitalization, as new data are used to refine and update treatment planning.

Planning, the second step, involves the formulation of a well-organized action plan linking the data gathered by the various disciplines. The plan pulls together basic diagnostic assessments in an effort to support or refine the admitting diagnosis and to identify specific treatment interventions and expected outcomes. This phase allows the nurse to discuss how nursing can provide consistent support for identified treatment team goals during the entire 24-hour period. The nurse contributes to the formulation of the diagnosis in several ways. Her identification and description of patient behaviors provide a data base for comparison, while the description of the quality and quantity of patient interactions assists the physician and other treatment team members in viewing the patient from a variety of perspectives. It is important for the nurse to understand psychopathology and the various schools of psychotherapy used in current practice, but it is more critical that the nurse and physician agree about the philosophy of treatment and the interventions necessary to bring about effective change.

In some hospitals, the department of nursing may choose to develop a specific nursing care plan based on extrapolation of information from the overall treatment plan. This provides more specific identification of presenting nursing needs and more precise direction for nursing personnel. For example, in the case of an acutely suicidal patient, the needs of the patient necessitate continual revision of nursing interventions.

The third phase, *implementation* of planned treatment interventions, includes several substantial tasks for the nurse. Some of these interventions depend on the development of the nurse-patient relationship, the milieu, and other structured activities. A major portion of the implementation phase is carrying out nursing tasks related to physician orders. In doing so, the nurse is responsible for the administration and supervision of ordered treatment, which may include medications, basic monitoring of vital signs, and ongoing assessment and monitoring of the psychological status of patients. Included in medication distribution is the documentation of the patient's reaction to scheduled as well as unscheduled medications.

In the process of carrying out identified treatment and nursing plans, the nurse carefully documents in the medical record: any change in behavioral patterns; physical status; the quality of interactions of the patient with staff, other patients, and significant others; and any unusual occurrence. The nurse is also responsible for assisting the patient in understanding the treatment being carried out and helping the patient communicate concerns and issues related to the plan.

Evaluation, the fourth component, is concerned with the effect of active treatment on the patient's progress toward identified goals. It demands a careful and thoughtful review of the effectiveness of planned nursing and treatment interventions and provides the nurse with feedback regarding which problems have been resolved and which need to be reevaluated.

The following case example illustrates the application of these phases.

> Katherine, a 67-year-old widow with a diagnosis of major depression, was transferred to a psychiatric hospital after a three-day stay in the intensive care unit of a local community hospital following a lethal dose of barbiturates. She had been diagnosed with lung cancer a year previous and had undergone two lengthy courses of chemotherapy. Two weeks prior to the suicide attempt, she had been told by her oncologist that the cancer was in remission.
>
> Fourteen months previously, Katherine's husband had died unexpectedly of a heart attack. He had been a successful business and community leader. They had been happily married for 45 years and had two children, a married daughter with two children living 60 miles away and a recently married son on the west coast.
>
> The information provided by the admitting physician described a well-dressed female appearing to be younger than her stated age, coherent, and a

good historian. According to the patient, the past year had been "holy hell," and she was "tired of coping." The overdose of prescribed sleeping pills was spontaneous, and she had not considered the effect of her actions. There was no previous psychiatric history, and she had come for treatment because her oncologist thought she needed to talk about the past year's events.

As part of the nursing assessment, the nurse learned that Katherine had been in good health throughout her life and the diagnosis of cancer had come as a complete surprise. She had gone to the doctor on her daughter's urging because of a persistent cough of two months' duration. Diagnostic tests including x-rays revealed lung cancer, and treatment was initiated immediately. At the time of her husband's sudden death, she and her husband had been planning a trip to Israel. For the past 20 years, she had served as the bookkeeper for her husband's profitable cleaning business. Both she and her husband were active in community projects and volunteer groups.

When asked about her eating habits, she revealed that she had not been eating well for the past year and had lost over 40 pounds. Part of this loss was due to the course of chemotherapy, but the basic reason was that her husband had done all of the cooking and food shopping during their marriage. He considered cooking his hobby and had entered several cooking contests. Katherine, on the other hand, loved puttering around the house and took care of all cleaning and maintenance work related to the house and yard.

Katherine stated that she had always perceived herself to be in good health and enjoyed playing tennis and swimming. She and her husband often walked two miles after dinner and she expressed some dismay that this had come to an abrupt halt after his death.

Her involvement in community and volunteer activities had been suspended during the past year. During her initial course of chemotherapy, she had withdrawn from groups; after that she made no effort to revive her former ties. She wondered if she had the energy to do it. She and her husband had been active members of the local church for many years. Since his death and her illness, she had not participated and expressed "feeling isolated and cut off." When asked about significant losses in her life, she identified that her mother, father, and most recently her husband had all died in an unexpected fashion. She seemed grateful that none of her loved ones had suffered before death but regretted that they had all died without any opportunity to bid farewell to her or other loved ones.

Planning for this patient based on presenting data focused on assisting her reintegration into society. Because of her diagnosis of cancer, she had disengaged herself from all activities; she seemed to welcome dying and joining her husband. However, the news of remission signaled a change in her belief that she was going to die and was the precipitating factor in her impulsive decision to overdose.

A major focus of the plan was to involve her in decision-making regarding the direction of her life. No longer could she be a passive participant in her life, because her remission had placed her in charge. It was necessary to identify activities that to use her strengths of communication, past experience, and willingness to take risks. At the same time, linking her up with past activities and support groups that she enjoyed would enable her to anchor and reintegrate herself in a deliberate and successful fashion.

A number of interventions suggested themselves on the basis of the case history and nursing assessment. First was the issue of safety; the patient was placed on special observation (see Chapter 8). Next was a concern about her ability to care for herself. Staff contracted with the patient to set up a schedule for participation on the ward. She was urged to become involved in her own hygiene and grooming. Because of her severe weight loss, a weight increase program was devised in conjunction with the dietician.

Nursing staff met with recreation therapy and suggested that the patient join a cooking group. This was dynamically important because her husband had previously been the family cook and subverted his wife's desires and abilities in these areas. Because the patient had been very active in church activities, nursing staff suggested a volunteer position with the chaplaincy service.

Antidepressants were prescribed, but nursing staff observed several episodes of orthostatic hypotension and conferred with the physician about dividing the dose. The primary nurse met with the patient and instructed her on how to deal with drug side effects. As the patient became more trusting and began to confide in her primary nurse and other staff, she was able to discuss her own fears and anxieties about her situation. As the psychotherapeutic alliance became stronger, the primary nurse worked closely with the therapist in implementing strategies to support the overall goals of treatment.

Nursing staff focused on strengthening independent functioning. The assigned nurse and other nursing staff worked with Katherine to coordinate her participation in cooking, values clarification, and widow groups. It soon became evident that Katherine was able to demonstrate initiative in planning for herself, as she started several of her own projects. Several family sessions were held by the therapist with Katherine's nurse and her daughter to discuss her progress and future plans following discharge.

Strong communication and support networks on the outside were established by Katherine as part of the discharge planning process. Outings with friends were used as a method to evaluate her level of comfort, acceptance, and ability to return to her environment. Specific aftercare plans included weekly therapist appointments, day treatment for three days a week for one month, antidepressant medication, and a volunteer job at the local library. The daughter also planned to see her mother regularly and to take a week's vacation with her in early summer.

Evaluation of Katherine's treatment is ongoing; at last report she had started her own cooking group for widows and widowers.

MODELS OF NURSING PRACTICE/STAFFING

The role that the nurse plays in a psychiatric institution significantly affects the determination of nurse staffing requirements. Such variables as patient level, intensity of treatment (length of stay), and type of treatment services are other factors to be considered.

An examination of organizational nursing models assists us in describing how nursing levels are calculated. Our intent is not to evaluate or endorse any of the three models but to show how the models affect evaluate staffing patterns used for delivery of psychiatric nursing services. Three basic models of nursing care delivery are primary, team, and functional. Each of the models calls for different numbers of R.N.'s and allocation of nursing resources, because the *direct care* nursing requirements depend on the planned involvement and coordination of activities by the professional nurse in response to identified needs. According to Hegyvary,[16] the essential elements needed to deliver direct nursing care include: accountability, autonomy, coordination, and comprehensiveness.

In a *primary* nursing model, the nursing role combines case manager functions with direct care functions. In this capacity, the primary nurse is responsible for coordinating all aspects of care on a 24-hour, seven-day-a-week basis. The role encourages a meaningful collaboration with the physician and other members of the treatment team by promoting ongoing, consistent, and effective monitoring of all patient activities. The central focus for the nurse is the establishment of a strong nurse-patient relationship, beginning with admission. While ideally the primary nurse carries out all activities, including the initial nursing assessment, this is sometimes not possible and does not seem to affect the overall quality of care delivery.

In a primary nursing model, the nurse usually carries several primary patients and may serve in an associate or other backup capacity for the others. The ongoing objective of this model is to assist patients in understanding their illnesses and in participating in activities relevant to identified goals of treatment. The nurse-patient relationship is based on consistent interactions with emphasis on reality orientation. In the 1970s, the nursing profession was active in promoting the establishment of primary nursing model systems in acute care hospitals. Psychiatric units within these hospitals implemented this organizational model, and the patients benefited from this trend. Large private psychiatric hospitals with adequate staffing levels have also implemented primary nursing models and have reported positive responses by both patients and staff.

The second model, *team* nursing, is essentially a plan which places the professional nurse in charge of nursing care for a selected group or number of patients. Other nurses and nursing personnel are assigned to assist with such care. In this model, the professional nurse is the individual responsible for care and for coordination of assignments of other team members. The chief benefits from this type of organization are the availability of supervision to other team members and the continuity of care to the patient.

In a *functional* nursing model patient care is divided into discrete tasks. Nurses and other personnel are assigned particular tasks, such as escorting patients, medication distribution, taking and recording vital signs, and distributing food trays. This method does not require ongoing communication among health professionals, nor does it promote development of accountability for nursing care.

Each of these methods require different levels of staffing. In the functional method the number of nurses needed is small because the major focus is on task rather than person. In the team method, more nurses are required because of the need to balance the ratio of professionals to paraprofessionals. The primary nursing model requires the largest number of professional nurses because of the level of accountability, autonomy, and authority assigned to the role.

The new era of cost containment in the 1980s has affected levels of nurse staffing, but it is still not clear what the impact will be on primary nursing implementation models. Debate over whether or not a reduction in the number of R.N.'s significantly affects the continuity of care is now underway in most circles, although the effects of reduction on treatment are still not well researched. Most experts acknowledge that patient feedback is positive and supportive of a primary nursing model, but qualitative and quantitative benefits have not yet been clearly demonstrated.

ADJUNCTIVE ROLES

Paraprofessionals are important in the delivery of psychiatric care. Persons in this role are usually directed by a registered nurse, because of the nurse's overall accountability for care. The majority of a paraprofessional's time is spent interacting with patients. These frequent and intense contacts between patients and nonprofessional staff contribute to the development of therapeutic alliances.

The role of the paraprofessional in the delivery of psychiatric nursing care is to provide monitoring, reality orientation, and ongoing feedback to patients about their behavior. Basic communication skills are required in carrying out this role because the tasks involve balancing a humanistic, caring approach with realistic maintenance of boundaries. It is not uncommon for patients to speak fondly of these nonprofessional staff members and to express gratitude for their involvement in the treatment process. Paraprofessionals need additional training, as well as clear direction and monitoring by professionals, so that they can maximize the effects of their contacts with patients and avoid either under- or overinvolvement with boundary-setting.

Because paraprofessionals are recruited from a variety of educational backgrounds, providing orientation and supervision is challenging. Nevertheless, the richness of their diverse backgrounds serves to enhance their representation of the realities of the outside world, to bring to the clinical setting a practical orientation, and to provide a balance of inputs to the nursing and treatment teams.

STAFF DEVELOPMENT

Training for professional nurses and other support nursing personnel is a prerequisite for delivery of quality care. Institutions approach orientation and staff development in different ways. Some hospitals have specific training programs within nursing staff, conducted by nurses at the graduate level, while other facilities have general staff development personnel, with nurses involved in programs specific to them.

For the new graduate nurse, the focus of orientation is on supplementing the educational foundation of psychiatric nursing. Nurses who come with either past psychiatric or other types of nursing experience are carefully evaluated to determine their learning needs, taking into account past experience and skill, roles, and type of program. Pretesting and other methods provide data for planning appropriate learning experiences.

Since most paraprofessionals have little or no formal patient care experience, a major focus of orientation is development of communication skills and documentation. Even those paraprofessionals with baccalaureate degrees in psychology or social work usually lack practical experience or exposure to inpatient psychiatric treatment and the entire active treatment process. It is imperative for the paraprofessional to be given opportunities to learn about psychopathology, presenting patient behaviors, and application of safe and effective interventions. At the same time, nursing administration must carefully balance this knowledge with realistic involvement and expectations for the paraprofessional within the team and unit functioning.

Documentation, crisis management, and familiarity with policies and procedures require continual update and review for all staff. Ongoing programs on aggression management, as well as emergency medical, fire, and safety training, are also part of basic education offerings, although those without previous psychiatric experience often do not appreciate the importance of aggression management during orientation.

ROLE STRESS

Provision of direct care in a psychiatric hospital is stressful. As part of a helping profession involved in close ongoing intense contacts with patients, psychiatric nurses are vulnerable to stress. According to Dawkins et al.[17] stress is costly to the individual, as well as the organization, and jeopardizes the ability of the individual to provide care and feel satisfied with life. While it may not be possible to eliminate all the factors producing stress for the psychiatric nurse, health care organizations, administrators, managers, and nurses themselves should work to devise methods to improve the quality of life within the psychiatric setting.

Regular staffing patterns and schedules, programs to ensure patient safety and limits on aggression, and work schedules that allow for adequate rest and time away from the job reduce stress for the nurse. Open lines of communication, support for decision-making at the level closest to the patient, and rewarding financial and benefit packages that demonstrate valuing of staff create an environment in which competent, humanistic and enthusiastic patient care delivery can occur.

FUTURE DIRECTIONS

Future psychiatric nurses will need to be flexible and take the lead in role development. In an era marked by a continuing dual emphasis on psychosocial and biologic treatments, nurses must stay abreast of current knowledge in both fields. Nurses must carefully examine current organizational systems, utilize technological advances and research findings, and design practice models which promote autonomy and professionalization of the role. The value of the psychiatric nurse in the inpatient setting will continue to increase if nurses are able to address the issues of accountability, recruitment and retention, stress and job satisfaction in a timely and productive manner.

REFERENCES

1. Leininger, M (Editor): Contemporary issues in mental health nursing. Boston, Little, Brown, 1973
2. Richards L: Reminiscences of America's First Trained Nurse, Boston, Whitcomb Barrows, 1915

3. Leininger M (Editor): Contemporary issues in mental health nursing. Boston, Little, Brown, 1973
4. Peplau H: Interpersonal Relations in Nursing. New York, Putnam's, 1952
5. Tudor GA: Sociopsychiatric nursing approach to intervention in a problem of mutual withdrawal on a mental hospital ward. Psychiatry 1952; 15
6. Weiss MO: Attitudes in Psychiatric Care. New York, Putnam's, 1954
7. U.S. Surgeon General's Consultant Group on Nursing: Toward quality in nursing. Washington, DC: US Public Health Service, 1963
8. American Nurses' Association Committee on Education: First position paper on education for nursing. Am J Nursing, 1965; 65:106
9. U.S. Department of Health and Human Services. Proceedings of Two Conferences on Future Directions, Rockville, Md. NIMH, 1986
10. American Nurses' Association, Division on Psychiatric and Mental Health Nursing Practice: Statement on psychiatric and mental health nursing practice, Kansas City, MO, 1976
11. American Nurses' Association, Division on Psychiatric and Mental Health Nursing Practice: Statement on psychiatric and mental health nursing practice, Kansas City, MO, 1982
12. American Nurses' Association, Division on Psychiatric and Mental Health Nursing Practice: Statement on child and adolescent nursing practice, Kansas City, MO, 1985
13. Remen S: Planning psychiatric hospitals—Human design considerations, Psychiatric Hospital, 1987; 18:11–16
14. Lion JR, Reid WH: Assaults Within Psychiatric Facilities. New York, Grune & Stratton, 1983
15. Yura H, Walsh M: The Nursing Process. New York, Appleton-Century Crofts, 1983
16. Hegyvary S: Primary Nursing. Boston, Little, Brown, 1983
17. Dawkins JE, Depp FC, Selzer NE: Stress and the psychiatric nurse, J Psychosocial Nursing, 1985; 23:9–15

14
Inpatient Psychiatric Research Units

John J. Boronow

The history of research on inpatient psychiatric units is coextensive with the modern era of psychiatry since Pinel. Because of the need until quite recently to treat psychiatric patients in hospitals, and the self-evident ignorance of early clinicians about the nature and treatment of psychiatric illnesses, the distinction between clinical treatment and research has often been blurred. One has only to think of the work of Charcot at the Salpetriere, Bleuler and Jung at the Burghoelzli, or Meyer at Phipps Clinic.

Today, with the widening gap between university and private hospitals and the increasing financial pressure from state and private funding agencies to expedite discharge, there is a danger that less and less research will be done in any but the most specialized inpatient settings, such as clinical research centers. This is unfortunate, since the inpatient unit provides a unique clinical laboratory for the observation and controlled treatment of psychiatric patients. More than any other medical specialty, psychiatry requires detailed, longitudinal observation of its subjects and the prevailing environmental variables, which often cannot be adequately accomplished with a few cross-sectional repeated measures. Short of an "in vivo" ethological approach, where the investigators live with the patients in their own outpatient environment, the inpatient unit provides an irreplaceable source of clinical data. And clinical questions about such data are the heart of any clinical research investigation.[1]

There are several kinds of problems which the inpatient unit is particularly suited to addressing. Any study of severely psychotic patients whose behavior cannot be managed in an outpatient setting must perforce be done in hospital. More common is the study of psychotic patients whose behavior can be managed on drugs as an outpatient, but where the protocol calls for a drug-free period, which may not be so easily managed. Protocols where the "active treatment" turns out to be ineffective may also lead to decompensation and are therefore more safely done in hospital. Management considerations may lead to an inpatient preference, as when a need to insure accurate medication compliance, avoidance of substance abuse, or implementation of a detailed behavioral protocol overrides the relative advantages of keeping the subject in his so-called "natural" outpatient environment.

Even if placebo-controlled medication trials or targeted complex behavioral interventions are not the goal, inpatient research may be preferable to maximize careful observations. This includes observation in its broadest sense, meaning anything from intensive behavioral ratings to highly technology-dependent methods requiring close proximity to a hospital. Examples of the latter include continuous video recording, telemetered EEG or activity recording, or longitudinal biological sampling, as with twice daily venipunctures for several weeks. Any serious study of the interpersonal behavior of psychiatric patients, as well as their behavior in groups, may also benefit from an inpatient setting, where the more subtle vicissitudes of relationships over time can be studied without having to infer what might have transpired between the patient and others in the interval between outpatient visits. Finally, for those very sick patients who cannot get beyond chronic institutionalization, the inpatient unit provides the identical milieu in which to study those factors which seem to keep the patient trapped in the hospital.

MOTIVATIONS TO CONDUCT RESEARCH

Before describing in greater detail the nature of inpatient psychiatric research, we would do well to reflect on the various reasons both patients and staff agree to participate in such an endeavor. For patients, consenting to be a subject in psychiatric research is often a highly complex decision based on a wide variety of motives. For some, it is merely a way to earn money, as with those protocols which actually reimburse patients for their participation. Others may harbor wild delusional beliefs which coincide with their perception of what the research means. For example, several patients at NIMH have specifically consented to CT or PET scans because of their conviction that they would finally see what they had "known" all along, namely that their brain had rotted away. Some patients cooperate out of a pathological passivity and wish to please authority figures. At its worst, this amounts to a kind of identification with the aggressor, and sensitivity to the patient's relationship with the therapist and investigator is called for. Such passivity can be particularly influential in an academic setting, where the therapist may be the investigator. In such cases, the patient may actually confound his therapy with the research and respond to it (for better or worse!) in terms of the vicissitudes of the ongoing therapy.[2] For example, a patient who is aware of the importance of the research to his therapist's professional goals may participate because of a wish to please and be like the therapist. Similarly, patients may be swayed by peer pressure and a wish to conform with the milieu norm. Just being admitted to a research ward can tilt an otherwise uncooperative patient toward consenting to research.

Of course, one always strives to inform the patient about the rational reasons for participation. The establishment of a genuine cooperative alliance based on the patient's understanding of the protocol and realistic wishes to benefit is the cornerstone of successful involvement. Benefits that involve direct improvement in the patient's lot, as with a successful trial of a new drug, are the most obvious. However, one should not discount more subtle benefits to the patient, such as the gratification of healthy altruistic wishes, which may be quite therapeutic to patients' self-esteem. To be able to say, "I have helped others, I have contributed something, I have real worth despite this awful illness," can be a wonderful boost to an otherwise apathetic and depressed patient. The job of the investigator and the Institutional Review Board is to try as best as possible to disentangle these conflicting motivations so as to ensure the least abuse of any patient. We shall say more about informed consent later.

Professional staff have a different set of motivations for doing research, and a variety of dynamics is relevant to a full understanding. On the negative side, it may be assumed that the intrusive, invasive, pressured, and oftentimes painful qualities of research can stimulate sadistic and voyeuristic impulses (in the psychoanalytic sense of those terms). This is not unique to research, to be sure, as the same can be said for many aspects of the practice of medicine in general.[3] Such impulses are not necessarily all bad, however, since the lack of, or reaction formations against, such impulses can eliminate otherwise talented people from doing this kind of work.

I am reminded of several young and idealistic residents with whom I trained. They complained about and even refused to participate in a well-designed, multicenter, collaborative, placebo-controlled protocol for their patients because it was "unethical." They objected to the randomized crossover design, which might lead a patient to remain unmedicated and therefore quite tormented for as long as an additional month. Their characterological makeup made it quite difficult for them to accept socially sanctioned and supervised procedures which could result in this prolonged suffering, informed consents and review boards notwithstanding. Clearly these colleagues were rendered ineffective as researchers in the presence of perceived sadism in others (and in themselves perhaps?), despite safeguards agreed upon by senior clinicians and by the patient himself! There is nothing pathological about such a stand, to be sure; however, if all physicians dealt with their conflicts over sadism in that way there would be a lot less research done throughout medicine.

Researchers, on the other hand, may be motivated by desires to avoid regular clinical work. Many gifted people with much to contribute are simply not happy with the demands of routine patient care. They prefer what can often be a more intellectually stimulating and less emotionally taxing research environment. Such individuals may be temperamentally or characterologically uncomfortable with psychiatric *patients*, being more at home at the micro level of neurotransmitter receptors, on the one hand, or at the macro level of abstract systems, on the other. This uneasiness, well-known to residency training directors, is usually overdetermined and may derive from a variety of factors, not all of which are problematic. After all, some people really are better thinkers than doers!

When there is a problem, however, the potential danger is that hypertrophied intellectualizing defenses may blind the researcher to the more subtle emotional, interpersonal, or countertransferential aspects of a situation. Such an investigator may do poor quality research because of a defensive need to constrict inappropriately his scope of inquiry. In the worst cases, he may also render suboptimal clinical care to his patients, discharging them hastily at the end of a protocol with the rationalization that "the research efforts were a sufficient replacement for regular clinical care and that more could not be done for the patient anyway." This pseudoboredom with routine clinical work may coexist with a certain disdain for ordinary clinicians, who can be trivialized as "touchy-feely," unmedical, or technically incompetent. Such attitudinizing may in fact be a defensive projection of the researcher's own guilt over his abandonment of difficult and intractable patients after their brief fling on the relatively safe and contained research setting. Researchers whose private practices consist primarily of consulting to other therapists may have quite a hard time escaping such stereotyping. Biological researchers in particular are vulnerable to this kind of distortion, although the best, like Robert Post,[4] John Docherty,[5] and the Strauss and Carpenter collaboration[6] are outstanding examples of a more synthetic and clinical approach to patient care.

Along these same lines may be an investigator's wish for fame. The narcissistic wishes underlying research are often extreme, if not grandiose. The "Nobel Prize" fantasy can be a powerful impetus to many researchers, especially biological ones, where the prizes may indeed be given some day for a major breakthrough in our understanding of the brain. Such fantasies, coupled with the other characterological traits mentioned above, can undermine good research through excessive competition or secretiveness. The pressures to publish in what *Science* has called "Least Publishable Units"[7] and to change research topics quickly so as to be always on the "cutting edge" are hazards of such narcissism. A fantasy of omnipotence is another closely related trap that can lead the researcher to devalue the observations and efforts of clinical colleagues. Clearly, the academic environment may predispose to such behaviors as well. Nevertheless, these traits can be quite adaptive if the extremes are controlled.

The best possible motivation stems from a genuine curiosity coupled with healthy altruism and a wish to help others. Such attitudes need not be merely defensive and derivative of the above-mentioned character traits. It is important to recall that researchers often must make real sacrifices to pursue their chosen careers, including financial inferiority to many private clinicians, job insecurity in the form of competition for tenure and grants, and bureaucratic constraints attendant on working in large institutional contexts. The decision to go into a research career is thus quite complexly determined and can call on the best and worst aspects of a caregiver's personality.

Finally, a word should be said about the motivations for institutions like hospitals to sponsor what can often be a very expensive undertaking. In the clearest case of a university teaching hospital, there is a fundamental mandate to encourage and support research. This is not necessarily easy to implement, however, and for inner-city teaching hospitals facing an un- or underinsured clientele the funding can be an insuperable obstacle. Research can be seen as a superfluous activity which merely drains away resources from already limited teaching and clinical programs. On the other hand, an active research program can in fact help to overcome some of these problems. The impact of quality research on an institution's clinical care can be profound. University teaching hospitals often do provide the very finest caliber treatment, even in the midst of decaying facilities. The standard of intellectual excellence which researchers expect of themselves infuses teaching and attending staff with an extra commitment to quality, which shows in the thoroughness of their workups and the precision of their diagnostic and treatment thinking process. The desire to be at a center of learning where the newest treatments are being studied can also lure both patients and high quality professional staff and trainees to otherwise undesirable geographic locations. Similarly, public relations and marketing departments can use research, especially the more "glamorous" technologies like PET or NMR scans, as a magnet to attract private and public funds. In the end, the host institution's motivation for and commitment to research are as critical as that of patients and staff.

PREREQUISITES FOR CONDUCTING RESEARCH WITHIN A HOSPITAL

Above all, psychiatric research requires that staff possess very specialized knowledge. Professional staff (psychiatrists, psychologists, social workers, or activity therapists who are the principal investigators) must have sufficient background to be able to plan and complete a project successfully. This may seem a truism, but considerable resources have been wasted at times when well-meaning but naive investigators have embarked on projects for which they lacked the requisite skills. To begin with, an in-depth understanding of the area to be studied is called for, be it biological or psychological. Thorough familiarity with current diagnostic controversies and methodologies is paramount, as is experience in administering standardized assessment instruments such as SADS. A working knowledge of the rating scales or other measurements of change chosen must precede their indiscriminate use, as well as an appreciation of the rationale and methods for assessing their reliability. Principles of research design must be mastered in order to develop an appropriate approach to the problem at hand. Finally, a basic education in medical statistics is a sine qua non. Perhaps the single most common error committed by investigators is the construction of a project whose data cannot in principle be meaningfully analyzed because the data are not collected in a manner consistent with conventional statistical methods. Although early consultation with a statistician may obviate such problems, the investigator's own understanding of statistical principles is indispensable.

Training professional staff to develop the above skills is a major undertaking and cannot be lightly imposed as an afterthought or mere good intention. Psychologists tend to have a rigorous background in research methodology and may need specialized training only if they intend to study a biological area for which their education did not prepare them. Psychiatrists, on the other hand, are often woefully lacking in most of the necessary skills to do modern research. Most come from liberal arts undergraduate programs with little or no exposure to scientific research. Most medical schools spend little time on research methods, and statistics is usually not a requirement. Psychiatric residencies tend to be very service oriented, and research projects are frequently "add ons" in the last year. There is seldom time for actual additional course work, such as a statistics or methods class at a nearby university.

The solution traditionally has been the apprenticeship model, whereby the interested graduating psychiatrist stays on in an academic setting and "learns by doing" under the guidance of an already established investigator. More recently, specialized research fellowships have been offered which present selected trainees with a more formally structured didactic and experiential program aimed at bringing them quickly up to speed. For institutions considering beginning or upgrading their research programs, it is important to realize the extensive training and experience involved in creating seasoned investigators. The institution must be prepared to invest heavily in either training or recruitment, or both, if the professional staffing needs are to be met.

Training of nursing personnel requires considerable attention on an inpatient unit. Psychiatric nursing in particular tends to perceive the patient within the context of the belief system that pervades their local institution. Thus, one hospital may view most behavior as symbolic of unconscious conflicts, and thus pay little regard to physical parameters. In the extreme case, staff at such hospitals might be adverse to any research that entails invasive biological procedures, as even the hanging of a simple IV might be considered alien and beyond their professional scope. Similarly, a heavy emphasis on interpretive psychodynamics might discourage the staff from close and meticulous documentation of discrete behaviors, since the details of what a patient actually said or did might be seen as secondary to what the patient "really meant." Conversely, highly trained medical-surgical nurses might be superb at facilitating biological protocols but intolerant of regressed or acting-out behaviors inherent in the psychiatric population. In that case, their technical expertise would be of no use if they were unable to maintain a holding milieu. The point is not that one or another type of staff belief system is best, but that the underlying assumptions and limitations of a given belief system need to be clearly understood and taken into account.

It is important that the nursing staff have a grasp of what the general thrust of the research on the ward will be. It has been suggested at times that if staff know "too much" about the research, this will prejudice them in their ratings and so it is better that they be kept only generally informed. It seems to me that this is only thinly disguised prejudice, since the physician's bias is not questioned equally. Proper double-blind and control methodology should contain such potential bias in either nursing or physician staff. Much more important is the psychological boost given to nursing staff when made a genuine collaborator in the research enterprise. Staff can become understandably resentful when they are asked to manage and tolerate the oftentimes extremely regressed behavior of patients on placebo without being given the courtesy of being told why such extra work is vitally important. This goes doubly for unmedicated assaultive patients. The whole attitude can be transformed if the staff are included in the planning process and educated on an ongoing basis about the rationale for a particular course of action.

Ideally, nursing staff can actually participate in the development of discrete aspects of a research project. On our unit, after several weeks of struggling with the shortcomings of a particular rating scale, the staff began to make a variety of specific suggestions about creating a new instrument. Their clinical observation and daily contact with the patients made their comments invaluable, and a new form was created which was far superior to the previous one. And since they had to actually spend the time day in and day out using it, their motivation was enhanced because of their direct input into its creation. Similarly, feedback to staff about the results of ongoing work, even if only preliminary, can stimulate their enthusiasm enormously.

Staff must be properly trained to perform any ratings with which they are involved. This requires varying degrees of inservice training, depending on staff's level of education. At the NIMH, for example, all the staff are at least R.N.'s, and many have master's degrees. Their level of sophistication can at times be awesome; it may even require some tempering in order to maintain reliability with instruments which are fairly simpleminded. On the other hand, a mostly nonprofessional staff of mental health workers may require considerable training in order to reach agreement about even the most basic concepts, such as the difference between a disorder of thought form and content. One major benefit of such training is that it raises the clinical competence of the staff enormously, since accurate observation and assessment are as critical to good clinical care as to research.

In some settings, nursing staff may need additional training to develop proficiency in a variety of specialized procedures besides ratings. This may include highly technical competence in the performance of a patient procedure, such as maintaining a 24-hourly blood sampling IV apparatus. The entire area of skills needed to maintain the milieu while research is going on will be discussed in detail below.

In addition to the above personnel prerequisites, successful inpatient psychiatric research requires an available source of appropriate subjects. Certain settings are severely constricted or specially favored (depending on the interests of the investigator) in their access to a particular diagnostic or demographic group. It behooves the investigator to capitalize on the strengths of a particular setting and eschew projects for which their are few potential subjects. It makes no sense, for example, to try and study anorexia nervosa in an all male VA hospital! A more subtle kind of limitation on patients can come from the very process of selecting volunteer subjects. People who volunteer are not necessarily representative of the group under scrutiny. To illustrate, one of the hallmarks of chronic "negative symptom" schizophrenia is willful, stubborn oppositionalism. Although this may represent a behavior well worth studying, its very presence makes such study problematic. How does one get the patient to volunteer and cooperate with structured interviews, ratings, test procedures, etc., when saying "No" is at the very heart of his illness? At the very least modifications in conventional research methods may be called for (see below), and in the most extreme cases the subject must be excluded altogether. Other common and legitimate reasons for exclusion are unpredictable violence, suicidal behavior, or gross disorganization and disinhibition of primitive impulses.

Too much exclusion for one or several practical reasons can nonetheless generate a powerful bias in the actual sample studied, which in turn may undermine the very basis of the research.[8] At the Clinical Center of the NIMH a rather unique group of schizophrenic patients was selected. They were nonviolent, non-substance-abusing, too refractory to medications for ambulatory care, and passive enough to permit frequent invasive procedures such as lumbar punctures. One can fill a unit with such patients if you offer free hospitalization and have the entire United States as your catchment, but just barely! Large or small notwithstanding, such a skewed sample at the least raises the question of whether the study of such patients can be generalized to the broader population of schizophrenics. The answer to that rests with what exactly is being researched. If the investigators were studying behavioral or pharmacological treatments to be used with outpatients, then they would run a risk of their results being either falsely positive (as with behavioral interventions that would flop when tried on more oppositional or aggressive outpatients) or falsely negative (as with trials of medication that fail on inpatients who fail to respond even to known effective neuroleptics). If they were studying pharmacokinetics, neurotransmitter metabolism, or other presumably less behavior dependent variables, then the limitations on the cohort studied would have much less impact.

A final prerequisite for conducting high level inpatient research is adequate institutional support. This includes such areas as finance and administration, as well as the physical plant. It is beyond the scope of this chapter to detail the myriad considerations that go into providing appropriate financial and administrative support, but it should be clear that such mundane matters as indirect cost allocation, professional assistance in drafting budgets for grant applications, and secretarial/computational services can all have a major impact on the final efficiency of a research program. The physical plant is a topic which does deserve some additional elaboration, however.

The first architectural consideration in planning inpatient research is whether to house the patients on a single unit, perhaps a dedicated research unit such as 3 South at Payne Whitney Clinic at New York Hospital. The alternatives would be to have the beds consolidated on a single unit but constituting only a fraction of the census, or to have the beds more or less randomly dispersed throughout the clinical services. The latter approach requires that the other units be similar in patient mix and clinical orientation, a condition that is becoming less common in this era of specialty programs. The advantages of dispersing research beds are few, but one can argue that there is less stigmatization and mystification and better dispersal of professional expertise when research is somehow "integrated" into the everyday workings of the entire institution. On the other hand, such efforts run the risk of never becoming integrated and of being sabotaged by both professional and nursing staff who experience the occasional research bed on their unit as odd, a nuisance, and something to be avoided. The sheer magnitude of work entailed in training an entire hospital staff, even if only with regard to attitude, as compared with the more manageable task of developing a single unit, makes the relative advantages of consolidating beds evident.

In addition to these staffing considerations, creating a specialized unit also allows the architecture of the unit to be tailored to the unique needs of the patient population under investigation (within the limits of the budget!) For example, on our chronic schizophrenia unit at Sheppard Pratt Hospital, we have made several modifications to improve the physical plant. Carpeting has been replaced with linoleum in the bedrooms of the lowest functioning patients to prevent malodorous soiling from incontinent patients. Similarly, some furniture has been reupholstered with water-repelling vinyl. Sofas have been replaced with easy chairs to discourage daytime sleeping and to help maintain boundaries between disorganized patients. A linen room was converted into a patient store (for a token economy), and a large room with a pool table became an activity therapy room, so that activities could be brought to patients too regressed to leave the hall. Likewise a kitchen was upgraded to a dining area so that meals could be served on the hall. A bedroom was converted to a "time-out" room, a comfortable and furnished alternative to the seclusion room, which was kept unchanged. Since such patients need room in which to pace and distance themselves from others at times, an ajoining courtyard was fenced in to provide time off the hall with minimal staffing for supervision.

Many of these and similar alterations were modeled on the schizophrenia unit the NIMH Clinical Center. They reflect not so much direct needs of the research per se, but the decision to concentrate a group of highly regressed patients in a single location. Here again, however, the *clinical* payoff from a decision based on research considerations is significant, since most of these plant changes led to a better milieu in general.

Other plant modifications depend more directly on the specific projects being conducted. A second time-out or seclusion room may be necessary if aggressive patients are being studied. An extra hospital bed and refrigerator may be required if cold wet sheet pack is used frequently during drug-free periods. Rooms with one-way mirrors and/or video equipment may be important. Procedure rooms with ample space to perform lumbar punctures or venipunctures without making the patient feel exposed or claustrophobic are helpful for biological studies. Having some laboratory and computing equipment right on the unit can also facilitate the work; this, of course, requires additional space.

PRACTICAL, CLINICAL, AND ETHICAL CONSIDERATIONS

One of the first issues to be grappled with in establishing an inpatient psychiatric research program is the decision whether, and if so how, to routinely include drug-free periods. This is a particularly emotionally charged issue for certain nursing and professional staff, who perceive such maneuvers as at best unhelpful to the patient and at worst dangerous for all concerned. Untrained staff who have little experience with research or unmedicated patients are prone to regressive fantasies which imbue the unmedicated patient with magical destructive powers and the investigators with callous Machiavellian deviousness. The pressure to medicate the patient right away and to explain all clinical problems in terms of lack of medications can become irresistible at times, even from a staff that would otherwise consider itself to be psychodynamically oriented.

In countering such irrational fears, it is important to understand the scientific rationale for drug-free periods. For biological studies, where fundamental physiology is being investigated, such as with catecholamine metabolites, a normative homeostatic baseline needs to be established for comparison purposes. In more clinically oriented treatment trials, the drug-free period may be a kind of control design, namely using the subject as his own control. Clearly, some kind of controls are needed to account for such phenomena as placebo effect, spontaneous remission or exacerbation, effects of age, sex, etc. By withdrawing patients from drugs, rating them, and then treating them, the subjects themselves quite efficiently control for these phenomena, thus decreasing the number of subjects needed. It is an elegant approach, but not the only one, and when ethical issues are raised about vital treatment being withheld, it is reasonable to consider alternatives.

Some kinds of research, especially observational/descriptive studies, can forgo conventional controls altogether if the purview of their questions is limited to the patients' behavior in the clinical setting.[9] If larger groups of patients are available, especially in big outpatient studies, randomization to two different treatment regimens is a viable option. Or patients may continue as their own controls, but the active treatment can be piggybacked onto an already ongoing and efficacious treatment, with the researcher looking for an incremental benefit. This latter technique has certain clinical merit at times, since very often a new treatment will indeed be an addition to, rather than a replacement of, a conventional treatment.

It is often helpful to emphasize to concerned staff the legitimate clinical reasons for withdrawing patients from medications. While drug-free periods are a standard part of any clinical drug trial, that is not their only justification by any means. Perhaps most importantly, with any patients chronically on neuroleptics a drug-free period is essential for the accurate assessment of tardive dyskinesia (TD). This has become an increasingly important determination to make in the light of the recent rise in lawsuits over TD. Clinically, it is still believed important to identify TD as early as possible, so that alternative therapies and/or neuroleptic reduction can be pursued. Since neuroleptics mask TD in its early stages, drug-free periods remain the only definitive way at present to make an accurate diagnosis of the syndrome.

A more immediately compelling justification for drug-free periods can be made in those patients with complex courses, atypical treatment responses, and uncertain diagnoses. That group probably comprises half of all inpatients. Given the often poor quality of phenomenological description in past records and equally haphazard diagnostic practices, it is common for inpatient psychiatrists to have relatively little substantive past history upon which to base their assessments. Nowadays it is simply bad clinical practice to accept someone's old diagnosis of schizophrenia, for example, without extensive corroborating clinical data. Sadly, often the only way to get those data is to observe the patient drug-free for an extended period of time. That modern third-party payment programs usually do not provide adequate reimbursement for this kind of approach does not detract from its utility and necessity and is in fact, a rather sad commentary on the antiscientific attitudes latent in such bottom-line oriented programs. Fortunately, for those situations where drugs may actually be making the clinical situation worse (as, for example, in a tricyclic-induced mania or a lithium/neuroleptic neurotoxic syndrome), drug withdrawal is still seen as an appropriate intervention.

In these examples, the pressure to medicate stems from a primitive dynamic that stresses action in the face of adversity and values the resolution a present crisis over any future benefit. Perhaps one of the most lasting contributions of the scientific attitude toward patient care is the detachment and objectivity it brings to bear on oftentimes emotion-laden clinical dilemmas. Nursing staff may wish to have a difficult patient "sealed over" as quickly as possible in order to lessen their workload, maintain a stable milieu, or decrease the immediate suffering. Professional staff may also desire rapid symptomatic treatment in response to financial pressures for quick discharge. However, premature treatment which turns out to be merely palliative instead of definitive can actually do long-term harm to a patient. Obvious examples of this include: the misdiagnosed manic who is given only neuroleptics because he looks schizophrenic; the misdiagnosed psychotic depressive who is not given a tricyclic because his "schizophrenic withdrawal" will respond to neuroleptic; and the schizophrenic patient who is labeled "borderline" because he does not demonstrate psychotic symptoms *while on neuroleptics*. In these and many other instances, a drug-free period can be a critical intervention in the patient's course of illness, correcting well-meaning but hurtful misconceptions which perpetuate rather than resolve a pathogenic process.

Drug-free periods are not a panacea, but neither are they a dangerous intrusion into an otherwise perfect treatment program by clinically naive investigators. One maneuver that is often helpful in winning over staff to the reasonableness of such periods is to show clinically sensitive flexibility as to when such periods are instituted. Giving new patients a chance to accommodate to novel surroundings and personnel before subjecting them to potentially disorganizing increases in their psychopathology makes good clinical sense. Staff, too, need to get to know a patient in relative tranquility before "all hell breaks loose." This was standard procedure at the Clinical Center of NIMH. Similarly, it makes no sense to withdraw several patients from their medications simultaneously if there is already turbulence on the unit. Any milieu can eventually reach a critical level of psychopathology, such that a kind of chain reaction or contagion sets in. In such cases the thoughtless withdrawal of a patient from medications would only create a crisis and probably vitiate the potential usefulness of the maneuver anyway.

INFORMED CONSENT

Another area worthy of some discussion is the role of informed consent in the conduct of psychiatric research. As discussed above, psychiatric patients can often have a host of bizarre and irrational motivations for agreeing or refusing to participate in a research protocol. These must be carefully considered by any Institutional Review Board (IRB) in overseeing the conduct of a particular project to ensure that adequate safeguards are built in.

The pressures on investigators and potential subjects are manifold and at times quite powerful. Investigators may need to run a critical number of patients through a protocol in order to complete it by a certain deadline, perhaps so as to be the first in publishing some new finding. They may so genuinely believe in the therapeutic efficacy of their investigational treatment that they lose their capacity to empathize with a patient's fears. A scientific understanding of the actual risks and benefits involved may blind them to a patient's distorted but very real fears of what is involved. Their unconscious identification with the project and emotional involvement may also generate passionate enthusiasm. This can potentially lead to abuses, such as when the investigator proselytizes potential subjects, using his oftentimes considerable charisma to sway patients' decision. Subjects may be more vulnerable to this kind of covert coercion when they have already been admitted to a hospital unit and fear (all protestations from the investigator notwithstanding!) that refusal to cooperate with this powerful person will lead to retaliation.

Pressures on the patient may also come from family members, who may see the research as some kind of magical "last chance" for their loved one to be "cured." This is especially likely to happen in families where the patient has taken on a negative, devalued identity and the family has overidentified with the positive, idealized doctor. In such instances it is crucial to assess whether the patient is being subtly coerced into cooperating as part of a family's larger pattern of struggle over control. Needless to say, the investigator may not necessarily be in the most objective position to evaluate this, since he, too, may be open to countertransferences which reinforce the parents' idealization and foster a paternalistic view of the patient.

Another potential pressure on patients is a kind of financial blackmail by society. For the seriously disabled chronic patient, participation in state-supported inpatient research programs which cost the patient nothing may be the only alternative to institutionalization in a state hospital. Since most state hospitals continue to be overcrowded, understaffed, and in poor physical repair, the prospect of staying for several months in a small, well staffed, well maintained research program may be very appealing. Some patients find the tradeoff of participating in even very invasive procedures such as lumbar punctures to be preferable to state hospitalization. I have known at least two patients who systematically went from one research unit to another in Maryland in order to ensure what they perceived to be the best accommodations. There is nothing inherently wrong with such "professional research subjects," of course, so long as the patient genuinely understands the risks of whatever he is consenting to. The potential danger lies with the delusional patient who, although he really does not wish to be a research subject, may be so terrorized of state hospitalization that he will do "anything" to avoid it. Here again, the investigator is probably not the best person to assess the quality of the informed consent, since he already "knows" that what he is offering is safe and even valuable for the patient.

A larger issue lies in the capacity of the delusional and/or cognitively impaired patient to truly understand exactly what he is consenting to. Especially with contemporary biological investigations, the complexity of issues under study may be confusing even to nonpsychiatric medical professionals, much less a psychotic patient with a functional IQ of 85. The criteria for being "informed" are theoretically much more demanding than, for example, merely giving consent for voluntary commitment to a psychiatric facility. In the latter case, the patient need only demonstrate an understanding that he is signing into a hospital for the mentally ill and that once committed he cannot leave without following a well-defined procedure that may entail a hearing. There is no requirement that he understand that he may have any illness or that certain treatments may have adverse consequences. Even consenting to an invasive medical procedure, such as ECT or an operation, requires relatively little understanding. For example, in proving competence to refuse a necessary but non-life-threatening medical procedure, in many states patients must only demonstrate that they understand that they have an illness, that they comprehend rationally the risks and benefits of the recommended treatment, and that they comprehend rationally the likely outcome should they refuse the treatment.

By comparison, consent to participate in a research project may involve several more levels of complexity. The project itself needs to be described, even if in only rudimentary terms, to the patient, and this often entails several pages of print and/or concomitant discussion. Explaining the rationale for why you need a radioactive isotope to do a PET scan requires more elaboration than telling a patient that he needs to have his appendix out or it will burst. Moreover, any special procedures performed during the protocol require detailed explanation, often with quite detailed commentary. The consent to do a lumbar puncture as a medical procedure is far shorter than the same consent to do it as a research investigation. The patient must understand the potential consequences of consenting to no treatment, i.e., placebo trials, but it may be hard for the cognitively concrete patient to envision the absence of something. Assurances of confidentiality, especially when videotapes are made, often stir up a whole new area of concern, especially in paranoid patients, that is simply not as big an issue in a nonresearch setting, even though confidentiality is just as important. The difference is that confidentiality is not usually explicitly highlighted in the clinical settings unless the *patient* brings it up.

A final dilemma in obtaining informed consent from psychiatric patients is a sort of converse twist on the nature of being informed. Rather than protecting the patient from misinformation propagated by the researcher, it sometimes occurs that patients must be screened for possible disinformation they may have about a particular treatment under study. Patients may arrive convinced that a novel therapy, such as hemodialysis for schizophrenia, is an already proven cure for which they will do almost anything. While such patients might superficially appear to be a researcher's dream, they in fact pose a real challenge. Uncritical acceptance of such patients into a protocol without a serious effort to reeducate them about the actual risks and benefits can lead to both an excess of placebo responses and difficult clinical situations at the end, when patients in fact realize that they have not benefited.

In general it is fair to say that truly informed consent is probably not realistically possible in at least half of the most severely ill patients who participate in research protocols. The legal repercussions of this are much less important than the ethical issues. After all, the pages of single-spaced print are usually adequate protection against the more flagrant lawsuits. The fundamental issue is: How does society protect the interests and rights of severely impaired mentally ill research subjects, or must their participation be prohibited altogether? First of all, family or close friends should always be involved as coparticipants in the informed consent procedure. In spite of the potential for family coercion, most families have their loved one's best interests at heart and they are almost always able to understand rationally the proposed protocols. Occasionally the family, or a single member, may be so disturbed as to be almost as impaired as the patient, thus diminishing the family's helpfulness, but in my experience this is quite rare. Moreover, having the family well informed and in alliance with the researchers is as facilitating of ongoing work on a research unit as is their cooperative involvement in a conventional treatment milieu. It just makes good sense.

Besides insisting on family involvement, the institution can and should bring further objective safeguards to bear on research participation. The IRB, which always has members from the community and professionals uninvolved with the project at hand, has a serious responsibility to review protocols in light of all the factors we have been discussing. Any doubts should always provoke further inquiry, interviews, and site visits as necessary, and problematic aspects of the protocol should be revised. At times, a periodic renewal of a subject's consent, either verbally or in writing, has been suggested, especially in long-term inpatient studies. This can, unfortunately, "put ideas" into the heads of some of the more suggestible patients, whose ambivalence is a hallmark of their illness.

A more elegant and probably more informative procedure was devised at the Clinical Center of the NIMH.[10] A weekly research meeting was instituted which brought together all the patients, nursing and professional staff, as well as many of the outside technical staff who performed various procedures but were not part of the treatment milieu per se. During these meetings a systematic review of each patient's involvement in any research procedures that week was made, and discussion of their thoughts and feelings about it ensued. Often delusional misinterpretations (e.g., "They took out all my blood and replaced it with plastic" = plasmapheresis) were aired and corrected publicly in an atmosphere of trust and genuine interest. Ideally, other patients helped reality test the delusion or gave believable reassurance to a peer because they had done the same thing themselves. In addition, at the completion of a patient's tenure on the unit, his overall stay in the program was reviewed. A graph showing his ratings was shown to him, with the periods when he was on placebo or active compounds indicated. This helped to demystify the confusing world of placebos, strange experimental compounds, and ratings, and to put the stay into a more conventional and rational framework. This kind of elaborate procedure might not be necessary on a unit studying chronic depression, but was an invaluable contribution to the ethical *and* practical functioning of a chronic schizophrenia research program.

This ethical question of how informed the potential subject can or needs to be is in part based on the tacit assumption that being on a research unit ipso facto results in less than optimal care.[11] The realistic concern that a patient may be deprived of a therapeutic modality temporarily is confused with a more general prejudice that any patient in research is being denied more thorough clinical treatment. This issue has been addressed by several thoughtful investigators, and the counterargument has been made that research units may actually deliver superior care because of the extra time and care devoted to patients.[12-14] While it is certainly possible that patients may be taken advantage of in *any* setting, there is really little evidence to suggest that research units are especially prone to deliver inferior clinical care. Accepting this may require considerable education of families, patients, and even some staff.

Before leaving this topic, a final word should be said about research with the involuntary patient. Many programs refuse to consider such subjects outright, and when the research involves invasive and potentially harmful treatments or procedures, their position is understandable. Nevertheless, many involuntary patients are surprisingly cooperative and nonoppositional and actually spontaneously volunteer to participate in research. For some patients, involuntary certification is a kind of face-saving maneuver in an ongoing struggle with their parents (or with immediate authority figure displacements). Once certified, the patient feels free to participate in the clinical treatment program because, after all, they are "making" him do it, and no one can accuse him of passively going along. In such cases it would be a mistake to exclude the patient from research a priori, since such patients are common and their absence significantly distorts the sample one is targeting. Informed consent remains crucial, and it may be wise to explicitly include a statement to the effect that participation in the research will not per se have any direct bearing on the patient's release.

MAINTAINING A THERAPEUTIC MILIEU

Managing an inpatient unit of psychiatric patients is a complicated and delicate task in and of itself. Doing it on a research unit requires even more planning, coordination, thoughtfulness, and experience. One of the most taxing additional demands on the treatment team is the increased effort required to elicit from the patient cooperation with the research procedures. It is hard enough to get a psychotic patient on a conventional unit to participate in the treatment program; on a research unit, there is often a host of extra interviews, tests, procedures, etc., for the patient to refuse, in addition to the usual treatment activities. Helping the patient maximize his cooperation requires a concerted effort from the entire treatment team.

A consistent, rational, nonjudgmental, and supportive approach to the patient is a key ingredient of such an effort. The patient is under stress from his illness and is also stressed from the very fact of being in a research program. He is also doing the researchers a favor, even if for his own reasons. It is therefore incumbent upon the researchers to do everything possible to help the patient feel protected and appreciated for his efforts. Positive, praising compliments for every instance of appropriate cooperation are very helpful in this regard; threatening or blaming criticisms for oppositionalism are not. An open attitude toward performance that acknowledges that there will be good days and bad, and that validates the reality of the patient's inhibitions and fears, fosters trust and a capacity to compromise. Willingness to spend extra time with the patient, even to the extent of having a favorite nurse or even a therapist participate in the procedure along with the patient, can further extend the limits of what even a very regressed patient can tolerate. Time spent clearly explaining, often repeatedly, the exact nature of the procedure or test is also effective. Sensitivity to a psychotic patient's short attention span can be shown by breaking up lengthy assessments such as a neuropsychological battery into many brief sessions. Liberal use of oral reinforcement such as cigarettes and soda are often facilitating, not because patients are being "bribed" but simply because they need frequent opportunities to relax and reorganize when asked to perform at a high level for long periods of time.

Persistence is critical to any successful outcome. If one were only to do research on patients who agreed to things on the first go-round, there would be much less known in psychiatry today! The team must be prepared to repeat some efforts over and over again, be it explaining a protocol, attempting a lumbar puncture, or inquiring about delusions. The first "No!" should always be met with neutral curiosity and friendly exploration, followed by a genuine (not feigned) willingness to try again another day. After much discussion, cajoling, or leaving alone, it may sometimes pay to simply try and begin a procedure with a patient without stopping over the formalities of yes and no.

Obviously, I do not mean to suggest here that one would ever impose any invasive procedure or treatment on a research patient without his consent. But, for example, there are times when a patient is so caught up with the very process of saying no that he no longer is aware of the content of what he is refusing. This can occasionally be circumvented by going directly to that content, as when a patient is engaged in a soft-sign battery directly by tossing a ball to him. He may catch it, toss it back, laugh, and proceed cooperatively with the assessment without realizing that he would have said no had he been asked.

As a last resort, one may have to set a firm limit. Unfortunately, that often has the quality of a threat, even if based on legitimate reality constraints. After all, if the patient refuses altogether, he cannot be kept in the research project, and yet the alternative for him may be transfer to a state hospital. This is a sad development which makes all involved uncomfortable, and in my experience rarely works for very long. At that point it may be best to cease the struggle with the patient, terminate his participation on a friendly note, and reframe the problem in terms of what can be done to help the patient now that the research is completed.

The demands of nursing staff in such an environment are considerably more than on a conventional unit. The staff must not only be familiar with the characteristic ways psychiatric patients may misperceive the goings-on around them, but also have the time and experience to respond supportively as described above. It requires enormous patience and extra manpower to have the luxury of working quietly and persistently with oppositional patients until they come round. Completing ratings, helping with procedures, and explaining procedures to family all take additional time as well. Managing an excess of impulsive and disorganized patients, especially if off their medications, adds yet another, at times extremely taxing, extra duty.

The modern psychiatric nurse has been trained in the era of psychopharmacology and has learned to expect that the assaultive, self-destructive, or impulse-driven patient can be contained with medications. It is therefore guite an adjustment to cope with the fact that the patient cannot be given *anything* during a drug-free period. Staff must learn to respond routinely to severely regressed behavior with techniques that are nowadays usually reserved for brief crises requiring temporary management while waiting for medications to take effect (seclusion, restraints, one-to-one close observation). Another modality which is rarely taken advantage of in other settings is the sedative cold wet sheet pack. This treatment, which involves wrapping the patient in layers of cold wet sheets mummy-style, dates back to the pre-phenothiazine era. If helpful, it has a rapid calming effect on the agitated patient, and as it gradually warms up, can soothe the patient to sleep. The sheetpack usually requires three people with a cooperative patient and many more if the patient is combative, and necessitates one-to-one supervision until the patient comes out (two to four hours later). It is thus a highly labor intensive procedure and highlights the special demands placed on the staff of a research unit.

Maintaining a therapeutic milieu on a research unit requires additional attention to matters which may not be as carefully scrutinized on a conventional unit. For example, there are always strangers on any psychiatric unit, be they delivery personnel, repairmen, or administrators. The research unit may have many more, however, in the form of laboratory technicians, research assistants, audiovisual personnel, visiting researchers, etc. Patients may develop delusions about these people, some of whom they may have occasional contact with for various procedures, and staff must be constantly helping patients reality test these misperceptions.

Confidentiality may be of special concern to certain patients in a research setting, what with all these extra personnel, audiovisual recordings, ratings, and other potential invasions of their privacy. Although the patient may have given truly informed consent, recurrent fears about loss of privacy may crop up from time to time, particularly in patients with already impaired boundaries. Here again, skillful staff can intervene early on with reassurance, anticipating the patient's fears and explaining, or even demonstrating, how the patient's identity is coded and not revealed in the research publications.

If the patient's therapist is his rater, there may be times when the patient will tell the therapist one thing as his confidant and yet deny it the next day when being interviewed for a rating. Often this has less to do with fears of the patient that what he says might be used "against" him than with the fact that the therapeutic context is conducive to more self-revelation and less concern about appearances of being "crazy." Using data from therapy is crucial to accurate ratings, which are otherwise prone to being based on an artificial and stilted interview situation.[15] I have rarely come across a clinical situation where the patient protested that what he said in confidence to his therapist could not be included as data for research ratings. The key, of course, is to handle *all* privileged communications, psychotherapeutic or research-based, with the respect and dignity they deserve.

In maintaining a safe and supportive milieu in the face of often frightening procedures and technology, it is often helpful to flaunt the process publicly so as to desensitize the patients to it and thereby normalize it. Patients with indwelling catheters should be encouraged to walk about with the IV pole rather than stay in their rooms; venipuncture and ratings can be done in the dayroom just like any other therapeutic encounter; staff meetings to discuss interrater reliability can be held in the midst of the patients, so they can see for themselves what the researchers are talking about. Even sedative wet sheetpack can be demystified, such that the patient can literally be brought into the dayroom and participate in the community meeting. Patients can then see concretely the efforts of staff to help the (presumably) unmedicated patient and be reassured that he is all right.

Finally, the experience and sensitivity of all the staff cannot be overemphasized in its importance in the successful creation of a genuinely therapeutic milieu. All the sophistication in the world cannot replace the love and wisdom shown by staff who have worked long years with patients who have problems disabling enough to bring them to a psychiatric research unit. Cultivating a cohesive staff with low turnover and high morale pays off with a more focused and reassuring milieu. High turnover, even though it be of immensely gifted personnel, takes a toll in milieu stability and ability to cope with adversity. The attitude of the staff will also ideally encompass the whole person. A too biological approach, even though motivated by the highest ideals, may undermine the efficacy of the milieu and thus, inadvertently, of the entire research enterprise. If the staff, nursing or professional, lack the necessary warmth and emotional commitment to the patients, the group process of the milieu may become regressive, oppositional, and not conducive to research or treatment.

PERCEPTIONS OF THE RESEARCH UNIT WITHIN THE HOSPITAL

The research unit reflects many common experiences of specialized treatment settings in medicine at large. For the staff working within the specialized program, there is always a dynamic tension between the hubris of feeling valued as doing something important and the shame of feeling that no one cares about such esoteric work at all, or between the confidence of being perceived as powerful, the patient's "last chance," and the rejection of only getting the "incurables," the ones no one else wants anyway. Often staff cope with this by identifying with the wider scientific or professional world at large, leaving their relatively isolated programs from time to time to mingle in a community of peers who truly understand their work. Nursing staff are just as vulnerable to this kind of isolation and also need such refueling from like-minded peers, either vicariously through the researchers, or better, by engaging themselves in activities outside of the institution which foster supportive contacts.

During the creation of a new unit for chronic schizophrenic patients at Sheppard-Pratt, there was much concern about whether the hospital was subverting its traditional and honored role as a humane asylum in the name of some cold and unfeeling research. There was initial reluctance to transfer patients from within the institution, for fear of subjecting them to a dehumanizing treatment. Residents were explicitly barred from routinely rotating through the unit because of concerns that the experience would not provide the kind of psychodynamic education in which the institution took justifiable pride. Many of the nursing staff requested (and were given) transfers to other units when they discovered just how unfamiliar the approach to the patient was.

As time has passed, however, the unit has attracted the interest of many professionals from varying disciplines, and staff members have been asked to consult or give presentations throughout the hospital. The consulting role has been particularly expanded in the area of psychopharmacology, where the unit has developed a reputation for agressively medicating refractory patients with care and safety, and occasionally success. The severity of the patients on the unit is notorious throughout the hospital, and the entire staff is regarded as dedicated and hardworking. There is no envy that as a research unit we are somehow "getting away" with something. In fact, most of our colleagues wonder that we can stand to work day in and day out with such severely regressed patients and are often relieved to be able to transfer cases to us. The envy, when there is any, is over tangible manifestations of institutional attention, such as a hall based computer, extra staff, and a video system. Outpatient therapists carp that all our elaborate inpatient efforts are not generalizable to the aftercare setting, but, if true, that is probably the case for most intensive inpatient endeavors and is not specific to a research setting.

In summary, any specialized unit represents a potential administrative and financial drain, a round peg in a square hole. Nevertheless, such programs should continue to be developed and nurtured, for they do return a great deal in other ways to the life of the institution. As places of training, they educate staff of all disciplines, exposing them to a kind of clinical experience which cannot be reproduced in any other setting. As a source of expertise, they provide the hospital with consultants who can share their experience with other staff. As a research environment, they generate curiosity and encourage study, thus serving to stimulate the intellectual life of the entire professional staff. And finally, as a testament to the devastation of mental illness and society's commitment to respond to the challenge, they represent hope, both to the patients themselves and for our profession as a whole.

REFERENCES

1. Strauss JS, Hafez H: Clinical questions and "real" research. Am J Psychiatry 1981; 138:1592-1597
2. Park LC, Slaughter R, Covi L, et al: The subjective experience of the research patient: an

investigation of psychiatric outpatients' reactions to the research treatment situation. J Nerv Ment Dis 1966; 143:199–206
3. Menninger K: Psychological factors in the choice of medicine as a profession. Bull Menninger Clin 1957; 21:51–58, 99–106
4. Post RM, Ballenger JC: Models for the progressive development of psychopathology: sensitization to electrical, pharmacological, and psychological stimuli, in Handbook of Biological Psychiatry, Vol. II. Edited by van Praag HM, Lade MH, Rafaelsen DJ et al, New York, Marcel Dekker, 1981
5. Docherty JP, Marder SR, van Kammen DP et al: Psychotherapy and pharmacotherapy: conceptual issues. Am J Psychiatry 1977; 134:529–533
6. Strauss JS, Carpenter WT, Jr: Schizophrenia. New York, Plenum, 1981
7. Broad WJ: The publishing game: getting more for less. Science 1981; 211:1137–1139
8. Miller RD, Strickland RN, Davidson J, et al: Characteristics of schizophrenic and depressed patients excluded from clinical research. Am J Psychiatry 1983; 140:1205–1207
9. Kramer DA, McKinney WT: The overlapping territories of psychiatry and ethology. J Nerv Ment Dis 1979; 167:3–22
10. Sacks M, Fink E, Carpenter WT, Jr: Functioning at the clinical-research interface: the clinical research meeting. Am J Psychiatry 1975; 132:919–923
11. Reich L, Weiss B: The clinical research ward as a therapeutic community: incompatibilities. Am J Psychiatry 1975; 132:48–55
12. Epstein R, Janowsky D: Research on the psychiatric ward: the effects of conflicting priorities. Arch Gen Psychiatry 1969; 21:455–463
13. McGlashan T, Carpenter WT, Jr: Does research interfere with patient care? Am J Psychiatry 1975; 132:975–976
14. Braff DL, Bachman J, Glick I, et al: The therapeutic community as a research ward: myths and facts. Arch Gen Psychiatry 1979; 36:355–360
15. Carpenter WT, Jr, Sacks MH, Strauss JS et al: Evaluating signs and symptoms: comparison of structured interview and clinical approaches. Br J Psychiatry 1976; 128:397–403

15
Regulation, Insurance, and the Medical Record

Robert W. Gibson
Lynn Flanigan

The encroachment upon psychiatric care in the modern psychiatric hospital by third-party payers—primarily through a paper review—is perceived by clinicians as at best a wasteful nuisance and at worst a mindless exercise that has run amok. Indeed, the process does at times feed upon itself. A popular slogan to mobilize clinicians is, "If we don't do it, 'they' will, so we must get into the process." We agree completely with this proposition but believe it misses the mark.

Utilization review in its various forms does encroach on the autonomy of those of us who provide services. But it also reflects the concerns of our times. Health care costs have increased at a staggering rate. In response there has been a demand for accountability by consumers, payers, legislators, and others. And we believe there are opportunities for alliances—rather than adversarial confrontations—that can constructively serve our patients, the payers and subscribers, the constituents of legislators, and we the providers. This chapter is not for or against regulation. It is a description of what exists, the dynamics, ways to respond, and suggestions for constructive alliances.

REGULATION

Psychiatric hospitals today are regulated directly and indirectly by a formidable array of agencies. The new demands for accountability pose especially difficult problems in the field of mental health, where outcome studies are inadequate, standards and criteria are still being developed, humanistic concerns are difficult to balance against cost-effectiveness, and the sensitivity of much of the information poses a serious threat to confidentiality.

Health care is being strangled by regulations that dig into every aspect of treatment through utilization review, determinations of medical necessity, standards for medical records, and even control of specific treatment modalities. Still other controls are aimed at protecting patients' rights, ensuring a safe environment, fixing hospital charges, and eliminating discrimination. Although well-intentioned, the controls often overlap, at times are contradictory, and contribute to the rising cost of care.

Acknowledging that government has the right to regulate hospitals, a New York State Hospital Association Task Force studying the impact of regulation wondered why 25 separate agencies must review hospital admitting procedures, 33 agencies protect patients' rights, and 31 agencies ensure patients' safety.[1] The task force found that during the preceding ten years, while the total number of employees in the state health departments went from 2,000 to 3,500, the number of accountants went from two to 170, and the number of attorneys went from three to 30, but the number of physicians declined from 69 to 60. The state's austerity budget called for 568 new regulatory positions in the department!

Furthermore, third-party payer review and increased regulation add to the cost of care. As new review requirements are added, staff manage for a time by working longer hours but ultimately must steal time from clinical assignments. As this begins to compromise the quality of care, more staff must be added to offset the regulatory demands. It is difficult to put an exact dollar figure on these added costs. Not only must new positions be added to handle the added administrative load, but clinicians and others throughout the system must also spend more time generating the documentation.

About ten years ago, Sheppard Pratt had an all-inclusive daily rate that did not break out services for specific charges. A major insurance carrier insisted on itemized billing for all services. For accurate cost accounting, the billing for specific services had to be recorded for all insurers. To do this required an added cost of $35,000 a year which, in today's dollars, would be closer to $100,000. Ironically, the insurer that had insisted on itemized billing had to pay more than under the all-inclusive rate.

In 1982 at Sheppard Pratt, we were forced by escalating costs to request a rate increase of 13% above and beyond inflation. Some of this increase was necessitated by shortening lengths of stay, more admissions, and more severely ill patients. But all clinicians found that the percentage of their time that could be devoted to direct clinical care had been significantly eroded.

Almost half of this 13% increase was caused by added requirements of documentation: more frequent treatment plan reviews, administrative hearings for involuntary admissions, more unit clerks to process paperwork for nursing staff, utilization review specialists to comply with federal and state legislation, and a great deal more. Some of this added documentation may improve the quality of care. Possibly, in the long run it may reduce the total costs of care even though the per diem is increased. But much of the added work is designed for one purpose only—to generate data that will provide a ready audit trail for accountants and others to use in their financial reviews.

Although regulators now espouse efficacy, patient satisfaction, and cost-effectiveness, the major target in years past has been safety. State and federal requirements have focused on physical standards—fire walls, width of doors, square feet per patient, sanitation, sprinkler systems, alarm systems, disaster drills, and the like—all of which are important. As treatment modalities have become more complex, the emphasis on safety standards unrelated to therapeutic values has become more irritating. Preoccupation with the multiple regulatory requirements can divert mental health professionals from their main goal of providing high quality treatment services appropriate to patients' needs. In exasperation, we protest that it has become more important to document that some arbitrary requirement has been met than to provide treatment that will be really helpful to the patient.

Should hospital accreditation by state, federal, and JCAH standards focus on whether there are thermometers in the refrigerator or on the quality of the treatment plans for specific patients? A safe environment is essential, but it should be a given—the modern psychiatric hospital can and should be safe. The regulatory thrust focused on safety should not be allowed to overshadow the more important issues of efficacy, patient satisfaction (including patients' rights), and the judicious use of resources to achieve cost-effective treatment.

CURRENT REGULATORY APPROACHES

For two decades the *utilization review* of psychiatric hospital treatment has been designed to control costs. It has included a wide variety of approaches by Medicare, CHAMPUS, Blue Cross, other commercial insurers, and more recently, self-insured employee plans.

At the very outset, in 1965, hospitals were required to establish utilization review programs to be eligible for reimbursement under Medicare and Medicaid. Utilization review as applied under Medicare and Medicaid was at best marginally effective. In an attempt to strengthen this system, Professional Standards Review Organizations (PSRO's) were developed in 1972 to provide timely review of services and to identify medically unnecessary admissions and services. On balance, the PSRO's failed to meet expectations.[2]

The utilization review approach was given new life in the Peer Review Improvement Act of 1982, which established Professional Review Organizations. The duties and functions of these organizations include implementation and operation of a review system to eliminate unreasonable, unnecessary, or inappropriate care to Medicare beneficiaries and to promote the quality of services.

Unfortunately, relatively few of the criteria relate to psychiatric hospitalizations; they are designed for general medical and surgical treatment. Indeed, the psychiatric hospital criteria proposed by the Maryland Foundation for Health Care (the statewide PRO up until October 1986) established standards only for admission, intensity of services required, and the need for continued stay. The maintenance of quality will rest upon the judgment of psychiatrists treating the patient. These same psychiatrists must simultaneously struggle against pressures to limit the scope and duration of treatment.

The review by third-party payers, for better or for worse, has had a major influence on hospital psychiatry. In the 1960s, when increases in the cost of health care accelerated, third-party payers tried various measures to contain costs: limitations on facilities to be paid, on the number of hospital days, on specific services; deductibles; higher co-insurance for psychiatric treatment than medical and surgical; exclusion of specific disorders, such as alcoholism; dollar limits per calendar year and for lifetime benefits. These restrictions were easy to administer. Professional review was not needed; a clerk could deny a claim.

Professional care providers objected to arbitrary limits that were based on a fixed number of days, deductibles, and co-insurance. Professionals argued, quite correctly, that these techniques did not address the needs of individual patients. A system that addresses the needs of patients requires the professional reviewer to decide if the hospital admission was medically necessary, if each specific service was medically necessary, and if the service was appropriate for the specific case and provided in accordance with accepted standards of practice. In addition, documentation that inpatient treatment was truly necessary and that day treatment or outpatient care would not be adequate for the particular problem is required.

In essence, the peer review approach requires standards and criteria for: medical necessity for hospitalization, appropriateness of the treatments provided, and the judgment that the patient will improve within a reasonable length of time. A clerk cannot make such judgments. Insurers are reluctant to accept this approach. When challenged, denials of payment based on such criteria create adverse publicity. Defending such denials in court is difficult. Nonetheless, the American Psychiatric Association (APA), after more than a decade of supporting peer review, has succeeded in getting many third-party payers to accept it.

THE INFLUENCE OF INSURERS ON HOSPITAL PRACTICE

An early example of how insurance decisions can influence the nature and quality of treatment occurred in 1972. The Federal Employees Program (FEP) Blue Cross Plan had been viewed by psychiatrists as a model program, because it provided coverage for mental illness on the same basis as medical and surgical conditions (inpatient psychiatric hospitalization when medically necessary was covered 365 days a year, and there was a correspondingly liberal outpatient benefit).

In 1972, when newspaper accounts suggested that the Blue Cross FEP might in a single year, lose some $60 million, denials, of psychiatric claims skyrocketed. The most common reason given for denials was that the treatment was primarily for milieu therapy. But milieu therapy was never defined. Blue Cross had accepted recommendations made by a consultant[3] that some treatment modalities, such as psychosurgery, insulin coma, electroshock treatment, and high-dose drug therapy, should be favored. The consultant had recommended denial of treatment approaches that stressed individual and group psychotherapy and low-dose drug therapy. These latter therapeutic approaches were equated with milieu therapy.

Paradoxically, the very programs the Blue Cross consultant advised against were advocated by the JCAH standards for psychiatric hospitals. Cost overruns, not patient need, were the driving force for the Blue Cross denials. Cost and quality were confounded in such a way as to give the impression that quality was the issue. In actuality, raising quality as an issue was a device to contain costs.

Again, in the mid-1970s, Blue Cross FEP was confronted by accelerating costs. This time, however, the claims review technique was not used. Instead, a sharp reduction in benefits was instituted, bringing the virtually unlimited inpatient benefit in any calendar year down to 60 days for the high option plan and only 30 days for the low option plan. In discussions involving officials of the Blue Cross FEP Plan and officers of the American Psychiatric Association, the fundamental distinction between the arbitrary limit approach (exclusively cost containment), and the medical necessity and appropriateness of care approach (utilization review to achieve cost containment and assure quality) was articulated.[4] In an effort to preserve quality while containing cost, the 60-day limit was withdrawn, with a return to the prior benefit capped by a $50,000 lifetime limit. An agreement was reached by Blue Cross and the APA to develop guidelines that could be used for peer review. This gave added impetus to the development by the APA of a system for peer review with standards by which reviewers could judge practice.

In 1977, the Department of Defense contracted with the American Psychiatric Association and the American Psychological Association to develop a peer review system that would deal with both quality assurance and cost containment. In developing the criteria and the system of review, the APA National Advisory Committee recognized that elimination of unnecessary or prolonged hospitalization would not only reduce costs but also improve quality. Elimination of medically unnecessary hospitalization not only saves money but assures that treatment is provided in the least restrictive environment.

In the APA CHAMPUS Peer Review Program, quality issues were dealt with directly. Reviewers did not simply approve or deny claims. They examined the specific treatment plan, progress notes, consultants' notes—sometimes, the whole medical record. Many professionals protested the imposition of what they called a "paper review," arguing that quality cannot be judged from the medical record alone. Experience has shown that quality can be assessed by a review of the medical record, but only after documentation has been focused on the critical issues.

ASSESSING QUALITY BY REVIEW OF THE MEDICAL RECORD

Quality can be assessed by reviewing the medical record in light of its inclusion of pertinent professional observations and treatment geared toward the specific nature of the individual's problems. Components of the medical record that are particularly important to comprehensive, quality medical records are the master treatment plan, treatment plan review, and progress notes by the various disciplines. In reviewing for quality, the flow of treatment is observed; it should lead directly and clearly from the master treatment plan, identifying problems and treatment approaches, through the progress notes, as a record of the efforts made by staff according to this process design, to the treatment plan review which evaluates and makes changes in the treatment approach. It is particularly important to establish a consistent approach to the treatment of an individual patient and to have this consistency established among the disciplines providing different elements of the treatment according to the master treatment plan.

The medical record is a good tool for the review of quality care but does have limitations; these are primarily associated with time constraints on professionals and ethical dilemmas related to confidentiality. Historically, the medical record was a repository for basic identifying and clarifying information regarding appointments and the dates that they were established and kept. In today's climate, the medical record must provide specific and legally defensible information regarding not only the professional assessments but also the treatment and follow-up of recommendations made by the primary caregivers, as well as any consultants involved in the treatment of a particular patient. The limitations of a written record are compounded by the unwritten assumptions of members of a treatment team and the failure to document what are thought to be obvious facets of a specialty program that are part of the basic program design. The dilemma for today's practitioner is that of trying to balance time spent with the patient delivering service with time spent with the record documenting each detail of the service offered.

The medical record can be a useful tool for assessment of quality care by documenting that recommendations by the treatment team have been carried out. It is essential that all treatment members follow a consistent plan for treatment based on the assessment of the patients needs. Denial decisions may stem from a lack of adequate documentation rather than differences in professional opinion. In the following case denial resulted from the peer reviewer's perception that the medical record documentation was inadequate to support continuing treatment as an inpatient.

> A middle-aged divorced male was referred for treatment of substance dependence. On intake, he presented with a significant history of substance dependence and emergent symptoms of depression, with decreased sleep and appetite and suicidal ideation. The symptoms of depression abated but new issues regarding his level of functioning at work and in social relationships emerged. Because continued stay criteria require documentation of symptoms and treatment of psychiatric problems in addition to the substance dependency, these emergent issues were recorded. When the case was referred to the physician advisor of the peer review agency, hospitalization was denied after detoxification due to inadequate documentation of psychiatric symptoms in addition to the substance dependency. The denial was appealed but upheld, and the patient was referred to an outpatient therapist and community support groups. The treatment team members were frustrated because they assessed the severity of non-substance-dependency problems as sufficient to warrant inpatient treatment and attempted to document this. The patient was not able to complete the inpatient program and establish a link with the outpatient therapist

prior to discharge. While the denial was based on inadequate documentation, there was also the issue of defining severity of symptoms to allow for congruent interpretation.

IMPACT OF ARBITRARY LIMITS

It is impossible to judge the full impact of the elimination of benefits for long-term (beyond 60 days) psychiatric hospitalization. Prior to the 1983 Blue Cross FEP and the 1983 CHAMPUS cutbacks, knowledgeable professionals guessed that 20–25 million individuals in this country had financial resources through insurance and personal funds to support psychiatric hospital treatment beyond 60 to 90 days. The Blue Cross and CHAMPUS cuts reduced this number by several million. Cuts by other insurers may have reduced to less than 2% of the population those individuals who can afford private psychiatric hospital care beyond 60 days.

What will happen to those patients who need but cannot afford long-term hospital treatment? Presumably, severely ill patients who fail to respond to short-term hospitalization will be referred to public mental hospitals for treatment. But the deinstitutionalization programs vigorously pursued by most states have reduced costs by eliminating the opportunity for long-term treatment. Admittedly, the length of treatment of less severely ill patients can be shortened by more rapid diagnostic workup and more intensive treatment. Psychiatric units in general hospitals are treating more patients on a short-term basis; their programs are often limited to symptom relief and stabilization. Some patients can be discharged from the hospital earlier if partial hospital services supported by transitional living and psychosocial programs have received only modest support to date from third-party payers. And in the end, some patients are resistant to treatment and will need longer periods of treatment within a hospital setting.

THE IMPACT OF CLAIMS REVIEW ON HOSPITAL PRACTICE

In general, when arbitrary lengths of stay are imposed and treatment is confined within narrow parameters, quality is compromised. Conversely, when a third-party payer permits longer stays monitored by peer review for medically necessary and appropriate treatment, the opportunity for quality is greatly enhanced. Whether it is considered quality assurance, utilization review, claims review, or managed care, the review process by a third-party payer will have a decisive influence on patterns of practice. The usual process for the review of a claim is as follows: An individual seeks help; a provider renders a service; the provider submits a request for payment to a third-party payer; an administrative review is made to determine if the treatment is medically necessary and appropriate; payment is either made or denied. The critical step in this review is the judgment of appropriateness of treatment. Over a period of time, pay/no-pay decisions about specific patients will shape patterns of policy. Reimbursements encourage, and denials discourage, the use of specific treatment modalities.

In treating a specific patient, psychiatrists can be relied upon to provide the treatment that in their clinical judgment is best for the patient despite an adverse decision by a third-party payer. Over a period of time, however, a continuing stream of denials dictated by cost will inevitably modify physician behavior. Claims review, driven solely by cost cutting, will not improve the quality of treatment; more likely, quality will be sacrificed. For example, denials are often based on a bias unrelated to the merits of the treatment. Adolescents are seen as troublesome delinquents, alcoholics as morally weak, and drug abusers as criminals. Claims review dictated by cost alone does not reflect or reinforce contemporary, state-of-the-art opinions about quality psychiatric care. It is not intended to promote quality. It is designed to reduce costs in response to the economic needs of the payers.

If judgments are made by administrators concerned primarily with cost containment or practitioners who do not represent the mainstream of professional thinking, the quality of psychiatric practice will be eroded. The APA Peer Review System for CHAMPUS was developed to maintain and improve quality by using reviewers judged by their peers to be outstanding practitioners. This system not only assures that clinical judgments about the treatment of individual patients are made by leaders of the psychiatric profession but also validates their judgments by using more than one reviewer. Utilizing outstanding psychiatric practitioners creates a dynamic system in which judgments will be responsive to changing patterns of practice. These safeguards are essential to assure that psychiatric practice will be shaped by day-to-day decisions made by competent professionals.

Many states have passed legislation requiring utilization review of all the admissions of all hospitals.[5] Large insurance carriers, Blue Cross and Blue Shield, for example, have also established utilization review programs for their own beneficiaries. Again, the review process focuses on medical necessity of admissions and continued stay.

With the emergence of multiple reviews by the hospital, the peer review agent, and the third-party payer, disparate criteria and rationale for review decisions have proliferated. Particularly since many hospitals receive patients from surrounding states, there is great potential for conflicting review opinions. While many programs utilize professionals to perform reviews, the diversity of psychiatric practice and the difficulty in establishing psychiatric practice standards have contributed to the complexity in arriving at concurrence regarding the best treatment approach and setting for a given patient.

An out-of-state adolescent male was referred for long-term treatment from a state hospital following four short-term hospitalizations. His insurance plan required preauthorization and concurrent continued stay review by telephone. The severity of the patient's symptoms met the admission criteria for both the hospital and peer review agent, so he was admitted. While continuing to demonstrate bizarre self-destructive and aggressive behavior meeting the diagnostic criteria for a diagnosis of schizotypal/personality disorder, he clearly met the continued stay criteria for the hospital. However, in continued stay requests with the peer review agency, continued hospitalization was denied after three weeks on the basis that the reviewer believed the patient could be treated in residential care and that he was not responding to long-term hospitalization! This decision was appealed to the medical director of the insurance carrier who upheld the denial decision and further stated that long term hospitalization would not be approved for treatment of any personality disorders. The patient was discharged following a family meeting which focused on discussion of other means of support for hospitalization (which were unavailable) and post-discharge treatment options.

THE MARYLAND EXPERIENCE

In Maryland, the private psychiatric hospitals and Blue Cross have established a closer collaborative relationship through a joint utilization review program. Psychiatrists for the hospitals and Blue Cross staff have jointly developed standards and criteria for review. At regular meetings, there is mutual feedback on the findings. This kind of dialogue has provided an opportunity to balance quality considerations against cost-cutting. Criteria for admission and continued stay have been developed for specific population groups commonly admitted to the private psychiatric hospital setting. These include criteria for substance dependency, adult admissions, and child and adolescent admissions (see Table 1, 2, and 3). As specialty programs, such as those for eating disorders, evolve, additional criteria targeted toward these specialty populations may be needed.

There are two primary ways of approaching review for care rendered, one being a concurrent review process, and the second being retrospective. The Blue Cross program in Maryland has been designed to be primarily a concurrent review whereby medical records are reviewed during the stay of a patient beginning with the fourteenth day of care and repeated on a 30-day interval for each case. This has allowed for ongoing current discussion with a physician advisor, when necessary, and has changed the third-party role from that of a paper-oriented adversary to a collegial consultant. This has

Table 1
Psychiatric Hospitalization Criteria for Substance Dependency

Admission to a psychiatric hospital is appropriate for alcohol and/or drug dependency of a severity which requires intensive intervention by a multidisciplinary health care team including physicians, nurses, counselors, social workers and other therapists. Severity of the illness is evidenced through the following criteria.

I. *Criteria for admission*
   A. Patient requires treatment for alcohol and/or drug dependency and has additional psychiatric symptomatology as documented by his or her ability to meet one of the criteria in Sections I or II of the Adult Psychiatric Hospitalization Criteria or the Child and Adolescent Psychiatric Hospitalization Criteria.
   B. Patients admitted for detoxification of alcohol and/or drug dependency shall be medically cleared by a physician.

II. *Criteria for continued stay*
   The treatment plan should include documentation, for both the substance dependency disorder and the psychiatric symptoms, of individualized goals of treatment and therapeutic modalities. The medical record should include, at a minimum, weekly patient progress notes by the psychiatrist or psychologist.

   While weekly documentation may justify the need for continued hospitalization, Blue Cross and Blue Shield expects that each service rendered by a physician or other provider of care and reported to the Plans for payment be documented in the medical record.

   In addition, criteria A through D from Section III of the Adult Psychiatric Hospitalization Criteria or the Child and Adolescent Psychiatric Hospitalization Criteria apply.

Copyright, Blue Cross of Maryland, 1986.

greatly enhanced the acceptance of the review program by practitioners within the hospital and has enabled ongoing communication and feedback to and from Blue Cross regarding the appropriateness of their professional assessments vis-à-vis those of the providers within the hospital setting.

Many hospitals are still dealing with the retrospective review mode as established by the peer review organizations for Medicare. This remains a difficult, after-the-fact type of review, whereby cases are often reviewed months after the treatment has been concluded, and there is no opportunity for discussion that might improve the treatment as it is delivered. From the provider's vantage the difference between these two programs is that of being put at risk for all days of care rendered in a retrospective review versus being liable for smaller portions of the treatment, particularly for a long-term type of facility, in a concurrent review.

Under the Maryland Blue Cross system, the medical records of all patients covered by Blue Cross are reviewed at the hospital every few weeks by a utilization review specialist from Blue Cross. Questions related to documentation, treatment plans, discharge plans, and the like can be discussed with

Table 2
Adult Psychiatric Hospitalization Criteria

Medical necessity of psychiatric inpatient admission must be documented based on conditions defined under either Section I or Section II.

I. *Criteria for admission based on severity of illness*
   A. Patient makes direct threats or a reasonable inference of serious harm to self or to the body or property of others.
   B. Violent, unpredictable or uncontrolled behavior, including patients with organic brain impairment and functional illness.
   C. Lack of insight, unwillingness or inability to adequately care for one's physical needs. Acute cases may include starvation or failure to take essential medications accurately and safely.
   D. Lack of response to previously attempted outpatient management of medication and/or psychotherapy.
   E. Mental or emotional impairment of the degree which severely interferes with social, familial or occupational functioning.

II. *Criteria for admission based on intensity of service*
   A. Need for continuous skilled observation (such as, but not limited to):
      1. to confirm diagnosis;
      2. to initiate medication regime;
      3. to regulate dosage of potent medication; or
      4. to withdraw potent medication.
   B. Need for electroconvulsive shock therapy.
   C. Where diagnostic assessment or treatment is not available or is unsafe on an outpatient basis.

III. *Criteria for continued stay*

The treatment plan should include documentation of diagnoses, individualized goals of treatment and therapeutic modalities. The medical record should include, at a minimum, weekly patient progress notes by the psychiatrist or psychologist.

While weekly documentation may justify the need for continued hospitalization, Blue Cross and Blue Shield expects that each service rendered by a physician or other provider of care and reported to the Plans for payment be documented in the medical record.

   A. The persistence of the problems that necessitated the admission, despite therapeutic efforts, or the emergence of additional problems consistent with the admission criteria.
   B. Severe reaction to the medication or need for further monitoring and adjustment of dosage.
   C. Attempts at therapeutic re-entry into the community have resulted in exacerbation of the psychiatric illness.
   D. Psychiatric evidence or rationale indicating the need for stabilization of patient's condition to a point where stress of community re-entry does not substantially risk an exacerbation of the psychiatric illness.

Copyright, Blue Cross of Maryland, 1986.

Table 3
Child and Adolescent Psychiatric Hospitalization Criteria

Medical necessity of psychiatric inpatient admission must be documented based on conditions defined under Section I or Section II.

I. *Criteria for Admission Based on Severity of Illness*
   A. Patient makes direct threats or a reasonable inference of serious harm to self or to the body or property of others.
   B. Violent, unpredictable or uncontrolled behavior, including patients with organic brain impairment and functional illness.
   C. Lack of insight, unwillingness or inability to adequately care for one's physical needs. Acute cases may include over- or undereating, running away, sexual acting out or failure to take essential medications accurately and safely.
   D. Lack of response to previously attempted outpatient management of medication and/or psychotherapy or to previous short-term psychiatric hospitalizations.
   E. Mental or emotional impairment of the degree which severely interferes with social, familial, scholastic or occupational functioning.

II. *Criteria for Admission Based on Intensity of Service*
   A. Need for continuous skilled observation (such as, but not limited to):
      1. to confirm diagnosis;
      2. to initiate medication regime;
      3. to regulate dosage of potent medication; or
      4. to withdraw potent medication.
   B. Where diagnostic assessment or treatment are not available or are unsafe on an outpatient basis.

III. *Criteria for continued stay*

The treatment plan should include documentation of diagnoses; individualized goals of treatment; and therapeutic modalities. The medical record should include, at a minimum, weekly patient progress notes by the psychiatrist or psychologist.

While weekly documentation may justify the need for continued hospitalization, Blue Cross and Blue Shield expects that each service rendered by a physician or other provider of care and reported to the Plans for payment be documented in the medical record.

   A. The persistence of the problems or maladaptive behavior that necessitated the admission, despite therapeutic efforts, or the emergence of additional problems consistent with the admission criteria.
   B. Severe reaction to the medication or need for further monitoring and adjustment of dosage.
   C. Psychiatric evidence or rationale indicating the need for stabilization of patient's condition to a point where stress of community re-entry does not substantially risk an exacerbation of the psychiatric illness.
   D. Attempts at therapeutic re-entry into the family, school and community have resulted in exacerbation of the psychiatric illness as manifested by regression in behavior and return to the maladaptive behavior and symptoms.

Copyright, Blue Cross of Maryland, 1986.

the hospital utilization review specialist or, if necessary, with the patient's doctor.

Some themes have emerged from our experience with the concurrent review process to date. Commonly identified elements of treatment that must be documented include:

1. initiating discharge-planning early in treatment;
2. establishing consistency throughout the treatment relating progress notes to the master treatment plan or treatment plan review;
3. demonstrating communication among the various disciplines so that differences in observations are identified and promptly resolved;
4. clearly identifying the rationale for absences from the therapeutic setting, such as the use of sign-outs or leaves of absence;
5. demonstrating that such experiences outside of the therapeutic setting will be used to determine whether additional stay is justified and;
6. clearly identifying the plans of the treatment team in response to specialty consultations or reevaluations done by a practitioner outside of the treatment team. These chart reviews have highlighted the need to develop standardized information for specialty programs so that the practitioner can focus on the specific needs of the patient rather than spending time documenting the basic elements of a specialty program.

If these observations are included in the record looked at by a nurse reviewer, there is generally a straightfoward continuity of process established and a clear understanding by an outsider of the evolution of treatment and the changes necessitated by the progress or regress of a given patient. When the nurse reviewer is able to locate all of the information regarding the questions identified above, there is generally no need for the record to be referred to a physician adviser for consultation with the treating therapist.

If the Blue Cross utilization review specialist has a question about a patient's treatment, the case is referred to the Blue Cross psychiatric consultant, who in turn will consult with the treating therapist. As long as denials remain under 2% of the patient days for the three-month review period, all claims are paid. If denials exceed 2%, the denied days exceeding 2% are not paid, and the hospital does not seek payment from the patient. During the seven months of the program to date, hospitals have remained under the 2% denial. Most importantly, the process has moved away from an adversarial confrontation toward a collegial consultation.

Frequently, the Blue Cross consultant and the therapist discuss plans for discharge in an attempt to reach a mutually agreeable approach that will stay within the constraints of the patient's insurance policy. This type of interaction has some elements of what is now being called "managed care."

MANAGED CARE

There are many programs being developed today to address the concept of managed care, including an individual case management program put together by several of the major insurance companies. Generally, these programs are designed to assist with contract revisions or exceptions that may offer a patient the opportunity to have services which are not ordinarily covered under a basic contract but which are cost-effective for the employer who is the purchaser of the contract. An example might be the funding for halfway house or residential placement instead of inpatient intensive treatment. The working relationship usually involves the primary caregiver and a nurse affiliated with an insurance carrier, who considers the former's recommendations regarding the patient's ability to move to a lower level of care and the time frame, within which this would be appropriate. This individual case manager then takes a proposal back to the employer outlining how an exception to a basic contract would be cost-effective and save money in the long run.

One of the more common new product structures in response to cost containment has been the involvement of a peer review agency or *fourth party* as a gatekeeper for contract benefits. Usually, this type of arrangement requires preadmission approval and ongoing concurrent monitoring, usually conducted via telephone review, with a member of the hospital staff collecting data to relate to the peer review agent at the time of the telephone contact. This off-site review has the potential difficulty of requiring information that is not present in the medical record documentation. Our experience suggests that the contacts with external review agencies should be centralized to ensure that information is taken directly from the written documentation rather than from a verbal report by a practitioner unfamiliar with the process. This is essential, since these review programs usually provide for spotchecks of actual documentation to verify that what was reported through the telephone review process was accurate.

Most hospitals are now dealing with the issue of on-site versus off-site review. In on-site review, a representative of the peer review agency (fourth party) or the insurance carrier actually visits the facility, reviews records directly, and possibly interacts with staff. For psychiatric facilities, on-site review must be conducted in a way that protects patients' privacy and provides a quiet atmosphere for the reviewer. In our experience, this has been managed by having work space available in the utilization review department. Medical records personnel pull the charts from the patient hall according to a schedule that has been coordinated with the halls and bring them to the reviewer. The original order sheet and most recent progress note sheets are left on the hall in a folder with a note indicating that the case is being reviewed and listing two telephone numbers so that the chart can be located and returned to the hall in the event of an emergency. Charts are returned to the patient halls as soon as possible after the reviews are completed.

Off-site review is traditionally managed by having a request for copies of documentation, which are then sent to the review agent; feedback is delayed due to the mail process and time for the review itself. As mentioned above, much off-site review is now conducted by telephone. Many cost containment contracts require preadmission authorization and concurrent review by telephone. The frequency of contacts is determined by the length of stay assigned by the reviewer and may be as often as every three days. For most of these programs, written verification of the approved days is sent to the beneficiary with a copy to the provider. Such frequent review has had a subtly negative impact on the therapeutic relationship, since many patients are anxious about the potential discontinuation of approval and the short length of stay approved. Some patients have experienced such an increase in stress due to the potential financial burden if the recommended continued stay were not approved that they have not been able to invest in the therapeutic alliance or to benefit fully from the treatment offered.

Telephone review has posed some new problems for the psychiatric provider, particularly regarding confidentiality. The provision for preadmission contact and exchange of demographic information has been obtained. Most insurance contracts with preadmission requirements assign the responsibility for this interaction to the beneficiary. This poses problems for psychiatry in that the beneficiary becomes the patient whose symptoms impair judgment and management of basic responsibilities. If the provider of care is unable to make this contact on behalf of the patient, many contracts have financial penalties which increase the deductible or decrease the percentage of coverage for services.

This problem is minimized when it is recognized that psychiatric admissions cannot be planned or anticipated. Psychiatric crises are often life-threatening and treatment cannot be delayed for planning of financial coverage. State laws mandate treatment regardless of payment, and contracts with preadmission requirements make provision for telephone contact within 48 hours following an urgent or emergency admission. This allows time to secure a written release of information and the demographic and clinical information necessary for approval.

For those cases where the admission can be delayed, a preadmission interview is recommended. During this interview the potential patient can be asked to sign a release of information permitting the provider to make the necessary contacts without breaching confidentiality or violating the patients' rights. A preadmission interview also provides an opportunity to discuss the preadmission requirement and assign the responsibility for making the required notification.

It is recommended that the responsibility for making phone contact for preadmission and concurrent review be centralized through the utilization review staff. When this is not permitted by the peer review agent, who may insist on speaking with the primary therapist, it is important to have a utilization review coordinator monitor the case and remind the therapist when contacts are due and that the verbal report must agree with the written documentation.

PROSPECTIVE PRICING SYSTEMS AND HOSPITAL PSYCHIATRY

Amendments to the Social Security Law in 1983 established a prospective pricing system for treatment provided under the Medicare program. Prospective pricing is designed to reward hospitals which keep their costs below Medicare's present prices. At the heart of this is a methodology known as Diagnosis-Related Groups (DRG's); these establish norms for total costs of the treatment of a specific group of diagnostically related conditions.

The DRG approach has had a profound impact on the occupancy of general medical-surgical hospitals. Free-standing psychiatric hospitals and psychiatric units of general hospitals meeting certain requirements have received waivers pending further study. The limited experience with DRG's in the psychiatric hospitals makes it difficult to anticipate the full impact if the prospective pricing system comes to be applied to all psychiatric hospital treatment. It is reasonable to assume, however, that DRG's as proposed would virtually eliminate long-term hospital treatment. It appears that norms for the length of stay and costs of the psychiatric conditions may be established largely through experience in psychiatric units of general hospitals. Lengths of stay under the DRG's currently used in general hospital units are exceedingly short: depressive neuroses—9.4 days; psychoses—10.8 days; alcohol dependence—8.1 days; and childhood disorders—15.4 days. Absolute cutoff dates range from 24 to 35 days.[6] For practical purposes, treatment beyond 30 days would be eliminated.

In some measure, the present norms are adequate for symptom relief and stabilization. Most patients, even those who are severely ill, respond to neuroleptics in a relatively short period of time. Long-term reconstructive and rehabilitative treatment designed to achieve increased capacity to tolerate stress, improved impulse control, and greater coping abilities usually takes longer. Improved intrapsychic and interpersonal functioning is essential. Such changes require ego growth and psychological maturation achieved through acquired interpersonal and adaptive skills. Conflict resolution is not enough. It takes time and therapeutic milieu to establish the psychotherapeutic relationship essential to reconstructive, rehabilitative treatment. Psychiatric hospitals offering intermediate to long-term care have programs specifically designed to achieve significant change and lasting results.

The prospective pricing approach utilizing DRG's has strong economic incentives to provide less intensive and shorter-term care. Such a system relies heavily on the commitment of professionals to preserve quality care despite economic disincentives. Given the varied opinions about what constitutes quality psychiatric care and the inherent methodological difficulties in evaluating it, psychiatrists are concerned that the DRG approach, if applied to psychiatric hospitals as it now is applied to general hospital units, will seriously undermine quality.

The National Association of Psychiatric Hospitals,[7] the American Psychiatric Association,[8] NIMH through a contract with Macro Systems,[9] and other organizations have conducted extensive studies on psychiatric DRG's. Using different data bases and different methodologies, all of these studies arrived at the same conclusions:

1. The existing psychiatric DRG's explain only 3-7% of the variance of length of stay and resource utilization for the treatment of psychiatric patients.[9] Introducing additional elements into the system can improve the predictability of resource utilization but only marginally.

2. Application of the present psychiatric DRG system would result in a systematic redistribution of resources. Specialized psychiatric facilities, larger general hospitals with discrete psychiatric units, and teaching hospitals would be penalized. There is no evidence to suggest that application of the psychiatric DRG's to all hospitals would improve the psychiatric delivery system. Indeed, the studies all indicate that universal application of the DRG's would cause a serious erosion in the quality of care.

3. Whatever approach is ultimately utilized, it will be essential to have utilization review programs that can truly measure whether the pressure for cost containment erodes quality. The assumption that erosion of quality will be prevented by the clinical judgment of individual practitioners is absurd. Such an assumption ignores the complex interplay of variables outside the control of the treating physicians, as well as the economic and political dynamics of the health care system.

Although the DRG's apply only to payments under Medicare, they are being expanded. Maryland has applied the DRG limits to Medicaid patients in general hospitals, while some states have applied DRG limits to all payers.

This is understandable, because Blue Cross and commercial carriers fear that they will be expected to subsidize losses incurred under Medicare. We must assume that all inpatient psychiatric care will be affected by prospective pricing utilizing DRG's. The outcome of future studies of DRG's by DHHS, NAPPH, and the APA is critical to the quality of all inpatient psychiatric treatment. In addition, there is likely to be a spillover to outpatient and partial hospitalization treatment.

It is generally believed that capitation would be more effective than prospective pricing. Under such a system, the provider of services agrees to deliver all necessary services to a defined population for a fixed charge. This creates an economic incentive to provide services at the lowest cost. It also creates an incentive to provide as few services as possible. The assumption is that professional and ethical integrity will prevent clinicians from undertreating. This proposition has yet to be conclusively tested. In fact, there is a growing concern that financial pressures have led to discharges that are "sicker and quicker."

THE FUTURE

The pressure to cut costs by reducing the length of hospital stay the amount of outpatient services is of concern to all medical specialties, but it poses particular difficulties for psychiatry. Medical necessity for psychiatric treatment, whether inpatient or outpatient, is difficult to define. There is little clamor by the consumer for psychiatric services; those who have not suffered a psychiatric illness deny that they ever will. Those who have had psychiatric treatment are reluctant to come forward because of the stigma.

Health maintenance organizations (HMOs) have minimal benefits, ranging from 30 days inpatient and 20 outpatient visits to virtually none. In addition, they add co-insurance payments, exclude patients with prior illness, and have relatively low lifetime limits. Obviously, the HMO is not for the person with a severe mental illness. Such individuals may now be able to get coverage by a carrier that provides adequate mental health benefits. But as HMO subscribers increase in number, this will lead to adverse selection, pushing more of those needing psychiatric treatment to a dwindling number of carriers providing adequate mental health benefits. In time, these carriers will have to reduce benefits to remain competitive.

With fewer and fewer individuals able to afford private treatment for long-term illness, private psychiatric hospitals will move away from the more intensive treatment programs for the severely ill. This will place an increasing burden on the public hospitals, which are already under great pressure to reduce occupancy with programs of deinstitutionalization. Clearly, the moves toward greater regulation and various devices for changing the delivery system to reduce costs will place increasing demands on the psychiatric hospital.

REFERENCES

1. Hospital Association of New York State Task Force on Regulations, 1976
2. Medical World News. HEW, too, says, PSRO's don't save money, Nov 28, 1977
3. Lahar E: Psychiatric Care Manual. Chicago, Blue Cross Association, 1973
4. Westlake, RJ (Editor): Shaping The Future of Mental Health Care. Cambridge MA, Ballinger Publishing Company, 1976, pp 78–79
5. Maryland State Department of Health and Mental Hygiene, Maryland Register Vol 12, Issue 8
6. Federal Register, Rules and regulations. 48, 171, Washington, 39885, 1983
7. The National Association of Private Psychiatric Hospitals' Prospective Payment Study Final Report, Rockburn Institute. Lewin and Associates, 1985
8. American Psychiatric Association. Findings and Conclusions of the American Psychiatric Association Study & Evaluation of the Medicare Prospective Payment System-Diagnosis Related Groups and Psychiatric Patients, 1985
9. Health Economics Research, Inc., Health Data Institute, Inc., Marco Systems Inc. A Study of Patient Classification Systems for Prospective Rate-Setting for Medicare Patients in General Hospital Psychiatric Units and Psychiatric Hospitals, 1985

16
Forensic Issues

Jonas R. Rappeport

In any society human rights and human freedom are of major importance and must be kept in balance with the general needs of the state and society. No other medical specialty comes as close to invading as many of the inalienable rights of man as psychiatry does. The right to be left alone, the right to think, and the right to act within certain limits are a part of this freedom.

These freedom issues arise in hospital psychiatry with reference to admission, release, and the rights that the patient has in the hospital vis-à-vis clothing, mail, contact with attorney, right to treatment and right to refuse that treatment, confidentiality of patient communications and records, and use of restraint and seclusion. The rights of the hospital staff to carry out their duties without unnecessary controls and restrictions and without placing them at risk of both physical and legal (malpractice) harm are also important.

This chapter will discuss those areas in which the law touches upon hospital psychiatry, covering the major issues and including some recommended solutions, as well as further readings should there be a need for more information.[1,2]

HOSPITALIZATION

Voluntary

The majority of patients admitted to a psychiatric hospital enter on a voluntary basis in the same fashion that they would enter any hospital for care. However, unlike general hospital patients, voluntary *psychiatric* patients must sign an agreement that they will give notice of their desire to leave. Although this is in a sense a contract, it is not really enforceable in a court of law. The purpose of the voluntary commitment agreement is to allow the hospital time (usually 72 hours) to decide whether or not to release the patient outright or against medical advice (AMA) or to arrange for commitment according to appropriate local laws. When a 72-hour or three-day notice is presented, the doctor must assess the situation clinically. Some considerations are: Is the patient suicidal or homicidal? Is the patient likely to be a danger to himself or to the person or property of others? Is the patient in such need of continued hospitalization that it would be "wrong" to allow him to leave? These are some of the criteria of "dangerousness" to be considered for commitment. Only when a psychiatrist is convinced that the patient *must* remain in the hospital would a move for commitment be made. Before undertaking such action, the family or others to whom the patient may listen should be recruited to try to convince the patient to withdraw the three-day notice and remain in the hospital voluntarily. Failing all efforts to have the "dangerous" patient remain voluntarily, the appropriate involuntary commitment process would then be undertaken. This scenario can of course occur at any time during a hospitalization, but usually occurs early, before a therapeutic alliance has been established.

Patients who submit a three-day notice are usually released. On rare occasions the psychiatrist may be faced with a patient who is believed to be particularly dangerous and yet demands immediate release "at the moment." Such patients may assault staff members if the door is not unlocked. Firmly believing (with the aid of consultation from a colleague) that the patient cannot be safely released, the psychiatrist in charge must utilize emergency action by staff and, if necessary, assistance from hospital security, depending on previously established hospital policy. As stated, the need for such extreme action is rare. In fact, when such a situation does occur, staff should evaluate what went wrong to create such an impasse.

Certain types of voluntary patients frequently give three-day notices: alcoholics, addicts, some paranoid schizophrenics and manic patients. Hospital policy will determine whether or not to ever admit such patients voluntarily. Patients with personality disorders may use the three-day notice in a manipulative or controlling fashion which must be appreciated by the clinician. As a means of dealing with these patients who abuse voluntary commitment, some hospitals have the patient sign a "contract" to stay a specified time. While some of these patients will adhere to the agreed-upon time, others may disregard the contracts they signed and demand to leave. Since these patients do not meet the involuntary commitment requirements, it is wise to allow them to leave. (Clinical problems associated with the patient's abuse of the three-day notice are discussed in Chapter 6).

Involuntary — Two Physicians' Certificates

Every jurisdiction has some form of involuntary commitment. In all 50 states this involuntary commitment requires that two physicians (or one M.D. and one Ph.D.) who have examined the patient document that the patient suffers from a mental disorder that requires inpatient hospitalization as the least restrictive alternative because the patient represents a danger to himself or others or is unable to care for himself adequately. While the exact wording of the requirements in a particular state may vary from this, the concept is essentially the same.

Involuntary commitment is based on two legal concepts: *parens patriae* and the police power of the state. Under the *parens patriae* principle, the state has the duty to protect its citizens who are unable to adequately care for themselves. This would apply to the infant, the orphan, the blind, the severely handicapped, and the mentally retarded, as well as the severely mentally ill. Although such protection is primarily a family's duty, for various reasons the family may not be able to assume this responsibility; thus, the duty falls upon the state: *parens patriae* — the state is the parent. Under the police power principle, the state has the duty to prevent one citizen from harming another, that is, to prevent the dangerous or violent individual from harming others and/or destroying others' property. This is a part of the state's duty to maintain peace and protect its citizens from harm.

Under *parens patriae* the patient is a danger to himself or herself, as in suicide, or is unable to adequately care for his or her own welfare as to food, clothing, and housing or (more liberally interpreted) unable to accept the treatment he or she needs to become well. Under the police power principle the patient is a danger to the person or property of others (assault, malicious destruction, etc). The specific legal meaning of the word "dangerous" for the purposes of involuntary commitment varies from state to state based upon the actions of courts and legislatures. Such criteria attempt to balance the community's concerns about taking away certain human freedoms with the protection of the community. Applicable commitment requirements should be available at all psychiatric hospitals. An excellent compendium of most mental health laws has been published by the American Bar Association.[3]

Involuntary commitment by two certificates is now limited to a brief period of time (3-14 days), following which a hearing is required before either a specially designated administrative officer or a judge of the probate or district court. At such a hearing the judicial authority determines whether the patient should be kept in the hospital for an additional period of time (15 days to six months). It is necessary to consult the specific law applicable, as such laws vary. Some jurisdictions require a hearing prior to any hospitalization, except in extreme emergencies. At these hearings the patient is usually represented by counsel and the hospital should also be so represented. However, in most cases the hospital is represented by a social worker or physician, who presents the clinical evaluation to the hearing officer. The patient's attorney closely scrutinizes the commitment papers to be sure that they are in order. On occasion, just because a date is wrong or there is an improper signature or inadequate information, the hearing officer has released the patient. This is more likely to happen if the patient's attorney is very aggressive in presenting such deficiencies. After carefully hearing the evidence, most hearing officers utilize good "clinical judgment" and attempt to work out an arrangement so that the patient receives care and is not placed at risk.

The following example illustrates a hypothetical commitment hearing:

> A 47-year-old female patient has been committed on two certificates as a danger to herself following an overdose of aspirin in an apparent suicide attempt. The commitment hearing occurs after five days of hospitalization. At that time she says that she is ready to leave the hospital: "It won't happen again." However, when the doctor testifies, he says that this is the third time she has overdosed and each time has been more serious. On the two previous occasions that the patient was hospitalized, she was released by a hearing officer and did not follow through with her promise to seek outpatient treatment. The doctor believes that with 30 more days in the hospital it may be possible to establish a therapeutic relationship and assist the patient in recognizing the need to continue treatment.

The hearing officer must decide what is in the patient's best interest. She is not a threat to the community (police power), so this is a *parens patriae* issue. What decision will best protect the patient's freedom and individual rights and at the same time prevent her suicide? These are not easy decisions for the hearing officer. The patient's attorney may argue strongly for the patient's right to determine what she does with her life, and he may try to assure the court that the patient will, this time, follow through with outpatient treatment. This then places a burden on the doctor to convince the hearing officer that continued hospitalization is "best."

Since physicians (and other mental health professionals) are not trained to advocate their positions, participation in such hearings may require the development of new talents. Therefore, it is incumbent upon the hospital physician to learn how best to participate in this adversarial process. A good way to learn is by carefully observing colleagues and attorneys and the subtle techniques they use.[4] It could be argued that we should do no more than present our diagnosis and the reasons why we believe continued hospitalization is necessary. However, some psychiatrists believe that the physician's duty requires that all reasonable and ethical efforts be exerted to convince the hearing officer of the need for continued hospitalization. Otherwise the system is out of balance because the patient's attorney is ethically obligated to present the patient's wishes as strongly as possible.

Emergency Commitment or Detention On occasion a disturbed patient may be totally uncooperative and refuse to even be examined or to allow friends or relatives to provide transportation to the doctor's office or hospital. Under these circumstances, all jurisdictions have a means of obtaining police help to get the patient to a place where he can be examined and/or have an immediate hearing. Again, states vary quite a bit as to particulars. For example, in Maryland a relative, friend, psychiatrist, psychologist, police officer, or judge can petition a judge to issue a warrant in order to allow the police to transport the patient to a designated facility, usually an emergency room, if this person can convince the judge that the patient is an imminent danger to himself/herself or others. At the designated facility, two clinicians will evaluate the patient. If the patient still refuses to enter the hospital voluntarily and meets the requirements for involuntary hospitalization, the two physicians sign certificates and the police or family can then transfer the patient to the hospital. There the patient will be treated as any other involuntary patient and have a hearing in five days.

Testifying at a Commitment Hearing

The law is interested in specifics and not in vague, loose, ill-defined, unproven concepts. The hearing officer must make decisions based on as many facts as possible. The decision is a subjective one and therefore calls for considering as much information as time will allow. The role of the person testifying is to do his best to educate both the attorneys and the hearing officer. They do not understand mental illness and must be helped to appreciate what various signs, symptoms and diagnoses mean. Psychiatrists are trained to evaluate the patient's illness, arrive at a diagnosis and develop a treatment plan. Issues of dangerousness and freedom are foreign to the doctor and not essential for the treatment goal. As stated, the hearing officer must balance issues of freedom and self-determination versus detention and loss of freedom based on a vague concept called "dangerousness." While the physician might think that the loss of freedom is best determined medically, the hearing officer might not believe that the doctor's opinion best determines the legal issue. Most commitment laws require the hearing officer to more or less base the decision solely on the issue of dangerousness and not on what the hearing officer might think is best for the patient.

There are ways by which the physician testifying can try to clarify facts about the patient's illness and how it will affect the patient's behavior. A hypothetical example:

> A 25-year-old male, after ingesting an overdose of a tricyclic antidepressant which had been prescribed by his physician, was committed on two certificates from an emergency room five days earlier. He had been depressed for two months following problems arising from his father's dislike of his girlfriend. At the hearing he says he is sorry and will never do such a thing again and now recognizes that his father is right. His attorney says that the patient and his father have a new understanding about the girlfriend and the patient and his father agree. The psychiatrist believes that the patient continues to love his girlfriend and that the family conflict and his patient's inability to deal with it will continue unless the patient receives psychotherapy. This would best be started by a longer period of hospitalization.

What the hearing officer needs to understand from the psychiatrist is as much about the patient's personality structure as is necessary to allow him to estimate the risk to the patient of discharge at this time. The hearing officer would like to know how the patient's dependent relationship with his father might affect the patient's future behavior. What likelihood or what degree of certainty is there for a repetition of the suicide attempt given all that is known? The psychiatrist may need to quantify the chances of the father not continuing his need for control. The hearing officer needs to have an understanding of why inpatient treatment is necessary and why outpatient treatment is not yet appropriate. Will the treatment plan reduce the chances of further suicide attempts, and how likely is it that these efforts will succeed? Obviously, information on other aspects of the problem would also help the hearing officer make a decision — one, we would hope, in agreement with the psychiatrist's opinion. All of this needs to be said without professional jargon and while the patient is present.

If testimony is given in a speculative fashion, the hearing officer may reject such testimony as being vague, inconclusive, and speculative. The hearing officer wants to hear examples of the patient's past dependent behavior. The hearing officer also wants to hear about articles published in the last 10 years in accepted psychiatric journals and in the recognized textbooks which support the psychiatrist's views and not the plan proposed by the patient's attorney. It is difficult for the patient's lawyer to negate clear, concise, and convincing testimony. The hearing officer wants to hear facts, specifics, important details, etc. Although this does place a heavy burden on the physician, many believe that it is a part of the treatment responsibility.

Many times in hearings psychiatrists have the feeling that patients have managed to fool hearing officers. Such patients have been able to present themselves in a fashion that sounds quite reasonable to anyone who is not clinically sophisticated, as in the case of the previously mentioned suicidal woman who said, "It won't happen again." This may be particularly true of paranoid, hypomanic, or suicidal patients. Doctors need only to remember early in their careers when they were fooled by such patients. Hearing officers similarly lack clinical experience. Fortunately, they have the clinician to help them learn about mental illness and the need for inpatient care for certain patients.

It must be remembered that the only patients having hearings will be those involuntarily committed who refuse to stay voluntarily. It is important to have a good history in order to point out specific incidents to the hearing officer. Clinically the psychiatrist may not want to focus on the patient's past failures for therapeutic reasons and for fear of losing the patient. However, if he doesn't present the facts to the hearing officer, the patient may be released and never enter treatment.

For example, in rendering testimony the psychiatrist might describe a suicidal patient's actual statements at the time of admission: "I'll do better next time; you wait and see." To counter the patient's current claim of recovery with no future suicidal ideation, the clinician could quote from the literature that there is a proven clinical concept which states that a suicidal patient who suddenly shows indications of feeling better may be presenting in this fashion because a suicide plan has been developed, which of course is usually dependent upon discharge from the hospital.

Unfortunately, it is not always possible to furnish sufficient proof to convince the hearing officer that the patient is being put at undue risk, and the patient may be released. It is hoped that the doctor's concerns will prove to have been incorrect. This does not mean that the doctor was wrong. In fact, the doctor's extra effort, as well as the emphasis that was placed upon the patient's condition, may have been of some therapeutic benefit to the patient.

The hearing officer needs to obtain clinical experience and can best do this if furnished follow-up reports. In this way a hearing officer can mature in clinical acumen and make better decisions. However, the burden is still on the clinician to present sufficient evidence to overcome the presumption that everyone is sane, not a danger, and deserving of freedom. Experience has shown that hearing officers have trouble understanding such concepts as the borderline personality and the hypomanic patient. The therapist's skill as a teacher is put to the full test when trying to commit such patients.

DISCHARGE

When the patient has been treated to the point of discharge, discharge plans must be made in a detailed and understandable fashion. Some jurisdictions require a plan. It is important that the patient participate in the planning and that the patient's record reflect the discharge plan. The record should reflect the reasons why it is believed that the patient is ready to be discharged, as well as the risks and potential benefits. The fact that the patient's insurance has expired is not an adequate medical reason for discharge.

Risk/Benefit Note

There were good reasons for keeping the patient in the hospital. What are the reasons for now letting this same patient out? The following hypothetical example may clarify this issue:

> Mrs. Jones' depression has now improved. She continues to be shaky. However, the experience of caring for her children, with outpatient and family support, is most important in helping her regain her self-esteem. While there is some slight risk that she will regress and need hospitalization again, that risk is far outweighed by the benefits to be obtained by her resumption of responsibilities. She has already had weekend and longer trial home visits which have produced regular improvement, albeit with trepidation on her part. The risks and benefits have been discussed with her husband, who agrees with the plan and understands his responsibilities and the necessity for precautions and careful observation. All of this—the risks and benefits, the discussion and approval of the husband, etc.—should be clearly written in the progress notes.

The discharge note should also indicate when, where, and from whom the patient is to receive the next treatment, as well as the quantity of medication the patient was receiving at the time of discharge. This type of risk/benefit note should be written any time a major decision is made involving a patient's care. Such major decisions would include home visits, discharge, unusual treatments, etc.

AMA Discharges

Many patients will insist on leaving the hospital against medical advice. While the physician may disagree, the patient may not appear so sick as to require a commitment hearing, but is allowed to sign out AMA. Even then,

Forensic Issues 279

the record should clearly reflect the risk and the benefit of the action the doctors have taken:

1. Patient's stated reasons for wanting to leave.
2. Physician's reasons for not attempting to commit against patient's wishes.
3. Patient's family notified and given opportunity to dissuade patient.
4. Patient's plans.
5. Indications of patient's awareness of opportunities for further care and treatment.

The physician needs to exercise caution in his disappointment at the patient's rejection of his advice. The patient has a right to know about other options even if they are not recommended; the responsible medical practitioner will discuss these with the patient. It is useful to offer to arrange an appointment with an outside doctor who is willing to treat the patient. Medication to tide the patient over until the new doctor is seen is also desirable. If the patient throws the medicine at the doctor, then the chart should clearly reflect this.

This chapter will frequently mention that "the record should reflect," which means that the clinician should write specifically what has transpired in the hospital chart. This is important, as most lawsuits are won or lost on what is in or missing from the record. What is in that record will protect. Whether the decision proved to be incorrect or not, the record will at least reveal that the doctor gave serious consideration to the risks and benefits and made a well-founded decision. What is not in that record is assumed not to have been considered and will defeat the doctor in court.

Elopement

All hospitals have policies for dealing with patients who have eloped. At the very least this requires notification of hospital security and the patient's family or other responsible parties. In some situations it may require notification of the police. Is this a court commitment? If so, the judge, the patient's attorney and the prosecutor need to be notified. In all situations an estimate needs to be made of the patient's dangerousness to self and/or to the person or property of others. This appraisal will determine what action is necessary. For example, if a homicidal patient has eloped after making threats to kill his wife, it is imperative that his wife and the police be notified. There have been cases in which patients have eloped from the hospital, returned home, and murdered family members. Such unfortunate circumstances might have been prevented if timely efforts had been made to notify the authorities.

Once again, the record should reflect exactly what action was taken, who was called, at what time, what was said, etc. Hospital policies to be followed in the event of an elopement should be worked out with the hospital attorney. One should keep in mind that part of the duty of the hospital attorney is to see that the hospital is not sued. Therefore, the advice the attorney gives may not be consistent with the "caring" responsibilities of the physician. In cases where there are conflicts, many clinicians believe that the physician should make a decision based on medical rather than legal criteria.

Court-Ordered Patients

Most state hospitals and occasionally even a private hospital accept patients who are ordered to the hospital by the court. Such commitments are usually called court-ordered commitments. Patients may be so ordered for evaluations for competency and/or responsibility and sometimes even for treatment. It is imperative that the hospital clearly understand under what circumstances the patient has been ordered to the hospital, the limits of the hospital's responsibility, the limits of the court's responsibility and what authorities need to be notified when the patient is ready for discharge or if he elopes. The committing court must understand exactly how much security the hospital can provide before ordering the patient to the hospital. If the patient has already arrived and the doctor believes the security is inadequate, the court order improper, etc., the hospital's attorney or a psychiatrist familiar with the forensic issues should be called upon to intervene with the court.

Hospitals must exercise care to avoid becoming responsible for patients they cannot adequately manage. Some hospitals may not have sufficient security to manage a criminal who is an escape risk, while they can easily deal with a geriatric case who needs temporary custodial care and planning for long-term care. Attorneys, in their effort to help their client, may unknowingly misrepresent the hospital's capability. When possible, direct communication with the judge is useful in order to be sure that everyone understands the situation. After all, the doctor usually cannot discharge a court-ordered patient without the court's permission.

The contents of the report to the court is another area of frequent misunderstanding. There is generally no confidentiality for court-ordered patients, yet the court usually only needs to have medical answers to its legal questions, with sufficient supporting data, but not all of the personal details. Discretion is desirable.

Hospitals can contribute a great deal to the court's understanding and eventual disposition of many mentally disturbed offenders if they are careful and plan in advance. Even some private hospitals are willing to evaluate and treat a limited number of murderers and sex offenders. Such patients can be challenging and stimulating to the staff. Good care for such patients may make the difference between a useful future versus a destroyed one. The same may apply to accident victims with emotional problems or those accused of fraud, forgery, etc. Of course, in court cases records may be subpoenaed and testimony of staff required. The availability of an experienced forensic psychiatrist for advice and guidance is useful in managing these court-ordered patients.

PATIENT RIGHTS

Even though hospitalized, patients still have many of the rights they enjoyed as free citizens at home. In the hospital patients do not have freedom in terms of access to things that are taken for granted elsewhere. Physicians must therefore be sure to see that patients can communicate with their attorneys and that a telephone or writing materials and postage are available. Physicians also have the duty, as caretakers, to see that proper clothing, bed, food, etc., are provided. This does not mean that physicians can allow patients to order a truckload of chickens when that is not therapeutically indicated or to write threatening letters to the President of the United States. However, if physicians wish to limit patients from exercising their rights, the reasons for the restrictions should be clearly recorded. Time limits for such restrictions are determined by local laws, which require that all restrictions be reconsidered at reasonable intervals and that the patient clearly understands why his freedom has been restricted.

Right to Treatment

The right to treatment is a concept that received its strongest legal support in 1972 in the famous *Wyatt v. Stickney* case.[5,6] Judge Johnson stated that, if the state of Alabama was going to commit patients (take away their freedom), the patients had a right to adequate treatment so that they could recover their freedom. Since then there have been many right to treatment suits brought against various state hospital systems, claiming that the committed patients were not receiving adequate care. Because the public treatment of the mentally ill has only on rare occasions been adequately funded, it has always been quite easy to show that patients are not receiving adequate treatment. Right to treatment suits have not been filed against private hospitals as the dissatisfied patient can merely stop paying his bill and thereby be discharged or transferred to a state facility.

The individual treatment plan, as a measure of treatment adequacy, resulted from the *Wyatt* case, as have many other "paper rights" for mental hospital patients. To the patients' benefit, funding has improved, allowing better staffing. However, the major effect of the right to treatment movement has been the discharge of large numbers of patients from public institutions in order to meet court-ordered staffing ratios. Unfortunately for the large number of discharged patients, adequate community facilities for their care are not available. The literal dumping of many of the mentally ill into the community has not been a solution for these patients and continues to be the major reason for the presence of many severely mentally ill people sleeping in gutters and empty buildings throughout America. Stephen Rachlin wrote an aptly titled paper on this subject: "With Liberty and Psychosis for All."[7]

Right to treatment suits did benefit some individuals who did not require hospitalization on a continuing basis and who have been able to take advantage of the limited facilities in the community. All public mental health systems continue to attempt to supply an adequate patient/staff ratio and to fulfill patients' treatment needs. Despite the *Wyatt* decision, hospitals continue to be funded inadequately. The right to treatment movement had a tremendous effect on the care of the mentally ill, and this effect continues to be felt.

Right to Refuse Treatment

Having given the patient the right to treatment, the mental health system was then faced with the patient's right to refuse treatment. Forced treatment had been rather freely practiced on committed patients in the mental health system. The mental health bar, as a group of bright, young, devoted, and determined attorneys came to be known in the 1960s and 1970s, pushed not only for patients' rights, such as clothing and mail privileges, but also for the patient's right to refuse invasive treatment, such as brain surgery and electroconvulsive therapy (ECT), as well as psychotropic medications.

The Massachusetts Supreme Court, in the case of *Rogers v. Commissioner*,[8,9] referring to the use of antipsychotic medication, said "[antipsychotic] drugs are powerful enough to immobilize mind and body. Because of both the profound effect these drugs have on the thought processes of an individual and the well-established likelihood (*sic*) of severe and irreversible side effects . . . we treat these drugs in the same manner we would treat psychosurgery or electroconvulsive therapy."[10] The Massachusetts court equated psychotic thinking with the First Amendment right of freedom to think and said that if psychiatrists changed psychotic thought to normal thought they were interfering with the patient's rights. Doctors were unable to convince the court that a psychotic person is not a free person but is a captive of the psychosis, and that in fact psychiatrists with their medications are the freedom fighters.

Voluntary patients of course have a right to refuse treatment. Although they are in the hospital and doctors have control over their movements, doctors can only forcibly treat them under one circumstance, an emergency—an extreme danger to themselves or others. Again the record should reflect the reasons for determining that there is a danger. (Each state has its own definition.) Then and only then can psychiatrists impose the emergency conditions. These emergency conditions, for a voluntary patient, can only last for 24 to 48 hours (depending on local laws), at which time the patient must either be involuntarily committed or discharged. When the patient has been committed, psychiatrists again should not force treatment on the patient unless doctors believe that it is an emergency or unless they have complied with the special regulations for enforced treatment that exist within the jurisdiction.

In recent years almost every state in the United States has adopted rules and regulations for the use of forced medication. Generally these regulations establish the circumstances under which such treatment can be forced, by whom, and for how long. The conditions usually require something less than an emergency and frequently include a situation in which the patient's health would deteriorate without active treatment. Treatments allowed are generally limited to standard, acceptable forms of treatment that do not present a serious risk to the health of the patient; ECT is generally excluded. In no case is forced treatment allowed merely for the staff's convenience or as a punishment.

The regulations allowing treatment of refusing patients require a review of the patient's condition, usually by a panel from the hospital staff not involved directly with the patient's care or by an outside consultant. First psychiatrists must attempt to get the patient to agree to take the treatment; if that fails, the decision is whether it is in the patient's best interest to receive the treatment, even against his or her will. Such enforced treatment is generally limited to a few weeks; then the process to gain approval for further forced treatment must be repeated.

The following is a hypothetical example of the type of procedure used for the refusing patient in Maryland:[11]

> A 24-year-old paranoid schizophrenic male has refused to take the haloperidol prescribed in any form. When discussing this with his psychiatrist he says that he believes there is nothing wrong with him and that the intent of the staff is to experiment upon him with the medication to see if it will cause him to kill someone. He believes that they think he is the reincarnation of Pontius Pilate and that the gov-

ernment is trying to force him to kill so he can be prosecuted for murder. He has refused to eat or drink for three days, fearing medicine or poison in the food. He is dehydrated and has pedal edema from his constant pacing. The staff psychiatrist, being unable to convince the patient otherwise, notes these facts in the patient's chart and informs the clinical director of the situation. Since this is not yet an emergency (danger to life and safety), no treatment is started but the clinical director appoints a clinical review panel composed of himself, a staff psychiatrist, and a non-M.D. mental health care provider to evaluate the situation for the following factors:

1. clinical record
2. personnel — patient's needs
3. patient — why refusing?
4. decisional capacity of patient
5. risk/benefit of forced medication
6. acceptable alternatives

They then decide whether or not to force haloperidol, another medication, or some alternative. If they decided to force medication, it may be given to this refusing patient for 60 days. If at the end of that time he continues to refuse (a rare circumstance), another panel must be appointed and the process repeated. In this fashion, necessary treatment is not delayed.

It goes without saying that any patient who is treated must have a reasonably complete knowledge of the type of treatment, as well as of the risks, benefits, and alternatives available. Only in this way can the patient give an informed consent to the treatment. In some jurisdictions the procedure for forcing treatment is much more difficult than cited above, and it is necessary to have a full judicial hearing with the patient being represented by an attorney. This can be time-consuming and contribute to deterioration in the patient's health. However, the law takes a very serious view of forcing care or treatment on patients. Psychiatrists need to continue to try to help the court understand that cumbersome legal procedures which delay necessary treatment may cause more harm to the patient than a loss of freedom to decide against treatment. A Massachusetts study revealed a delay of two to seven months before a hearing occurred.[12]

In many states ECT has been listed as a dangerous treatment, requiring numerous legal steps for its use. Unfortunately, this rule has prevented many patients who could have greatly benefited from ECT from receiving it. This unreasonable attitude of the law toward ECT represents psychiatry's inability to convince some courts that ECT is beneficial. The same applies to the use of antipsychotic medications. They cause tardive dyskinesia, a fact which, when presented to some courts exaggeratedly as a common and irreversible condition, has led to a restriction on the psychiatrist's power to force such drugs on a patient. When a patient refuses treatment, it is imperative that the record be clear in delineating the factors that contributed to the decision to forcibly treat. The record should clearly show that the specific legal requirements that must be met before such treatment can be given were met.

Restraint and Seclusion

Much of what has been said about the right to refuse treatment also applies to restraint and seclusion. Here again, each jurisdiction has established its own rules and regulations about seclusion and restraint. Both should only be used for therapeutic purposes and not for the convenience of the staff, because there is a shortage of staff, or to punish the patient. Since restraint and seclusion are utilized so frequently in psychiatric hospitals, each institution has its own policy and procedure. An APA Task Force report discusses these issues very thoroughly and should be read by all clinicians.[13] Behavioral modification programs require special caution to ensure that they do not aggrandize punishment under the guise of behavioral modification. The seclusion room or restraints must be humane, so that such devices as four-point restraints are only used when necessary.

Confidentiality

Whenever a patient consults a doctor, the patient expects that what has been told to the physician will be held in confidence. This is particularly true when the patient speaks to a psychiatrist. However, there are many times when the communication is not held in the strictest confidence. As soon as information is put into a record, many others see it, and, although they are supposed to maintain confidence, their training may not be so intense and professional as to inculcate the need for absolute confidentiality. For this reason the clinician should be careful about what is placed in the psychiatric record. The clinician must be sure that what is there is of sufficient therapeutic importance and is the type of information that other staff will need to know in order to assist in the patient's treatment. Very personal information, such as statements that the patient has made about other patients, personnel, or family members, usually can be excluded from the record without interfering with the patient's care.

There may be a conflict between what is necessary for the documentation of adequate care and what is necessary to protect the patient's confidentiality. While the patient's care must be of utmost importance, sensitivity to the patient's privacy is also necessary. Pejorative statements should never be included nor should a therapist's negative opinions or attitudes about a patient be in the record. Many clinicians prefer to keep working notes of their own, which do not become an official part of the hospital record and are only of importance in the doctor-patient treatment relationship and in supervision. They are always kept separate from the patient's chart and are usually not subject to subpoena. (This should be clarified before making such working notes.)

Whenever the doctor is not clearly the patient's agent but is assisting an intervening party, such as the court, the employer, or the insurance company, this must be made very clear to the patient. Obviously, this situation will interfere with the level of confidentiality. For example, if a psychiatrist is examining an individual for the courts to determine competency to stand trial and/or responsibility at the time of the crime, it must be made very clear to the patient that the doctor may need to put in the report to the court whatever the patient says. This is particularly true if the doctor is going to say that the patient is not competent or responsible where supporting evidence is necessary, e.g., the patient is suffering from paranoid schizophrenia and told the doctor that God's voice commanded him to kill his neighbor who was poisoning the community. On the other hand, if the patient is competent and/or responsible, a doctor would not want to furnish proof of the patient's guilt, or to render a diagnosis of antisocial personality which could be used against the patient.

The same, of course, would apply if the doctor were evaluating a patient in the hospital at the employer's request and the employer wanted to have detailed information about the patient. The patient must know what will be held in strict confidence and what will not. In dealing with insurance companies, many problems concerning confidentiality are raised, particularly when the patient's employer sponsors the patient's insurance and the insurance forms are processed through the company. One can be sure that many people in the company will know about the patient's diagnosis. Usually DSM-III code numbers are used in an attempt to protect the patient. Further, because insurance represents a business, doctors cannot always be sure that some unknown business requirement will not override any attempts to maintain confidentiality. In truth, the only guarantee is the doctor's integrity. There are times when it is in the patient's interest to let the employer have some information. If possible, the therapist should discuss with the patient exactly what he will tell the employer. In many cases, for the clinician to "stonewall" and say nothing can cause the patient eventual harm. Frequently consultation with a colleague is helpful in maintaining a sensitive balance.

Privileged communication is frequently confused with confidentiality.

Privileged communication refers to the patient's privilege to prevent a psychiatrist from testifying under court order about what the patient has told the psychiatrist. It is important to be familiar with the laws applicable in the jurisdiction, as many states do not have a doctor/patient or psychotherapist/patient privileged communication statute. Confidentiality, on the other hand, is an ethical obligation of all mental health professionals and is part of the fiduciary relationship that every professional has with his or her patients.

It goes without saying that great efforts must be exercised in order to maintain patient confidentiality with reference to family and/or friends who desire information. It is particularly important to have a policy for the telephone operators and the information desk as well as the record room of the hospital. The record librarian in a general hospital must recognize that the psychiatric record is more sensitive than the general medical or surgical record of a patient, and procedures need to be established for treating psychiatric records in a special way.

TARASOFF—THE DUTY TO WARN

Tatiana Tarasoff's family members were the plaintiffs in the first case that involved the duty to warn a known victim of life-threatening danger. Tatiana was murdered by a young man who felt rejected by her. He had told his therapist he was going to kill her. The therapist tried to have him committed, but when that failed and the patient refused to return for treatment, the therapist did not warn Tatiana or her parents. In the Tarasoff case[14] the court stated that, although it recognized that confidentiality was important in a psychotherapeutic relationship, "The protective privilege ends where the public peril begins." The court said that a known victim must be warned.

This concept has spread so that several jurisdictions now recognize Tarasoff and have made various changes in the concept. Generally speaking, the duty is to protect from harm rather than to necessarily warn a victim when there is reason to believe that the patient might cause harm. The duty can be met by hospitalizing the patient or arranging for his arrest or by medicating the patient so the delusional beliefs no longer exist. It is a good idea to see that there are no weapons that the patient might use.

The conflict for clinicians is that they are honor-bound to maintain the patient's confidentiality; however, if the patient talks about killing the boss, and the therapist believes there is a chance that this might occur, the therapist has a duty to prevent this even if it means telling the boss and having the patient believe he was betrayed. The most difficult situation for the therapist is when the patient has made a threat but is no longer under the therapist's control, e.g., he refuses to return. Some jurisdictions require notification of the police under such circumstances. Regardless of the local rules, all therapists are expected to do their best to prevent harm by a patient, even if it means breaking confidentiality.

Generally, clinicians' experience has been that patients eventually appreciate reasonable efforts made to protect both the patient and a possible victim. Experience with Tarasoff has led most clinicians to discuss the problem with the patient when the issue arises, that is, when the patient makes a threat that the therapist believes might occur. The therapist should then point out to the patient that this cannot be allowed to occur and should state what the therapist would like to do or would like to have the patient do to prevent any such occurrence.[15]

Tarasoff considerations are particularly important at the time of discharge or when allowing a previously dangerous patient to go home on temporary leave, as this is a very vulnerable time in terms of homicide as well as suicide. It is therefore important to be sure that the therapist has a full and complete understanding of the patient's condition and of what is likely to happen when the patient is no longer under supervision. The risks and the benefits should be recognized, discussed completely, and recorded. When in doubt one should request a consultation and have this consultant's opinion recorded in the chart.

PREVENTING MALPRACTICE

No doctor wishes to be sued, but the chances of the psychiatrist's and even the hospital's being sued are increasing. It is imperative that psychiatrists attempt to develop a malpractice (therapeutic misadventure) prevention program. Rather than wait until someone on the staff has been sued, doctors should think about situations in which patients might be harmed and do what can be done to prevent that. It is important to communicate potential or actual harmful occurrences to others.

The incident report within the hospital is important and should be reviewed by someone who can then place the entire incident in perspective and do something to prevent a recurrence. If an incident of lost keys is reported, for instance, then this should alert the staff to reevaluate its key control program to be sure that it is sufficient for the hospital; the staff should certainly see that a similar incident cannot happen again. Doctors can become complacent and rarely look at certain patterns. For example, when someone looked at the number of broken hips suffered by elderly hospitalized patients from falls out of bed, it was discovered that these accidents generally occurred in the late night and early morning hours. Further investigation revealed that patients fell when they attempted to get out of bed to go to the bathroom. It then became relatively simple to see that patients were taken to the bathroom at 11:00 p.m. and, if necessary, again awakened at 3:00 or 4:00 a.m., so that they did not have to try to get up by themselves and suffer serious injury. In psychiatric hospitals risk management is very important. For example, the need for breakaway shower curtain rods and showerheads is something that may be overlooked. Many patients have hung themselves by tying a belt, sheet, or towel to the shower curtain rod or the showerhead.

Along these same lines, there should be a way of reporting to an appropriate staff member when a patient or his relatives are particularly unhappy about something that has happened within the hospital. A good prevention program will have a carefully selected and trained staff member available to discuss the dissatisfaction with all parties and attempt to resolve the issue before the anger or annoyance escalates into a lawsuit.

Whenever there is a doubt about a treatment, about overriding a patient's refusal, about a commitment, about a discharge – about anything – one should have available a colleague of equal or greater experience upon whom to call for an independent review of the situation and a recorded statement. It is highly unlikely that someone will say that two doctors carrying out independent evaluations are wrong. It is also important not to "second guess" what others in authority might do. A psychiatrist should not refuse to commit a patient whom the doctor thinks should be committed because the doctor believes that the hearing officer will discharge the patient. These are separate, unrelated decisions. When a doctor commits, it is done in good faith. When the hearing officer discharges, it is done in good faith. Both decisions may be absolutely correct because the decisions come from different directions at different times. If a psychiatrist believes that a patient is too suicidal to go home for a visit, that psychiatrist should not discharge the patient even though he knows that the patient's family is probably going to harangue the superintendent until the decision is overridden. The superintendent has to make his decision, but the psychiatrist must make his own decision.

When one is in doubt about forensic issues, it is quite proper and in fact important to consult with the hospital attorney or a forensic psychiatric consultant whom the hospital should have available. Each of these individuals will look at the situation from a different viewpoint and, although they may not agree, the decision maker will at least have additional options.

REFERENCES

1. Gutheil T, Appelbaum P: Clinical Handbook of Psychiatry and the Law, New York, McGraw-Hill, 1984
2. Halleck S: Law in the Practice of Psychiatry, New York, Plenum, 1980.

3. Brakel SJ, Parry J, Weiner BA: The Mentally Disabled and the Law, American Bar Association, 1985
4. Gutheil TG, Bursztajn H: Clinicians' Guidelines for Assessing and Presenting Subtle Forms of Patient Incompetence in Legal Settings, Am J Psychiatry 1986; 143:1020-1023
5. *Wyatt v. Stickney*, 325 F. Supp. 781 (M.D. Ala. 1971) and 344 F. Supp. 373 (M.D. Ala. 1972)
6. Jones RL, Parlour RR: Wyatt v Stickney, New York, Grune & Stratton, 1981
7. Rachlin S: With liberty and psychosis for all. Psy Q. 1974; 48:410-420
8. Rogers v. Commissioner of Mental Health, 390 Mass 498, 1982
9. Gutheil TG: Rogers v. commissioner: denouement of an important right-to-refuse treatment case. Am J Psychiatry 1985; 142:213-216
10. In the Matter of Guardianship of Richard Roe, III, 421 N.E. 2d 40 Mass. 1981
11. Annotated Code of Md., Health General-10-708
12. Valiz J, James WS: Medicine court: rogers in practice. Am J Psychiatry 1987; 144: pp 62-67
13. *Seclusion and Restraint, The Psychiatric Uses*, Report of the American Psychiatric Association Task Force on the Psychiatric Uses of Seclusion and Restraint, Report 22, American Psychiatric Association, Washington, DC, 1985
14. Tarasoff v. Regents (Tarasoff II), 551 P 2d 334 131 Cal Rptr 14, 1976
15. Appelbaum PS: Tarasoff and the clinician: problems in fulfilling the duty to protect. Am J Psychiatry 1985; 142:425-429

17
Violence and Suicide within the Hospital

John R. Lion

Violence is common within a psychiatric hospital. It can take two forms: violence against the self, and violence toward others. Patients may injure themselves or attempt suicide, or they may hurt other patients or staff. Both inward and outward aggression may also occur.

Although violence exists in hospitals, it is less often openly commented upon. Few institutions publicly review suicides committed by their patients and legal concerns force such discussions to be carried out privately. Aggression by patients is also often handled by denial.[1] Rarely does a hospital keep statistics about its assault rate, and underreporting of assaults is the rule and not the exception.[2] Suicides and assaults are an embarrassment to the institution and convey the stigma of mismanagement, despite the fact that many hospitals routinely work with suicidal and violent patients and are often able to satisfactorily devise successful treatment plans for them.

A suicide attempt within an institution is a major psychosocial event involving both staff and other patients. Kayton and Freed[3] have discussed the impact of such an experience. If the suicide is successful, the repercussions are enormous and inevitably lead to doubts about the facility's continued ability to treat such patients in general. Most hospitals try to talk about a suicide and promote staff and patient group discussions about the patient and his care, the errors involved, and the issues of blame and guilt; in reality, such openness is compromised by legal concerns about negligence.

A young woman had been hospitalized for almost a year for a depressive illness and after discharge killed herself. Her possible death had always been a consideration during treatment, but she had done quite well in the hospital and had evoked the optimism of staff and clinician. The suicide achieved some publicity, and the father of the deceased was an attorney; consequently, the treating doctor did not wish to hold a postmortem conference for fear of liability and exposure. Staff nonetheless prevailed upon him, and a brief one-hour meeting was held during which limited and cautious affect was voiced. The case was never openly discussed again.

In this instance, denial and fear played a large part in the avoidance of a public discussion, but concerns about an open case conference following a suicide are frequent, despite laws in many states enabling the review process to be exempt from the medical record. Krieger[4] has discussed the errors made in the management of a suicide case in an unusually candid article; his publication serves as a model for what should occur. Denial is particularly apt to be a response when the suicide occurred by a patient who was on leave home, freshly discharged, or "not really one of ours."

It is axiomatic that a hospital will have a prevailing suicide rate, largely determined by the nature of the risk cases it takes on. Unlike assaultive patients, a suicidal person is not usually refused admission to a psychiatric facility. But what may deter a hospital from accepting a particular patient is a critical mass of other hospitalized patients who are depressed or suicidal, thus tying up nursing staff who must "special" these patients through close observation periods. Even then, arrangements are usually made to handle the suicidal patient, for the hospital sees as its mission the acceptance of such psychopathology. This is less likely to occur with the aggressive patient who may be shunted to the criminal justice system.

In reviewing suicides in Los Angeles during the years 1967–1972, Schwartz and coworkers[5] determined that nine patients a year committed suicide within psychiatric facilities, but half of the patients were technically on leave from the hospital, thus highlighting the problem of gathering data on this subject. Depression is usually associated with suicide, but schizophrenic diagnoses were more common than depression among the authors' findings. Hanging was the most common form of suicide occurring within the facility. Although data exist which indicates the first week of admission to be a risk period for hospital suicide,[6] other statistics point in the direction of actual discharge or leave from the hospital as being the period associated with suicidal risk.[5]

In the management of a suicidal patient, most anxieties typically occur when the patient appears improved and is given some degree of freedom on the grounds of the hospital or a weekend home. Risk-taking in these ventures is usually shared through group discussions within the milieu; here the patient asks for a privilege and his peers comment upon the patient's readiness. Nursing staff, also, may join in. The hospital's confines are usually quite nurturant, and the risk of suicide may increase as the patient reenters society and goes home to face the stresses of the family and job. To take this risk in the service of the patient's improvement and growth is the hospital's mandate. But staff can err.

A woman with a psychotic illness was deemed to be better on antipsychotic medication, though still socially withdrawn. Her regressed behavior and poor socialization alarmed staff and they embarked on a course of activating her behavior. She was pushed into a variety of therapies and given passes outside the hospital. A few days prior to her suicide, she was noted to have command hallucinations again, and her medication was increased. On a pass outside the hospital, she escaped from the grounds and threw herself on high voltage lines.

Whether the patient's psychotic symptomatology worsened as a function of staff pressure was unclear; equally unclear was the determination of the nature of the patient's command hallucinations. Perhaps she should have been restricted to the ward and her condition reassessed. In any event, the staff took an unnecessary risk. Such errors in judgement occur and point up the difficulties involved in taking chances with patients and assessing their inner lives. To some extent, the clinician will never know everything about his patient, and the patient may encounter outside stresses that undo therapeutic gains in the hospital. The precariousness of some patients is so great that no amount of shelter can buffer them from self-destructive elements.

Some patients continue to remain depressed within the hospital and despite treatment succumb to their own internally directed aggressive urges.

A man with a depressive illness was admitted to a hospital for a long stay. He had been unsuccessfully treated for many years, and his treatments had included antidepressants and ECT. There was a strong characterological component to his condition, but superimposed on this were depressive moods unresponsive to drugs. He had lost his family due to illness, and was unemployed. He displayed frequent suicidal ideation and eventually hung himself on the grounds of the hospital. No clear precipitant could be determined for the suicide. His death seemed more the natural outcome of a decade of illness.

This is a severe example of chronic suicidal ideation whose actualization seems inevitable. Every hospital has such patients and more or less comes to reach some uneasy truce with the risk involved, so that it is no great surprise when the suicide occurs.

Sublethal forms of self-destructive behavior frequently occur in the hospital.

> A borderline patient with a history of self-mutilation was hospitalized after a romantic breakup. She initially expressed suicidal ideation, but this disappeared after a few weeks' stay on a psychiatric intensive care ward. Her former boyfriend, however, was also hospitalized and the patient then came to feel that she was responsible for his decompensation. While in the bathroom, she superficially cut her wrists and then promptly came to the nursing station to announce the deed.

Most clinicians have experience with these types of patients and the self-destructive behaviors they engage in. Wrist-cutting is not uncommon in a hospital setting and epidemics of wrist-cutting have also been reported. Other forms of violence at self include self-excoriation and head-banging, though such behaviors are seen more with regressed individuals who are organically impaired or suffer with mental retardation. On rare occasions, there may be admitted to the hospital a severely self-mutilative patient who attempts autocastration or autoenucleation, though these types of patients are generally quite psychotic. Conn and Lion[7] have reviewed the types of self-mutilating patients seen in clinical practice.

The use of knives or sharp objects to induce pain or lacerations is quite clearly self-aggressive; less obviously "aggressive" is a behavior such as an overdose with medication, though dynamics often reveal a vector of anger.

> A manipulative patient with a history of substance abuse and overdoses was admitted to the hospital. Though she was searched and placed on close observation, she was smuggled pills by a fellow addict. Following a stormy group therapy encounter during which other patients confronted her avoidant behavior in the hospital, she was found in an obtunded state in her room, semiconscious, with the pills in her dresser drawer. When confronted, she stated that she was furious with the other patients and in a fit of rage, overdosed.

How the introjection of aggressive urges leads to a momentary self-destructive act cannot always be clearly elucidated; for some patients, the "mode" of handling aggression is to channel it inwardly while other patients strike out or become externally violent. And both can occur, within the same patient.

A young man with organicity due to a head injury was prone to temper outbursts during which he would throw articles and furniture at home. He also overdosed on two occasions and frequently cut his arms with sharp objects.

This patient had temporal lobe epilepsy with marked affective lability. While it was difficult to predict his aggressiveness, he was prone to channel it internally when the object of his anger was not available. Bach-Y-Rita and Veno[8] have described this turning inward of aggression seen in incarcerated prisoners.

Hospital staff usually spend considerable time on the prevention of self-destructive acts. Caution is expended in the direction of privileges, and freedoms may be given and rescinded as a function of destructive behavior. Behavior modification may also be utilized, particularly with more primitive psychological conditions.[9] Head-banging, for example, may be amenable to a behavior modification schedule involving tokens for periods without such injury. Physical restraint appliances have also been used in such situations to prevent head injury. Generally speaking, the more stereotypic and repetitive the self-mutilation, the more it is approachable through a behavior modification program. In contrast, self-destructive actions such as overdoses usually reflect deeper intrapsychic difficulties which require psychotherapy.

Actual violence against other patients or staff confronts the hospital with different issues. Externally directed violence, when not associated with psychotic conditions, is often seen as deviant and indicative of behavior belonging outside the province of psychiatry. Although an institution may tolerate some violence by characterologically disturbed patients or those adolescents in turmoil, it still has thresholds and will discharge or transfer unmanageable cases, seeing them as beyond conventional psychological help. This is less likely to occur with self-destructive patients who, though they may engage in willful and repetitively self-mutilative acts, are still viewed as "mentally ill."

A borderline woman was presented at a hospital-wide conference because of severely intractable "suicidal" behavior. She swallowed objects and had undergone many surgical procedures because of her actions. The objects she swallowed were diverse and included razor blades, bed springs, a small spoon, and medication as well. Many exploratory surgical procedures had been performed. The patient appeared as a primitive character disorder without much insight; her self-destructive actions came following disappointments or perceived rejections from other patients but attempts to work therapeutically with her on these types of psychological issues had been to no avail.

In this case, staff unanimously agreed that the patient was a "psychiatric case," even though the point was raised regarding her prognosis and the wisdom of retaining her within the acute care division of the hospital as opposed to the chronic care facility on the hospital grounds. Staff were perpetually frightened of her, and this legendary case obviously consumed tremendous portions of staff time and anguish, highlighting the powerfulness of the patient. An attempt was made to keep her in physical restraints without success, and she ultimately again swallowed a foreign object and was transferred to a general hospital for surgical intervention.

Such cases confront caretakers with many theoretical and practical issues concerning the management of aggressive patients. Was this patient treatable? What was the precise etiology of this bizarre fascination with swallowing? What were the staff's obligations in the case of such intractable behavior? Just how controllable was this behavior of hers?

Sometimes staff become split over this mad/bad issue and large controversies swirl around a particularly aggressive patient.

> The patient, a borderline young girl with mild mental retardation, had been in both prison and psychiatric hospitals for severely aggressive and sociopathic behavior. She had assaulted police and hospital personnel and had also frequently cut her wrists. She had severe temper outbursts and volatile mood swings; in jail she had tried to hang herself, and in the hospital she was highly aggressive. She was viewed as cunning and manipulative, and dilemmas concerning her proper placement had reached the highest administrative offices in her state.

This notorious patient was alternately viewed as antisocial and psychiatrically impaired, and she had been shunted from one facility to another. Her case was championed by legal advocates who adamantly maintained that she needed "proper treatment." But hospital staff were dismayed by her continued antisocial and violent behavior. No resolution concerning appropriate placement occurred, despite many conferences and meetings. Which precise component of her behavior was viewed as "psychiatric" remained unclear, and the wrist-cutting and attempted hanging were perhaps the behavior which most disturbed public officials; her assaults appeared to be more universally agreed upon as manifestations of antisocial propensities.

Cases such as the one above clearly politicize caretakers and create an impossible ambience for any treatment. Yet even in "purer" illnesses of psychotic proportions, transfer and shunting to other facilities go on and reflect a political process.

A young schizophrenic man was severely aggressive and frequently assaulted staff and other patients. A rural state hospital, deeming him untreatable, transferred him to an urban security hospital for the criminally insane, where he was boarded. The rationale for transfer was that only this facility had the manpower and staff to handle his psychotic outbursts. Within the forensic unit, he quickly calmed and was managed with conservative amounts of medication. But when time came for his return to the psychiatric facility, the director of that institution refused, stating that the patient could simply not be managed. The director stated that the patient had assaulted members of his staff and such behavior would not be tolerated.

The milieu has a powerful effect on the aggressive behavior of patients. Control of behavior is a self-fulfilling prophecy, and if staff decide that they cannot manage a patient, it may well turn out to so be the case. Until skews in perception of management are dealt with, and until hopelessness or resignation comes to be discussed, no patient is easily managed. This "acting-out" of anger at the patient is an insidious process and may often occur after a patient has actually been violent within a hospital. At other times, immediate transfer is sought.

A deeply psychotic man attacked another patient. The private hospital staff were dismayed and perplexed over the assault as there seemed to be no warning and the assault was completely random. The patient again became assaultive and again showed no premonitory signs of intent or even anger. It was concluded that he became violent in response to covert command hallucinations and that intervention was thus ineffective; he could explode at any moment and hit someone. He was then placed in restraint devices to limit arm movements. His parents were pleased by this since they wished him retained in the private facility, but staff did not like the use of chronic arms restraints and were frightened of the patient. The consultant strongly suggested that such restraints be retained pending the use of different medication, as he feared that one more assault would lead the hospital to discharge the patient. At a meeting, staff seemed agreeable, but for unexplained reasons restraints were removed during a period of quiescence; he again struck a patient and was promptly transferred to a state facility.

In this instance, the staff somehow contrived to arrange events so as to lead to discharge of the patient. Strong psychological forces conspire in these matters of management. And competent management of violent patients requires experience and facility with many modalities of intervention, including restraint and seclusion. The recent publication by the American Psychiatric Association Task Force on Psychiatric Aspects of Restraint and Seclusion[10] highlights the ethical, legal, and clinical aspects of these parameters and furnishes the therapist with guidelines for their use. Still, training in the use of restraint and seclusion is haphazard in many hospitals and is often passed down by word of mouth; it is less likely to be taught in any systematic manner or endorsed by the physicians. Lion and Soloff[11] have advocated a profession-wide training program for all hospitals, modeled after one in Maryland where restraint and seclusion training is regularly taught in the state hospital system; other states, as well, have such training and have shown it to reduce assaults and lead to more effective patient management.[12]

Assaults on staff and other patients within a hospital is a function of such factors as the nature of the institution, staffing patterns, diagnoses of patients, and sex. Ekblom's classic study of this subject[13] showed the peak incident of assaults to occur when newly admitted male schizophrenic patients were mixed with older, feebler patients during a temporary period of understaffing within the hospital. Less obvious in the matter of patient and staff safety are such factors as the institution's alarm system, the role of its security force, spatial and architectural design, and the facility's attitude toward offenders. In regard to the latter, Hoge and Gutheil[14] have reviewed their own experience with the prosecution of assaultive patients, a complex endeavor but one which may well convey a message to the milieu of a hospital.

Nurses bear the brunt of injuries in hospital-based assaults, though psychiatrists have also been injured and even killed.[15] But few health professionals hear about these incidents in any professionally related way; organizations such as the American Psychiatric Association or the American Nursing Association do not disseminate data pertaining to the matter of injuries among their membership. Denial may play a major role here, for the subject matter is frightening and strangely alien to the more contemplative motives which lead most clinicians to become interested in mental health. Indeed, most nurses and physicians would state that the physical subjugation of mental patients is hardly what they trained for. There are no easy answers to these dilemmas. Rather, the profession must grapple openly with the fact that aggression management is part of the care of inpatients. Staff dealing with violent patients must acquire the fullest knowledge of all tactics and strategies, ranging from the physical restraint of combative patient and the application of a restraint device to the use of seclusion and effective titration of pharmacologic agents.[16,17]

REFERENCES

1. Lion JR, Reid WH (Editors): Assaults Within Psychiatric Facilities. New York, Grune & Stratton, 1983
2. Lion JR, Snyder W, Merrill GL: Underreporting of assaults on staff in a state hospital. Hosp Comm Psychiatry 1981; 32:497-498
3. Kayton L, Freed H: Effect of a suicide in a psychiatric hospital. Arch Gen Psychiatry 1967; 17:187-194
4. Krieger G: Management and mismanagement of a suicidal patient. Hosp Comm Psychiatry 1976; 27:411-413
5. Schwartz DA, Flinn DE, Slawson PF: Suicide in the psychiatric hospital. Am J Psychiatry 1975; 132:150-153
6. Copas JB, Robin A: Suicide in psychiatric inpatients. Brit J Psychiatry 1982; 141:503-511
7. Conn LM, Lion JR: Self-mutilation: a review. Psychiatric Med 1983; 1:21-34
8. Bach-Y-Rita G, Veno A: Habitual violence: a profile of 62 men. Am J Psychiatry 1974; 131:1015-1017
9. Wong SE, Slama KM, Liberman RP: Behavioral treatment of aggressive psychiatric and developmentally disabled patients, in Clinical Treatment of the Violent Person. Edited by Roth LH, DHHS Pub. # (ADM)85-1425, Rockville, MD, NIMH, 1985
10. American Psychiatric Association Task Force Report on Psychiatric Aspects of Restraint and Seclusion, Washington, DC, American Psychiatric Press, 1985d
11. Lion JR, Soloff P: Implementation of seclusion and restraint, in The Psychiatric Uses of Seclusion and Restraint. Edited by Tardiff K, Washington, DC, American Psychiatric Press, 1984
12. Infantino JA, Musingo S-Y: Assaults and injuries among staff with and without training in aggression control techniques. Hosp Comm Psychiatry 1985; 36:1312-1314
13. Ekblom B: Acts of Violence by Patients in Mental Hospitals. Stockholm, Scandinavian University Press, 1970
14. Hoge SK, Gutheil TG: The prosecution of psychiatric patients for assaults on staff: a preliminary empirical study. Hosp Comm Psychiatry 1987; 38:44-49
15. Madden DJ, Lion JR, Penna M: Assaults on psychiatrists by patients. Am J Psychiatry 1976; 133:422-425
16. Lion JR: Special aspects of psychopharmacology, in Assaults Within Psychiatric Facilities. Edited by Lion JR, Reid WH, New York, Grune and Stratton, 1983
17. Lion JR, Tupin J: The use of medication within the hospital setting, in Modern Hospital Psychiatry. Edited by Lion JR, Adler W, Webb W, New York, W.W. Norton, 1987

18
Treatment Considerations for Children and Adolescents

Donald H. Saidel
Richard M. Sarles

The existence of psychiatric hospital settings for children is a relatively recent phenomenon, dating back to the 1920s and 1930s, when units were established at Bellevue and Kings Park Hospital in New York, the Franklin School in Philadelphia, and the Bradley Hospital in Providence, Rhode Island. As knowledge has increased regarding the biological basis of childhood illnesses and as recognition of childhood psychiatric illnesses has improved, more hospital beds have been allotted to child and adolescent psychiatric patients. The largest growth in hospitals occurred in the 1970s, when facilities for the psychiatric treatment of children and adolescents sprang up around the country, partly reflecting a shift of care from the public to the private sector and increasing mental health insurance benefits.[1] The Joint Commission on Mental Health, in 1970, and the President's Commission on Mental Health, in 1978, both estimated that approximately .6 to 2% of children and adolescents are seriously enough disturbed to require some form of inpatient psychiatric hospitalization; this has also contributed to the increase in the number of hospital beds for children and adolescents.

Most communities in the United States do not have ready access to psychiatric hospitals. In these areas, hospitalization of a psychiatrically ill child or adolescent takes place on a general pediatric or medical ward and may represent a compromise in care; yet the mere removal of the child from a noxious home environment is often helpful. Placement of a child in a general hospital or medical ward may be useful if there is a good family support system or available outpatient care or if the patient is medically unstable or has a psychiatric condition secondary to a medical condition, such as asthma, diabetes, or ulcerative colitis.

OVERVIEW

Psychiatric hospitals are obviously needed for patients who require physical security, more intensive psychiatric services and the ancillary services of occupational and activity therapy, and a special school. The length of stay in the hospital is a function of several parameters, including the level of pathology, the availability and resources of the family, and the skills and orientation of the treatment team.

Short-term units often emphasize acute intervention, with a focus on stabilization and evaluation. A typical patient admitted to such a unit would be a teenager in acute turmoil with drug use and explosive tempers; once he is hospitalized and removed from his immediate environment, his behavior often quiets down, enabling the treatment team to make a diagnostic formulation and treatment recommendations. A very wide range of diagnostic groupings can be seen on short-term units, and as many as 20% of these cases are in need of long-term inpatient treatment.[2] The number transferred for such treatment is highly variable and is dependent upon available facilities and funding sources.

Intermediate-to-long-term hospital treatment for children and adolescents is usually prescribed for those patients who have impairment so severe that they cannot function normally in the home, community, or school, and who have failed to respond to a graduated intensity of psychosocial interventions in the community. Many of these patients have also had two or three admissions to short-term units. The pathology seen on a long-term unit is often characterologic rather than symptomatic, and may reflect behavior disturbances of childhood and severe adolescent adjustment conditions requiring milieu treatment and intensive individual and family therapy.

A typical patient referred for long-term hospital treatment would be a 15-year-old adolescent with a long history of poor peer relationships with declining academic performance. Sexual acting-out, poor appetite and hypersomnia, periods of intense sobbing and intermittent wide swings of mood had necessitated prior short-term hospitalization. Outpatient therapy following short-term hospitalization was unsuccessful due to erratic attendance and refusal to comply with medication.

Most intermediate and long-term hospital units are in psychiatric hospitals or specially designed units separate from a general hospital. Patients admitted to such units span the full range of diagnostic categories. On a children's unit, a large percentage of patients would fit the *DSM-III* diagnosis of pervasive developmental disorder, with affective disorders or severe attention deficit disorders also represented. Adolescent units would house a large percentage of identity-borderline disorders and affective disorders, with only a small percentage, perhaps 10%, of patients manifesting psychotic disorders. The treatment program usually addresses the psychiatric, psychosocial, and educational needs of individual patients through a multi-disciplinary approach. Various treatment modalities might include two to three times weekly individual therapy, twice weekly group therapy, daily recreational and activities therapy, and weekly family therapy, as well as medication when indicated. Obviously, the goals of long-term treatment are more ambitious than those of short-term treatment and generally involve reconstructive work with the patient and family. Eliciting change in a seriously disturbed family and patient requires sufficient time to permit the process of re-learning and rebuilding.

Residential treatment facilities usually offer intermediate-to-long-term treatment to children and adolescents with impairment insufficient to demand intensive hospital treatment but still too severe to permit outpatient treatment. Many residential centers grew out of orphanages. Gradually, however, it was recognized that many of the children and adolescents placed in residential centers had emotional difficulties serious enough to require a more comprehensive treatment orientation. A number of prominent clinicians, such as Aichhorn,[3] Redl and Wineman,[4] and Bettelheim,[5] have pioneered residential treatment facilities for behaviorally disturbed children. In these facilities, the methods of therapy have generally been based on the principles of the milieu, as a protective and nurturing environment with a "social model" philosophy of treatment.

STAFFING

Child and adolescent inpatient psychiatry programs generally require higher staff/patient ratios than adult programs. A National Association of Private Psychiatric Hospitals survey[6] showed that child psychiatry programs averaged 1.7 FTE direct care staff per child—almost twice that of adult programs. The staff must assume many functions of the parental role to insure that the child or adolescent follows the guidelines regarding proper hygiene, dressing, room cleaning, homework, and curfew.

Staff for most child and adolescent inpatient programs include child psychiatrists, child psychologists, social workers, occupational and activities therapists, psychiatric nurses, child care workers or mental health workers, and special education teachers. The exact number and concentration of these staff are dictated by the treatment philosophy of the institution, funding, and treatment programming. In general, short-term units require a higher staff-patient ratio than long-term units. In residential treatment centers, with the lowest staff-patient ratios, staff shift from direct care nurses and psychiatrists to child care workers and social workers. See Table 1 for recommended staffing guidelines.

ADMISSION CRITERIA

It is essential that each treatment program establish clear guidelines and criteria for admission. These criteria help define for the treatment staff, as well as for referral sources, the kinds of difficulties the program is designed to treat. The criteria for admission need to be related to the specific elements available in the treatment program. In a program that emphasizes the use of individual and group psychotherapy, it is important that patients who are admitted for treatment have some level of verbal capability and intellectual functioning above the retarded level. If a program is organized around the concept that treatment of children and adolescents requires active participation of the parental figures, then the latter's availability to the treatment process and team becomes an important criterion in determining admission of the patient. Furthermore, a facility may decide that only moderate behavior problems will be accepted for treatment due to limited staffing and lack of security. Or, a well endowed facility with a large staff may take on the labor-intensive treatment of schizophrenic children. Some facilities do well with hyperactive children who require medication, and other facilities focus on a psychotherapeutic model of intervention. Orientations vary considerably, even in this day and age.

Table 1
Staffing Guidelines

	12-BED COED UNIT		
	ACUTE UNIT	LONG-TERM UNIT	R.T.C. UNIT
Psychiatrist	2.5	1.8	.2
Psychologist	.5	.5	.1
Social Worker	2	.75	1.25
A.T./O.T.	2	.5	.25
Head Nurse	1	.5	
Staff Nurse	7	4.5	1.5
Mental Health Worker	8	7	4.5
Unit Clerk	.75	.25	

Unlike adult admissions, which often focus on symptoms, children and adolescents are usually admitted for developmental difficulties as reflected in poor school performance and social skills. Though somewhat vaguer and less acute than the adult counterpart, the child's pathology is viewed as nonetheless ominous, particularly if the patient has not responded to outpatient intervention. The following are two examples of patients referred for hospitalization.

> A 14-year-old boy was noted to be socially withdrawn at school with a distinct drop in performance. Outpatient evaluation revealed significant sexual conflicts, including masturbatory activity with mother's undergarments. Several months of outpatient treatment proved unsuccessful, as symptomatic difficulties continued and family stress increased.
>
> A 17-year-old girl begins her senior year in high school. She is described as a "model" student. Suddenly, she stops attending school and begins showing evidence of hallucinatory experiences. She reports voices are telling her "she is no good and should kill herself." A trial of medication does not reduce her distress or enable her to resume school attendance.

PRE-ADMISSION—ADMISSION PROCESS

The admission process for children and adolescents differs from that for adults. It is an essential element in establishing the therapeutic contract involving the hospital staff, the patient, and the patient's family. When patients are referred for long-term hospital treatment and a bed becomes available, the unit chief brings together the treatment team with the prospective patient and family. Often, the need to define responsibilities and set limits with a family begins with the scheduling of the pre-admission interview. While the hospital staff should not operate from a grandiose view of themselves, it is important that the family and prospective patient understand that there is a well-defined program and the staff bring clear expectations to their work with the patient and the family. During this interview team members describe their responsibilities in the treatment process and how they will work with the child and family. The family members then indicate why they believe hospitalization is indicated. Basic rules regarding patients' behavior, visiting, etc., are communicated. All parties to the treatment contract must be in some level of agreement. This means family members must then decide if they wish to proceed with the admission.

The pre-admission interview also allows the parents and child to observe the adaptive functioning of the "hospital family," the treatment team. Each individual on the team integrates his or her particular professional background and orientation with other professionals. The patient then has a model that reflects an ongoing treatment objective, the integration of his functioning. There are occasions when negotiations take place during the pre-admission process, when one or another aspect of the treatment program may prove unpalatable to the family or child. The team must determine with the family whether modifications can be made without compromising the quality and integrity of the treatment program.

Often, the referral material will provide indications of difficulties to be anticipated with the child and the family, and so, as a first step in the treatment process, the team focuses on these particular situations.

> Paul was a 14-year-old adolescent boy who had two previous short-term psychiatric hospitalizations. His mother had been suffering from severe psychiatric disorders for many years and frequently would be unable to set limits for Paul and would also engage in various forms of substance abuse with him. In the face of the difficulties with his wife and son, the father had become increasingly passive. He had been unable to accept the repeated recommendations for long-term hospital treatment for his son. When he finally did make the effort to provide long-term hospital care for his son, it was necessary to continually set limits with him in terms of when the admission needed to be scheduled. Finally, after many aborted admissions, he was told that the admission must take place at a designated time or it could no longer be made available. This type of intervention proved to be necessary in similar situations that occurred throughout the course of Paul's hospitalization. The patient experienced continued reduction of his internal tension and anxiety as he perceived the willingness of the team to continually provide necessary limits for him and for his parents.

The day of admission for a child or adolescent is a time of separation from the parents. Groundwork is necessary. The child should have seen the ward, and the pre-admission interview at the hospital should have prepared the child for the return visit during which he will be admitted. It is useful to encourage patients to bring those personal belongings with them that will help make the transition into the hospital less stressful. Often, the youngster needs to bring many personal belongings—stuffed animals, favorite posters, special records and tapes—in order to reduce the anxieties associated with the movement into the hospital.

PHYSICAL PLANT

In every aspect of work with children and adolescents, the developmental nature of their growth and developmental cycle must be taken into consideration. The primary characteristic of all child and adolescent inpatient hospital units is that they provide a safe, secure, and comfortable living environment. Colors should be bright and attractive, yet soft and soothing. Carpeting of the halls and individual patient rooms is desirable for softness and deadening of sound, but on school-age units, where a high proportion of children may be enuretic or encopretic, tiling may be preferable in individual bedrooms to reduce staining and odor. In general, child and adolescent psychiatric units require more square feet than adult units. A rule of thumb is a minimum of 300 square feet per child of on-ward space and 300 square feet of off-ward space (interview rooms, educational and recreational space).

Ward design should follow from the philosophy and treatment of the particular unit. It should reflect the active lifestyle of children and adolescents and be developmentally appropriate with the needs of the daily schedule in mind. For example, on school-age children's units it is often important to have a pantry and dining room for children to have their meals on-ward, in contrast to adult or adolescent units, where off-ward dining is more appropriate. Special washable walls may be constructed for hanging pictures or posters or for "special" graffiti. However, most units do not permit materials depicting drugs, alcohol, violence, or explicitly sexual scenes to be posted or written on walls. Each unit should be designed to have an adequate recreation space or day room for socialization. This area can also be used for group and milieu meetings or general free time activities. To emulate a home environment, the unit should also have a pantry and some form of cooking facilities so pizza can be heated and popcorn made, and rules and regulations for sharing, cleanliness and safety enacted.

Everything about the unit should be chosen for its therapeutic effect. The intent is to say, visually, to the child or adolescent, "You are safe here (from external and internal threats). You are welcome here and valued as a person. Your individuality and privacy are valued here. Your strengths are valued here. Your needs for comfort, help, activity, and fun are recognized here. Your ability for self-control is valued here and will be given scope to be exercised as you are able to do."[7]

Furniture should be sturdy and heavy to avoid breakage or throwing. Any damaged furniture or equipment must be quickly repaired or removed, since such disrepair invites further destructive behaviors. By using built-in furniture or two-way door latches, rooms may be designed so that patients cannot barricade themselves from within. Play spaces and group rooms are needed, and privacy on the hall needs to be respected. When hall policy allows bedroom doors to be closed, all staff and patients should knock and request admission before entering.

Nursing stations should be open to the ward, with closable half doors, and should be off limits to patients, but unbreakable glass partitions are seldom indicated. The nursing station should be located so as to command a clear view of the entire unit or hall and to monitor entrance to and exit from the unit of staff, patients, and visitors. Nursing staff should always be accessible, but should also have a private, quiet area for themselves.

The ideal unit has ready access to recreational spaces both within and without the hospital and easy access to school, which is always best contained within the same building as the inpatient units.

The number of patients on any unit is dependent on the geographic location of the hospital, the patient population served, and the general philosophy and length of stay. Thus, on an acute pediatric medical unit, one or two or three children with psychiatric disturbances may be housed, whereas in a large regional psychiatric hospital, up to 15 or 20 children or adolescents may be hospitalized on one psychiatric unit. When setting up a unit, however, the ideal range of adolescent patients is 10 to 12. If there are fewer than 10 patients, the milieu program lacks a critical mass for optimal functioning; more than 12 patients are difficult to manage to ensure patient safety and to provide individualized treatment. On children's units, eight patients appears to be an ideal number, because the younger child has less well developed ego structure defense mechanisms and capacity to delay gratification and modulate affect.

The question of locked versus open ward remains controversial but is best determined by the treatment philosophy of the unit, the type of patient, and the ability of the staff to maintain safety. For example, when a patient presents a suicidal or homicidal risk or a persistent risk of self-harm through runaway behavior or sexual, antisocial, or drug abuse behaviors, a locked unit is important. The decision to open or lock a door is usually made through an ongoing process of dialogue between patients and staff and depends upon issues of safety and trust. It is useful to enable the patients in a group to express thoughts and feelings regarding their ability to maintain control over their impulses. Often patients' anxiety regarding this ability will be expressed in their wish to keep the unit door locked. Other times they will express fears regarding the potential for self-destructive behavior of one of their peers and wish the unit door to be locked to protect this peer.

The locking or opening of doors needs to be seen in a broader context of the issue of control. The staff must emphasize that control of the unit is a means to help each patient control himself, with staff serving as models for the patient to foster inner controls by identification. Thus, control of children and adolescents on inpatient hospital units mainly results from the human relationship and has actually less to do with locks and doors, since an adolescent determined to leave the hospital will be able to run away from even the most restricted locked unit.[7]

AGE GROUPING

In general, it is best to maintain school-age children, 6 to 12 years old, on a separate unit because of their developmental needs and because of their size and vulnerability. On acute short-term units, it is reasonable to house adolescents age 13 to 18 in one treatment setting. However, in longer-term hospitalization, separation of younger adolescents (13 to 15 years old) from older ones (16 to 18 years old) is preferable. The developmental needs and tasks of these two groups are distinctly different; moreover, greater safety and comfort are provided for the individual and treatment team by distinguishing these age groups. Flexibility in these age groupings must be maintained. For example, a very physically mature and aggressive 12-year-old may be best housed on a younger adolescent unit, as well as a very physically and emotionally immature 17-year-old.

SEX GROUPING

Most short-term acute units are coed. On intermediate and long-term treatment units there is the option to have coed or unisexual units. There are advantages and disadvantages to both groupings. The advantage of a coed unit is that it provides a more natural social interactive environment; also, females on a unit tend to provide a quieter, less violent atmosphere. The disadvantages are that the chances for sexual acting-out are obviously increased, structurally two separate bathing and restroom facilities are needed, and admissions to the unit are limited by the availability of open beds for same-sex patients. A unisex unit avoids such problems but creates a potential for providing homosexual panic and also greater violence. In general, most adolescent intermediate or long-term units opt for a coed policy.

DIAGNOSTIC GROUPING

Except for specialized research units studying a specific diagnostic problem such as affective disorders or autism and pervasive developmental disorders, most child and adolescent units admit a full spectrum of diagnostic entities. A balance of various diagnostic categories provides the staff different therapeutic challenges and a broad spectrum of outcomes. This may minimize frustration and burnout of staff. However, the geographic location of the unit may lead to predominance of a certain population. For example, an inner-city hospital unit may attract patients with conduct disorders or drug-alcohol-related problems. If the unit functions as a tertiary care facility, specializing in long-term treatment or treatment-resistant patients, there may be an overrepresentation of the psychotic disorders, severe major depression, bipolar affective disorders, and borderline personality disorders.

ASSESSMENT/EVALUATION

Medical

The inpatient psychiatric unit provides an opportunity for the in-depth, continuous observation of the child and adolescent patient. Cycles of wakefulness and rest and activity levels may be monitored. Energy, mood, judgment, attachment to peers and staff, and areas of strengths and weaknesses are under constant observation. How the child functions in the activities of daily living in his own "life space" is equivalent to a mental status examination over time.

A thorough medical examination is required of all patients admitted to an inpatient psychiatric unit. This may be accomplished by a staff or consulting pediatrician or performed by one of the physician/therapists on the treatment team. A complete standardized physical examination must be accomplished with entrance of data onto a growth chart. There should be no routine laboratory investigations; all requested laboratory tests must be based on solid clinical judgment, for example, a strong suspicion of renal disease or brain tumor. The judgment of the physician should determine the use of the dexamethasone suppression test, EEG, CT, urine screening for abnormal metabolites, ophthalmological examination for cytomegalic virus inclusions, for example, or specialized studies or consultations in cases of suspected physical or sexual abuse.

A neurological exam beyond that in the standard physical should be requested only when history and physical examination indicate. It is clear that psychiatric inpatients have a higher incidence of learning disabilities than the general population and thus the history and physical should pay particular attention to the areas of attention deficits, short attention span, soft neurological signs, and clumsiness. Speech and language evaluations may be indicated.

Psychological

Generally, a standard battery of psychological assessment techniques proves useful in evaluating the functioning of child and adolescent patients. This would include measures of intellectual functioning, neurological functioning, and projective instruments such as the Rorschach and the Thematic Apperception Test. The psychological assessment aids not only in providing information regarding diagnosis but also in the elaboration of defensive operations, vulnerabilities, object relationships, and potential difficulties that might be encountered within the treatment process.

The psychological assessment should be completed on all adolescents admitted to the hospital for short-term treatment. Child and adolescent patients who are admitted for long-term treatment have often had psychological evaluations within the past several months. Unless there is question as to the validity or reliability of the findings, it is generally not useful to repeat the assessment. As treatment progresses, it may be useful to repeat all or portions of the assessment to provide another view of the patient's functioning. This is sometimes beneficial in providing a measure of change in functioning or when there is significant variation from the anticipated course of treatment. In some instances, when the admitting diagnosis is not clear, and after the acute symptomatology subsides, psychological assessment may be repeated for further diagnostic clarification.

Educational

The educational evaluation of the child and adolescent inpatient includes standardized achievement testing to ascertain current levels of educational achievement and also to assess the existence of learning disabilities. In addition, the educational assessment should include material from the most previous school experiences of the youngster as a measure of the current level of functioning. Many children and adolescents who enter hospitals for treatment are in need of special educational programming. For short-term patients, discharge planning may include varying levels of special educational services. The educational evaluation serves to identify the patient with these needs and to assist in assessing the required level of intervention, e.g., special education classes or a special education day program.

The Family

It is essential that a thorough psychosocial history of the patient's family be obtained. A high percentage of children and adolescents admitted to a psychiatric hospital comes from families where there are indications of significant pathology in one or both of the parents. This assessment information is invaluable in understanding the "natural history" of a child and in learning how the child has developed thus far. The family assessment also needs to address the parents' availability for treatment and their capacity to allow the treatment of the child to move forward. Often the resistance of the child or adolescent to treatment reflects the resistance of the parents to threats of their own pathology emerging.[8]

An integration of these various assessments should then provide a comprehensive understanding of the child's pathological functioning, as well as help in the ongoing process of treatment and discharge planning for the youngster. It allows for the anticipation of the course of treatment and enables the team to identify and prepare for disruptions and interferences as the treatment process unfolds.

TREATMENT PROCESS

Team Approach

The hospital treatment of children and adolescents exemplifies the importance of the multidisciplinary team providing multiple therapeutic approaches. Generally, it is beneficial to have one person identified as the team leader with the responsibility of coordinating and integrating the various treatment approaches. Regardless of the diagnosis of the youngster and the assessment of his or her various strengths and weaknesses, that youngster's pathology evolved within the context of relationships with others. The various members of the treatment team become the new figures, the displacement and transferential objects that the child reacts to and engages with as the treatment process recapitulates prior life experiences.

The beginning phase of treatment is the establishing of a safe and secure environment within which the patient's interactions with the staff may progress. In order for the patient to experience this sense of safety and security, it is essential that the staff be consistent and stable. Thus, it is preferable to have small treatment units with a small number of staff who are assigned responsibility of providing for the treatment to that group of patients. In this way, the patients deal with the same staff members day in and day out, while the staff members similarly deal with the same patients day in and day out. As such, the team engages in an ongoing struggle in order to help the patient relinquish previous pathological behaviors, which are nonetheless gratifying, in order to take the risk of developing new modes of interactions, new views of the self, and new views of the internal representations of people from the past that the patient brings into the treatment process.

It is possible to think of the treatment team as representing the executive ego, that is, the ego that observes, integrates, controls, and directs adaptive functions. One might also conceptualize the treatment team as representing different ego functions that gain integration through the communication process of the team members. For example, one member of the team may reflect dependency needs, another may reflect rules and regulations, and still another may reflect nurturance. It is through the integration and combination of these various aspects of the ego that the team demonstrates for the child integrated and adaptive functioning. The team must be able to experience stress and disagreement, as well as resolution of conflicts, just as the individual patient experiences internal conflicts—and slowly learns to resolve them. The team then becomes the symbol to the patient of the potential gratifications of healthy, adaptive functioning.

Initially, the treatment team must be willing to provide the necessary limits to the untoward behaviors of the patient. The acting-out of conflicts is continually thwarted, thereby increasing internal tension and anxiety levels; this produces the energy necessary for therapeutic work. Within the team it is important that each member feel valued, important and a contributor to the total effort of the team. It is essential that each discipline maintain respect for the integrity of the varying treatment modalities represented on the team. The individual psychotherapist may be struggling with the patient as they both explore issues related to anger toward parental figures. The therapist needs to recognize that at times some of these feelings are displaced onto nursing staff. Oftentimes, adolescent and child patients communicate with such intensity, with such fervor, that it is easy to be swept up in their distortions. The team must then provide checks and balances for its individual members so that acceptance of these distortions is minimized.

The treatment process should also include aspects of "normal" developmental experiences. Opportunities for both same-sex and opposite-sex peer interactions need to be integrated into the treatment program, as well as opportunities for physical exercise and the development of motor coordination.

The Milieu

The nursing staff has the responsibility for managing the milieu by establishing rules and guidelines. Attention is focused on routine tasks of daily living, including the wake-up time in the morning and the lights-out time at night. Throughout the day the activities of the patients need to be carefully monitored and programmed. At times, the nursing staff becomes the superego which confronts, limits and restricts the patients' behaviors; at other times the nursing staff represents the nurturant parent who provides the cup of hot chocolate to help the child in the transition from wake to sleep in the evening. The staff on the unit often become brother, sister, father, mother, policeman, and teacher to the patient. The nursing staff needs to have sufficient flexibility and self-awareness to allow these projective and displaced views in their interactions with the patients.

It is useful for the milieu program to include clear expectations and therapeutic activities that foster developmentally appropriate responsibilities for the patients. This might begin with a focus on the patient's responsibility for self-care, then for care of personal belongings, and finally for the general cleanliness of the unit and the well-being of one's peers. These expectations are always there. However, the assessment of each patient provides the necessary benchmarks that ensure that the patient will feel successful in his endeavors. Behavioral goals are individually determined and based on the needs of the particular patient.

Psychotherapy

Individual: Each child and adolescent patient needs to be provided with an individual psychotherapist. Oftentimes, the work in therapy seems solely to be the development of basic trust—the capacity for which is normally achieved in infancy. The disruptions in the relationships of those children and adolescents who require intensive, long-term hospital care is such that this basic trust, a very early phase of the developmental process, must be reexperienced with a more positive outcome than occurred initially. The psychotherapist must be able to withstand the onslaught of the anger and rejection while recognizing how important the relationship is to the patient. It is not uncommon for the therapist to feel that little is happening in the psychotherapy until, upon returning to the hospital from vacation, he is confronted by acting-out behaviors that reflect the anger and sense of abandonment that the patient felt during his absence. Patients often experience profound guilt related to this anger toward their therapists and may try to protect the therapist from these feelings. The skilled psychotherapist needs to provide a safe, controlled psychotherapeutic medium wherein these feelings can be verbalized.

It is essential that the psychotherapist not be seduced into allowing patients to act out their feelings. The prime focus of the psychotherapy must be to help patients increase their capacity for the verbal expression of feelings and thoughts. Interestingly, many adolescent patients do not begin the work of serious exploration until they have been discharged from the hospital. It is as if the experience in the hospital treatment represented a new beginning, a new foundation of a more stable ego; this provides the capacity for self-observation and exploration after discharge from the hospital. One might then think of the psychotherapy process in the hospital as helping the adolescent move forward until that time when the more traditional psychotherapy process becomes available to him.

Group Therapy: Group therapy is an indispensable part of the treatment program for adolescent patients. Early adolescent development includes strong allegiance to the group, with the group frequently becoming the substitute for the parents. The group becomes an important element in maintaining a positive treatment attitude among hospitalized adolescents,[9] with the better functioning members of the group interpreting to their peers their acting-out and treatment resistances. The development of the treatment group requires that patients continue living within the same treatment units throughout the course of their hospitalization. The group experiences a flow of patients, some entering in the beginning of treatment, some in the middle, and some at the final stages as they are ready for discharge. The group gains new members as old members move toward more independent functioning. The older members then become the source of role modeling for the newer patients, demonstrating that treatment can offer something positive, that the staff can be trusted, and that the maladaptive behaviors displayed by the new group members are not acceptable to the older members of the group. Within the group the internal struggle of each individual patient is manifested; that is, the struggle between the part that wishes to resist and cannot tolerate change versus the part that recognizes that change is necessary. In addition to its use as a psychotherapy medium, the patient group plays an important role in the treatment milieu. As the group demonstrates more adaptive functioning, it is given greater responsibility in the decision-making process affecting the lives of its members. This may range from decisions regarding activities to the locking or unlocking of doors.

In terms of the structure of group psychotherapy, various clinicians have found different approaches beneficial. There are some who believe it is useful to conduct all group therapy away from the patients' living units. On the other hand, the issues of living together often provide important material within the group therapy process, so that the day-to-day struggles become important thematic material within the group therapy; hence, the group sessions might best be held on the unit. It is essential that the individual and group psychotherapists maintain clearly defined meeting times and places with their patients, even when the latter reject therapy. If a patient chooses to resist by not attending a psychotherapy session, it is imperative that the psychotherapist still be available and keep the appointed time free for that patient.

Family Therapy

Family therapy is an important part of the treatment process. Hospital treatment represents a continued assessment of the role of the various family members in supporting the child or adolescent patient's pathological functioning or in dealing with the changes that treatment has induced in the identified patient. The family therapy process enables the child or adolescent to renegotiate the relationship with the parents and vice versa. Oftentimes hospital treatment uncovers a range of "family secrets" and it becomes necessary for the patient to confront the parental figures regarding these.

Level System

All hospital programs need to include some mechanism for monitoring the levels of responsibility individual patients may attain. It is useful to have clear behavioral requirements related to the degree of responsibility. Levels may be numerically coded, color coded, or otherwise labeled. All patients are begun on Level 1 or staff escort, whereby the patient is always with a member of the staff as he or she moves around the institution. As the patient demonstrates increased capacity for self-control, he is given a higher level of responsibility, which often enables him to travel from one place in the hospital to another with another patient and eventually on his own. Built into the system is the requirement that patients keep the staff advised as to where they are going and when they shall return to their units.

Sometimes the dependency needs of patients are so overwhelming that every time they move to higher levels of responsibility they must undo their newly achieved success by acting-out behavior, which results in a reduction of their level. With such patients, it may be best to eliminate the concept of increased responsibilities, lest failure ensue. Some of these youngsters are severely in need of the relationship with the staff and are often unable to verbalize this need; acting-out of anxiety occurs as soon as they are given some additional responsibility for themselves. As the process repeats itself again and again, it is important that the team members communicate to the patient that he will remain on the base level for an indefinite period of time. This treatment intervention is often sufficient to allow the patient to explore his fears of independence and his anxieties regarding relinquishment of his dependent status.

> John seemed to demonstrate improved functioning. However, each time he achieved higher responsibility levels, he would fail to maintain previously demonstrated behaviors. It was felt he was struggling with his need to feel close to staff. His treatment plan was modified so that improved functioning would not lead to higher responsibility levels thereby allowing him to remain on a level wherein contact with the staff was guaranteed. No longer needing "to ask" for contact with the "parental" figures through his acting-out behaviors, he was gradually able to maintain higher levels of functioning.

At times, adolescents' self-destructive behaviors become sufficiently severe so as to call for significant restrictions in their daily functions. The staff must be prepared to maintain patients on their living units sometimes for several days in order to help reduce these disruptions in daily functioning.

Medication

The philosophy of medication use varies widely, depending upon the orientation of the hospital. Some facilities use somatic treatment methods heavily, while others utilize a more psychodynamic or psychosocial approach. Some institutions receive more hyperkinetic or behaviorally aggressive patients, many of whom require medications. The use of psychotropic medications in children is beyond the scope of this chapter. However, it would not be unusual to find 50% of the patients on a long-term children's unit receiving some psychotropic medication, perhaps 50% neuroleptics, 30% antidepressants, 15% stimulants, and 5% Lithium.

School

The hospital treatment program for children and adolescents needs a special educational program and school. In addition to providing the normal developmental experience for the child and adolescent inpatient, a school also provides a window to the real world. Thus, the material covered in the curriculum represents a form of socialization of the child and adolescent patient, as well as an introduction and ongoing dialogue between that individual and the society in which he or she lives. At the same time, each child and adolescent needs to continue the tasks of mastering and achieving within the learning situation. The school must be perceived as an integral part of the therapy program and not as a separate, autonomous, free-standing entity. It is important that there be ongoing dialogue at staff and administrative levels. It is preferable that faculty members be employees of the hospital rather than teachers assigned from the local educational jurisdictions, as this allows for greater integration of the school into the overall treatment program. The school also needs to provide the range of special educational programming, including speech and hearing teachers, and the capability of participating with the team in the discharge-planning process by addressing the post-discharge educational needs of the child.

For patients on short-term units, the school experience is often best provided through the home and hospital teacher, who comes in for brief periods of time during the week to continue the educational process.

Activity Therapies

A broad array of activity therapies should be included in both short- and long-term programs. These include occupational therapy, therapeutic recreation, and art and movement therapies. In the short-term program, these modalities are important components of the assessment process, providing important information regarding what patients can do. As part of the long-term programs, these treatment modalities become important vehicles for patients to make up for deficiencies in functioning related to their psychiatric disorders. For example, the isolated adolescent with impaired peer relationships is gradually moved by the occupational therapist from one-to-one activities with the occupational therapist into a small group with a defined project.

Use of Quiet Room, Seclusion and Restraint

Removing the patient from the stimulation of his environment is an essential ingredient in the treatment of children and adolescents. One can think of certain child or adolescent patients as having failed to develop adequate mechanisms for defending against external stimulation or their own impulses. At these times, removal of the patient becomes important in helping him regain his own defensive controls. Therefore, such treatment interventions should be conceptualized and designed to help the patient with mastery and development of self-control.

Indications for the use of these treatment interventions include: (a) self-injurious behavior; (b) behavior physically dangerous to others; (c) destruction of property; and (d) disruption of the therapeutic milieu where the patient's uncontrolled behavior interferes with the treatment of others.[10] The intensity of the intervention needs to be determined by the severity of the loss of control experienced by the patient and also by the staff's knowledge of the patient. Thus, sometimes simply suggesting to the patient that he take 15 minutes in the quiet room is sufficient to enable him to regain control over impulses. However, staff may quickly place another individual behaving in the same way in locked seclusion because of staff's knowledge that, once an initial breakdown has occurred in this patient's control mechanisms, what follows may be an opening of the flood gates, with major and serious loss of control. Often, the staff must struggle with countertransferential feelings related to their "punishment" of patients. However, the failure to provide adequate external controls is often more punitive than their enactment.

A very useful technique with certain adolescent patients who experience significant disruptions in their control mechanisms is the use of cold wet sheet packs.[11,12] This procedure allows many severely disturbed patients to feel a sense of comfort and warmth, which may seem paradoxical given the fact that they are restrained on a table with sheets wrapped around them and straps holding them to the table. Often, material emerges during this process which the patient has been struggling with for a significant period of time and which has been seriously disruptive to his or her functioning. It has been useful with such patients for their therapist to conduct a psychotherapy session while the patient is in the sheet pack.

> Linda reported hearing voices directing her to do self harm. Indeed, over a period of years she had engaged in increasingly lethal self destructive activity. In the hospital, she had begun to run into walls with her head. This behavior was unpredictable and unresponsive to psychotropic medications. All the time she continued to report the "voices." She was begun on a treatment program including twice daily sheet packs. Her psychotherapist conducted many sessions with her while she was sheet packed. Gradually her delusional thoughts diminished and her self-destructive behaviors were eliminated. While Linda needed continued intensive hospital treatment, her new control over self-destructive behaviors provided a foundation for treatment to continue without the threat that she would permanently injure herself.

It is useful to minimize the extent of physical contact between staff and patients, regardless of the form of restraint. Thereby patients are removed from external stimulation and can begin to regain self-control. It is important for staff to be trained in techniques of aggression management to reduce the danger of physical harm to both staff and patients.

These techniques of restraint need to be considered as important components of the staff's efforts to maintain a safe and secure environment for all patients. Patients must believe and experience the security and safety of the treatment environment so that they can begin to recognize that external controls can be provided to them when they are faced with the onslaught of their own devastating impulses. Without the use of such mechanisms, it is impossible for treatment to progress and for patients to achieve higher levels of functioning.

The reevaluation

It is generally useful in long-term intensive hospital programs for children and adolescents to have a mechanism built into the program for periodically reevaluating the patient's progress. These reevaluations are best conducted by a member of the staff who is not directly involved in that patient's treatment. The reevaluation conference allows the treatment team to assemble with the staff consultant to review the course of treatment thus far. The consultant can then provide recommendations for impasses that have emerged in the treatment process or sometimes simply reinforce the treatment planning that has already taken place. Thus, these reevaluations provide the necessary feedback to the team members that they are on the right track or that they need to modify their goals and expectations of each other and of the patient. In addition, the treatment process with children and adolescents is so fraught with the potential for countertransference reactions that the reevaluation process serves to provide one of the means of checking such interferences in the treatment process. Often, the consultant needs to carefully ascertain the particular problems that have brought the team to this reevaluation conference. That is, why did the team choose one person over another to conduct the reevaluation? How does that help the reevaluator understand the treatment process and enable him to provide assistance and guidance to the treatment team in working with the patient?

Behavior Problems

Child and adolescent patients present a range of behavioral difficulties throughout the course of their hospitalization. Often it is the very behaviors that the child shows in the hospital that have led to the need for hospitalization itself. These behavioral difficulties often are experienced by the treatment team as well within the control of the patient. One of the countertransference issues the staff struggles with is the anger provoked by these behaviors interfering with the ability to identify their pathogenic roots. Treatment planning needs to include clear strategies for reducing the gratification the youngster experiences through the acting-out behavior. These behavioral problems range from patients' failure to manage their daily responsibilities on the unit, e.g., failure to clean their rooms, to more severe problems manifested through the impulsive acting-out of sexual feelings. Running away behavior is manifested by some adolescent patients and obviously represents a serious disruption to the treatment process.

> Jeff, a 16-year-old patient, intermittently refused to arise on time, attend to his personal hygiene and organize himself for the school day. He then became angry and seclusive when his privilege level was reduced. At the same time he seemed to gain great pleasure from arguing with the staff about how unfairly he was treated. The staff, aware of their anger, recognized that each time Jeff drew closer to independent privileges, his behavior deteriorated as a means of forcing staff to set limits. He was placed on a clear behavioral program including a behav-

ior sheet from each of his teachers and daily talks with a member of the staff. His performance was recorded on a checklist so he could monitor his functioning. In psychotherapy, it was possible to begin to work on understanding his anger and feelings of inadequacy and rejection by parental figures.

Usually patients do not manufacture new behaviors for treatment. Thus, one can look at the patient's history as an indication of how the youngster is likely to behave within the treatment environment. This enables the staff to anticipate behavioral problems, to develop contingency plans, and to intervene before behaviors reach serious levels. It is essential that the team members work in a prospective fashion in their efforts to anticipate the behavioral problems patients may present. On the other hand, they should not be disheartened by the need to continually set limits before old behaviors are replaced by higher level functioning.

THE DISCHARGE PROCESS

Criteria for Discharge

The discharge process is clearly dictated by the severity of symptomatology requiring admission, the ability to stabilize the patient and family, the resources within the home and the community, and financial limitations.

On short-term acute units, discharge planning generally begins with the admission process and proceeds actively within a predetermined time. On longer-term units, where personality restructuring is a goal of treatment, long-term discharge planning is required and is usually updated with periodic reevaluation of the patient's and the family's progress. Resolution of the presenting problems and the ability to function in a less restricted environment are indicators of the potential for discharge. In addition, the adaptive behavior on the unit and in everyday life gives some indication that the patient's strengths outweigh weaknesses and that the patient is able to tolerate stress and modulate affect. Of equal importance is the balance of the patient's inner thoughts against the visible, surface behavior. In general, on longer-term units a gradual reentry into the community is a part of the discharge process. Off grounds, out of hospital visits, home visits, and overnight or weekend visits are an important part of this process.

Post-Discharge Treatment

For most patients on either short- or long-term units, some form of aftercare is required. Careful integration with the patient's community school is an important part of such planning. Communication with the school and with the patient's therapist within the community is an important part of pre- and post-discharge care.

Regression at the time of discharge with return of original symptomatology is a common finding. This appears to be a defense mechanism to ward off the cultural shock of reentering the home, community, and school, where many of the problems which precipitated or created difficulties for the child or adolescent (drugs, alcoholism, troubled friends) are present. The return of symptoms may also indicate the fear of the loss of support and security of the hospital and the hospital staff. Sometimes, patients will wish to return to visit staff in the hospital many months after their discharge. These visits are positive experiences for staff and present patients, as well as for the visitor.

REFERENCES

1. Levinson AI: The growth of investor owned psychiatric hospitals. Am J Psychiatry 1982; 139:902
2. Sheppard and Enoch Pratt Hospital unpublished data
3. Aichhorn A: Wayward Youth, New York, Viking, 1935
4. Redl F, Wineman D: The Aggressive Child. Glencoe, Il, Free Press, 1957
5. Bettelheim B: A Home for the Heart. New York, Knopf, 1974
6. Gibson RW: Staffing Patterns Survey. National Association of Private Psychiatric Hospitals, Research Memo #512. Washington, DC, NAPPH, May 1981
7. Harper G, Geraty R: Hospital and Residential Treatment, in Psychiatry, Vol 6. Edited by Solnit AJ, Cohen DJ, Schowalter JE, New York, Basic Books, 1986
8. Rinsley DB, Hall DD: Psychiatric hospital treatment of adolescents: parental resistances as expressed in casework metaphor. Arch Gen Psychiatry 1962; 7:282-294
9. Lewis JM, Gosset JT, King JW, et al: Development of a pro-treatment group process among hospitalized adolescents. Adol Psych 1973; 2:351-362
10. Gair DS: Guidelines for children and adolescents, in The Psychiatric Uses of Seclusion and Restraint. Edited by Tardiff K, Washington, DC, American Psychiatric Press, 1984
11. Kilgalen RK: Hydrotherapy: is it all washed up? J Psych Nur 1972; 10:3-6
12. Singh H: Treating a severely disturbed self-destructive adolescent with cold wet sheet packs. Hosp Comm Psych 1986; 37:287-288

19
Inpatient Treatment Considerations of the Elderly

Barry W. Rovner
Marshal F. Folstein

There are currently 27 million people over 65 in the United States and this number will double in the next 50 years. This will confront psychiatrists with the care of many patients with dementia, delirium and depression.[1] These patients will often require hospitalization when ill, because their mental, physical, and social functioning tends to break down at once, overwhelming families and outpatient physicians. Once hospitalized, they require accurate diagnoses, multidisciplinary care and planning for rehabilitation from the onset.

Psychiatric disorders in the elderly often present with changes in cognition and mood, although symptoms in both areas can be part of different disorders.[3-7] For example, memory impairment combined with language disorder suggests dementia; memory impairment with depression suggests the dementia syndrome of depression; and memory impairment with alteration in consciousness suggests delirium. A similar differential diagnostic process applies to depression. Elderly persons can experience depression as an understandable response to loss, as in the case of grief, or suffer depression as the central feature of a pervasive and persistent syndrome. In the

---

The authors wish to thank Paul McHugh, M.D. for his review of the chapter and Colleen Gibson for preparation of the manuscript.

former case the mood is usually transient and unassociated with self-reproach or suicidal ideation; in the latter, negative self-attitude, disruptions in sleep, appetite and energy, and suicidal ideation can be present. Distinguishing depression as a transient and reactive mood from syndromal depression is important because they have different treatment implications. While counseling and supportive measures may suffice for the treatment of grief, vigorous somatic treatment is required for major depression.

Frequently, families may not be able to provide the necessary details about the history of onset, rate of progression, and relationship of symptoms to level of consciousness, mood, and intellectual capacity to enable outpatient psychiatrists to distinguish one condition from another. Furthermore, demented patients can become depressed or delirious, depressed patients may appear demented, and both demented and depressed patients can become delirious as a result of medications or other medical illnesses. The clinician must anticipate and recognize these various complications and be able to separate and treat them. This often requires hospitalization to permit continuous observation by experienced staff.

Delirium is a psychiatric syndrome defined by an alteration of consciousness and cognitive impairment. Although it occurs in 10–15% of medical and surgical patients, it is frequently undiagnosed. Risk factors for delirium include age, brain damage due to dementia, stroke, head injury, or seizure disorder, as well as medications. When delirium is readily apparent, the patient is drowsy, unable to remain alert, and exhibits a disrupted sleep-wake cycle. In a more subtle form, the delirious patient manifests only poor attention and inefficiency of thought. Associated changes include anxiety, restlessness, visual hallucinations, and paranoid delusions. Autonomic signs, such as tachycardia, fever, and temperature elevation, suggest an underlying metabolic or toxic process. Commonly medications, particularly those with anticholinergic activity, and urinary tract infections, anemia, electrolyte imbalance, and other metabolic disturbances are responsible.[8,9]

Diagnosing delirium and following its course can be assisted by using brief, quantitative clinical instruments such as the Mini-Mental State Exam.[10] Measuring cognitive capacity illustrates the patient's impairment and maintains awareness of the patient's limitations and need for supervision, assistance, and reassurance.

If cognition impairment is present in a non-delirious patient, depression must be ruled out as its cause. A past history of affective disorder, a subacute onset, a persistently low mood associated with sleep or appetite disturbance, and delusions of self-blame, hopelessness, or physical illness suggest an affective disorder.[11] It is important to recognize depression in this population because elderly men, particularly those physically impaired, are at high risk for suicide. Other risk factors for suicide include previous attempts, alcoholism, being unmarried, and having had recent surgery.

Not all depression in the elderly presents with cognitive impairment. In fact, more often the depressive symptoms are most prominent and cognitive impairment might be minimal. However, in patients with the dementia syndrome of depression, their low self-attitude, tendency to exaggerate failures, and hopelessness contrast with the generally good self-attitude and denial of symptoms of demented patients with Alzheimer's disease. While some patients with Alzheimer's do report their disability, they less often feel worthless or consider suicide.

Nevertheless, patients with Alzheimer's Disease can become depressed. Approximately 15% of these patients will exhibit a sustained change in mood and behavior characterized by dysphoria, tearfulness, feeling like a burden or suffering an abrupt decline in cognitive function superimposed on their preexisting impairment.[13] Because the depression often responds to treatment with tricyclics, it is important for clinicians to recognize and treat this complication.

Depression is known to follow stroke, particularly when the stroke results in left frontal damage. The depressive symptoms, their natural history, and their response to tricyclic antidepressants parallel those of depressions without known medical causes. Cognitive impairment associated with the depressed state in stroke patients occurs as well, and improves when the depression is treated. These findings emphasize the importance of recognizing the post-stroke depression syndrome and initiating appropriate antidepressant therapy promptly.[12]

Patients with irreversible dementia syndromes, such as Alzheimer's disease and multi-infarct dementia, are commonly admitted to inpatient psychiatric services. Because the diagnostic evaluation can usually be completed on an outpatient basis, demented patients admitted to inpatient units will be those whose cognitive impairment is complicated by behavioral disturbances, insomnia, depression, delusions or hallucinations. Table 1 lists the behaviors that cause the most serious problems for caregivers of demented patients, and Table 2 shows the problems caregivers report for themselves.[14,15]

Delusions or hallucinations complicate the dementia syndrome in one-third of cases seen in outpatient clinics.[16] Delusions are often present in relation to cognitive impairment. Individuals unable to remember where they place things may accuse others of stealing them. The presence of delusions or hallucinations alone, however, is not necessarily an indication for neuroleptics. Only when they are particularly frightening or lead to agitation might treatment be necessary.[17] Neuroleptics are also useful in patients

Table 1
Behaviors Cited as Causing Serious Problems

BEHAVIOR	NO. OF FAMILIES REPORTING	NO. (%) OF FAMILIES REPORTING IT AS A SERIOUS PROBLEM
Physical Violence	23	18 (75)
Memory Disturbance	37	25 (68)
Incontinence	21	13 (62)
Catastrophic Reactions	45	25 (56)
Hitting	16	8 (50)
Making Accusations	32	16 (50)
Suspiciousness	33	16 (48)

who are easily upset when minimally stressed, despite optimal approaches of staff or family.

The use of specific somatic treatment methods is beyond the scope of this chapter; however, a few basic principles will be mentioned. First, elderly patients may respond to lower than usual adult doses of medication due to physiological changes in absorption, distribution, metabolism, and excretion of drugs. However, a frequent error is to use excessively low and ineffective dosages. Antidepressant drugs are generally well-tolerated, although orthostatic hypotension and anticholinergic side effects can limit their use. Nortriptyline is the tricyclic least likely to cause orthostatic hypotension. Desipramine and Trazodone are among the least anticholinergic antidepressants and should be used for patients who cannot tolerate the anticholinergic effects of other tricyclics. Experience with newer antidepressants is limited. Until they are shown to have specific advantages, it is prudent to use agents of known reliability.[18-20]

MAO inhibitors may be useful for persons who are unresponsive to tricy-

Table 2
Problems Caregivers Cite for Themselves (N = 55)

	NO.	%
Chronic fatigue, anger, depression	48	87
Family conflict	31	56
Loss of friends and hobbies, no time for self	30	55
Worry that caregiver will become ill	17	31
Difficulty assuming new roles and responsibilities	16	29
Guilt	14	25
None	4	7

clics or who cannot tolerate them because of their anticholinergic effects. Ritalin is useful in the management of depression characterized by apathy, psychomotor retardation, and low mood that is worse in the morning.[21,22]

Lithium's utility in geriatric patients is established, particularly for the prophylaxis of bipolar disorder and the treatment of mania. However, lithium is more often associated with delirium in elderly than in younger populations, and lower levels are preferred, especially as kidney function declines with age.

The side effects associated with lithium include tremor, thirst, nausea, diarrhea and excessive urination. Because older persons are at risk for a variety of gastrointestinal and renal disorders, careful attention must be paid to any of these side effects. Also, because of the high prevalence of hypertension in the elderly, patients should be instructed about the interaction of lithium and diuretics to avoid lithium toxicity.[23]

When using antipsychotic medications, the clinician should anticipate the induction of parkinsonian side effects in a population already prone to such neurologic complications. Therefore, the use of low-potency agents such as thioridazine should be considered over haloperidol. Despite its higher anticholinergic activity, in our experience thioridazine is no more likely than haloperidol to impair cognition.[24]

Electroconvulsive therapy is often the most effective and rapid treatment for treatment-resistant depressive illness in the elderly. ECT should be considered for patients who cannot tolerate pharmacologic regimens for depression or who have delusional depression. Clinical experience suggests that ECT does not produce lasting memory changes in older patients. However, transient delirium following treatment is not uncommon.[25] Unilateral ECT is less likely to cause delirium. When ECT is used in patients with preexisting cognitive impairment, for example in those with Alzheimer's Disease, careful establishment of baseline cognitive function is necessary to detect superimposed impairment and the level of function the patient should return to following treatment.

While much of the care of elderly inpatients focuses on biological treatments, their care must also include psychological management. The goals of psychotherapy for these patients will depend on their illnesses, their cognitive status, their living situation (alone or with family), and the reality of certain losses of physical well-being, friends and family, and intellectual abilities. Therapy may be initially supportive, when the reasons for hospitalization, the purpose of treatment, and the nature of underlying disorders need clarification.

The psychotherapeutic process can often begin by helping patients make sense of the perplexing array of physical, emotional and social changes that beset them. Most patients require simple solutions to practical problems, and an empathic, supportive, and active therapist is valued. This approach encourages physicians and nursing staff to appreciate the patients' mental experiences as best they can and design strategies to improve their lives.

Hospitalization can also permit time for families to deal with the psychological issues of living with an impaired elderly relative. These might include redistributing responsibilities among family members and resolving conflicts reactivated by crisis.[26] Sadness and frustration over the losses already experienced and anticipatory grief over those to come are the most common issues in therapy. Effective treatment depends on a trusting relationship between the treatment team and the caregivers. Questions and expression of feelings are encouraged to provide information and emotional relief for family members. These allow hospital staff to assess the emotional strengths and needs of the family. Information about the patient's disorder, help dealing with specific psychological issues, and education regarding care enable families to adjust and to carry on care at home.

Care on the unit should be carried out by a multidisciplinary team under the direction of the neuropsychiatrist. The team might consist of the neuropsychiatrist, the head nurse and other nursing staff, a social worker, and occupational therapy staff. This team should meet daily and discuss each patient's mental status, behavior, medical problems, interactions with other patients, and performance in activity programs. Rounds should begin with a nursing summary of the patient's behavior, including sleep and appetite, over the preceding 24 hours. To obtain accurate information from the evening and night shifts, a convenient form, the "Evening and Nights Nursing Checklist" can be used (Table 3). The activities staff should report on the patient's participation and socialization. Focus should be on the patient's ability to attend to self-care and functioning in a simulated home setting. The psychiatrist should describe the patient's mental state and response to treatment, consider how the ward or home environment may be affecting the patient's behavior, and make pharmacologic and behavioral treatment suggestions.

Nursing care for elderly patients demands special expertise in medical and psychiatric skills. Nurses should be committed to working with aged patients because their care requires confidence with medical procedures such as IV therapy, frequent monitoring of vital signs, venipuncture, obtaining urine and stool specimens, and willingness to assist in activities of daily living such as eating, dressing, toileting and bathing. It is probably best to recruit nurses with this expertise rather than attempt to retrain other psychiatric nurses.

A primary nurse who devises and carries out a nursing care plan should be assigned to each patient at the time of admission. This encourages complete nursing assessment and regular follow-up care throughout the hospitalization. During the first days of a patient's hospitalization, the primary nurse must spend time assessing the patient's impairments and disabilities, self-care capacity, frustration tolerance, understanding of and compliance with directions, potential for violence, and tendency to fall. The nurse should document past history of falls, previous fractures, and the presence of risk factors for falls such as syncope and hypotensive medications.

The geriatric nurse should be able to recognize the signs and symptoms of various psychiatric disorders, the interaction of medical and psychiatric conditions, and medication side effects. Assessing patients accurately, having flexible approaches to care, learning from trial and error, and having patience are essential. Rigid adherence to a routine approach inevitably meets with resistance from patients who cannot comprehend nurses' instructions or who are not motivated to assist in their own care. Regarding this, nurses will find that one-step commands are more effective than elaborate explanations.

Certain management tactics can be related to specific diagnoses. Depressed patients tend to withdraw, are not communicative, and are not demanding in the way disruptive or wandering demented patients can be; care must be taken to prevent depressed patients from getting lost in the shuffle of a busy ward. Nursing staff should make special effort to engage these patients and encourage them to stay out of their rooms and socialize. The delirious patient requires frequent observation by nursing staff to prevent falls and wandering off the unit. The goal of treatment is to prevent the delirious patient from self-harm while guaranteeing the maximum amount of freedom and the minimum use of medication.

In general, patients with behavior problems such as agitation challenge the staff and illustrate the need for flexible care approaches. Sometimes agitated patients need restraints to prevent self-harm or harm to others, and sometimes they need space to defuse their anxiety. The optimal plan will vary with the intensity of the behavior, the kinds of patients on the ward, the atmosphere of the ward and the experience of the staff.

Management of behavioral disturbances begins with observing the person on the ward without medications. The staff attempts to identify the environmental factors and staff-patient interactions that likely precipitate behavior problems. Working with the patients as they dress, bathe, and interact with others provides valuable information about a patient's deficits and assets, and may lead to care approaches that meet with success. Identifying the specific cognitive deficits, such as aphasia or apraxia, that cause the patient's disability enables the staff to tailor their care plan to bypass these deficits and make use of retained capacities. This approach is superior to prescribing reflexively a neuroleptic for "a behavior problem" when the source of the behavior can be identified and treated precisely.

Wandering, combativeness, falls, and sleep disturbance are four problems that can be anticipated on any geriatric inpatient unit. The staff must decide when wandering should be permitted and when limited. It becomes a problem when patients disrupt the rooms of other patients or attempt to leave the unit or when they become agitated due to the restless pacing itself.

For some elderly patients, pacing or wandering throughout the day may lead to lower leg edema, which requires limitation of activity and elevation of the feet. To restrain a patient whose ardent pacing is disruptive to the ward, the Geri-chair is useful. It is a chair affixed with a table top that fits in front of a seated patient and slides back and forth to permit entry or exit. Patients so restrained should not be left unattended and need to be walked every two hours to maintain normal physical activity. It is useful to combine this exercise with regular toileting.

The second problem behavior is combativeness. Nursing staff have some sense of its likelihood from interviewing the patient's family at the time of admission. If combativeness was present before admission, it is important to control this disruptive behavior as soon as it occurs by adequately medicating or restricting a patient. In our experience, a short-acting neuroleptic such as Inapsine and a geri-chair are often as effective, if not preferable to, seclusion rooms.

The third behavior that nursing staff must anticipate is falls. Falls constitute the largest single cause of accidental death in the elderly and account for substantial physical disability. Factors associated with falls include decreased visual and auditory acuity, cognitive impairment, orthostatic hypotension secondary to medications or autonomic dysfunction, cardiac disease, sleep disturbance, gait apraxia, bradykinesia and physical frailty. Other factors include advanced age, postprandial hypotension, and transfer from wheelchairs.

Most falls tend to occur at the bedside during evenings and nights, with the greatest frequency occuring during nursing shift changes.[27,28] Nurses should regularly check on patients during the high-risk time periods when they are rising or retiring. Orthostatic blood pressure changes should be looked for routinely. Toileting schedules should be planned to assess the patient's ability to transfer. Assistance devices should be within easy reach of the patient, and the patient's ability to transfer independently should be evaluated by the nursing staff on admission. Items in a patient's room should be arranged safely and consistently; items should not be left on the floor. Simple measures such as providing proper footwear, using a night light and/or a bathroom light, and the use of the nurse call bell system should not be overlooked.

The evaluation of sleep disturbance begins with establishing a baseline sleep pattern during the first week of hospitalization. Often patients who had been unable to sleep prior to hospitalization sleep well once hospitalized because they participate in regular activities throughout the day and are tired by nightfall. In some cases, however, a sedative-hypnotic is useful. Chloral hydrate is a safe and effective agent that is started at 500 mgs at bedtime. It can be increased to 1500 mgs to treat a reversed sleep/wake cycle if lower dosages are ineffective. Our experience with benzodiazepines, even short-acting ones, is that they further impair cognition and are therefore not advisable.[29]

The multidisciplinary team should include a full-time occupational or physical therapist to direct structured rehabilitative programs emphasizing mental and physical exercise and stimulation. All patients are expected to spend the majority of their time while hospitalized engaged in activities when they are not involved in diagnostic or treatment procedures.

The names of all patients on the ward should be placed on an occupational therapy schedule located centrally near the nursing unit. This master schedule board can be laid out simply, with patients' names and activities clearly written. This allows the patient to see his or her name along with others and feel part a group. It also enables nursing staff to know the schedule and whereabouts of individual patients.

Through careful structuring of activities, therapists can find ways to make impaired patients feel productive and useful by engaging in purposeful activities.

A variety of groups are useful in this population:

- *Task group* focuses on activities where patients work on individual craft projects in a group setting. Patients will vary in their capacity to work independently, and patients who are least impaired can assist those more impaired. Many demented patients retain their social skills, will conform to the group behavior, and will sit and work on individual projects. This work provides a sense of mastery and encourages physical activity and socialization.
- *Sensory awareness group* uses exercise, group discussion, and sensory stimulation with varieties of textures, smells, and colors as treatment modalities. The type and extent of activities are individualized, depending on a given patient's temperament, quality of social interaction, and presence of behavioral problems.
- *Occupational therapy* focuses on activities of daily living in simulated home settings. This includes meal preparation, money management, telephoning, and mobility. Assessment of these activities complements the nursing assessment of dressing, toileting, and grooming and hygiene. The results of the activities of daily living (ADL's) evaluation may clarify for the primary caregivers what

individuals can and cannot do for themselves upon returning home. This is especially useful for caregivers who find it difficult to achieve the balance between providing necessary assistance and continuing to allow the patient maximal functional independence.[30]

The team should include a social worker familiar with community resources for elderly patients, such as home health agencies, senior citizen centers, adult day-care programs, nursing homes and sheltered housing. The social worker should meet with families to discuss the patient's illness and its effect on family life. These meetings are an essential preparation for care after discharge and may include coordinating follow-up medical and psychiatric care, community services, and various support groups like the Alzheimer's Disease and Related Disorders Association.

The goal for the development of the ward environment is the establishment of a therapeutic milieu (see Chapter 8).[31] A therapeutic milieu is a treatment setting designed to provide support for impaired patients, compensate for their deficits, and stimulate their remaining capabilities to achieve their highest level of function. The staff's approach to rehabilitation determines the milieu. The essential elements include working as a team, discussing patients' care plans regularly, and appreciating how the environment and the staff's attitude can shape the impact and meaning of patient's disabilities. A fundamental feature of the milieu approach is the recognition that a warm, meaningful and supportive environment promotes recovery and health.

Few data exist demonstrating the superiority or effectiveness of one setting design over another for geriatric inpatients. Most existing plans are based on experience with younger psychiatric inpatients, determined by economic considerations, or made intuitively. Some investigators reported on the advantage of open wards, finding that elderly patients showed a strong desire to be with one another and felt confined in private rooms. Open wards were thought to provide sensory and psychosocial stimulation when structured in a supportive environment. Spivak noted that "the elderly enjoyed watching the activities of others. Ward activity provides residents with visual stimulation and the opportunity for socialization."[32] Residents were supportive of and helpful to one another in this environment. However, any design for a geriatric patient population must consider their special nursing needs to provide care safely and efficiently.

The unit should include a nursing station designed to allow nurses to view the entire unit and into patient rooms. This can be accomplished by placing the patients' rooms opposite the nursing station in a semi-circular arrangement. An open day area is also important. This feature may prevent the adverse consequences of wandering while permitting maximal opportunities for unhindered walking and socialization, as well as adequate supervision. The area should be large and airy and, when possible, connected to an enclosed outdoor area where patients can wander and enjoy the landscaping, or even be able to garden during nice weather. Thus, a first floor ward has advantages. The staffing levels should be appropriate to prevent wandering without having to lock doors if possible. If not, then a variety of alarms can be installed to warn if patients are leaving unnoticed. Turn-proof handles should be used if cleared by the local fire marshal. Furniture should be soft-edged and modular, and handrails (in halls, rooms, and bathrooms) should be installed. Floors should be non-slip and easily washable.

Ideally, the unit should be self-contained and self-sufficient. It should include space for specialized group activities such as physical therapy, a dining area with family-style eating arrangements, and an area for socialization. These features reduce the number of environmental changes patients have to navigate (taking elevators to other floors for various activities), and minimize the stress of abrupt changes that elderly patients tolerate poorly.

In this chapter we have presented diagnostic and treatment considerations for the development of an inpatient psychogeriatric unit. The character of the ward, the problems that patients present, and the required training of staff will depend on the diagnostic mix of patients and the severity of their illnesses. Nevertheless, our hope is that a methodological approach based on accurate diagnostic, multidisciplinary, individualized treatment plans, and rehabilitation will advance the care of elderly inpatients. Ultimately, impairments must be recognized and carefully considered to identify potentially modifiable variables, which may include diseases, personalities, behaviors, and social circumstances. Until better treatments are shown to be effective, we believe these principles constitute an appropriate standard of care for elderly patients and their families.

REFERENCES

1. Kramer M: The continuing challenge: the rising prevalence of mental disorders, associated chronic diseases and disabling conditions. Am J Soc Psychiatry 1983; 3:1-12
2. McHugh PR, Slavney PR: The Perspectives of Psychiatry. Baltimore, Johns Hopkins University Press, 1983
3. Blazer DG and Williams CD: The epidemiology of dysphoria and depression in an elderly population, Am J Psychiatry 1980; 137:439-444
4. Mahendra B: Depression and dementia: the multi-faceted relationship, Psychological Medicine 1985; 15:227-236
5. Post F: Affective Disorders in Old Age, Paykel ES (Editor), Handbook of Affective Disorders, New York, Guilford Press, 1982
6. Roth M: The natural history of mental disorders in old age. Mental Science 1955; 101:281-301

7. McKhann G, Drachman D, Folstein M, Katzman R, Price D, Stadlan EM: Clinical diagnosis of alzheimer's disease. Neurology 1984; 34:939–944
8. Blass JT and Plum F: Metabolic encephalopathies in older adults, in The Neurology of Aging. Edited by Katzman R, Terry RD, Philadelphia, Davis 1983
9. Folstein MF: Psychiatric syndromes associated with brain disorders, in Clinical Medicine, Philadelphia, Harper and Row, 1982
10. Folstein MF, Folstein SE, McHugh PR: "Mini-mental state": A practical method for grading the cognitive state of patients for the clinician. Psychiatric Research 1975; 12:189–98
11. Rabins PV, Merchant A, Nestadt G. Criteria for diagnosing reversible dementia caused by depression. Psychiatry 1984; 144:488–492
12. Robinson R, Szetela B: Mood change following left hemispheric brain injury. Ann Neurology 1981; 447–453
13. Reifler PV, Larson E, Hanley R: Coexistence of cognitive impairment and depression in geriatric outpatients. Am J Psychiatry 1982; 139:623–626
14. Rabins PV, Mace NL, Lucas MJ: The impact of dementia on the family. J Am Medical Association 1982; 248:89–91
15. Wilder DE, Teresi JA, Bennett RG: Family burden and dementia, in The Dementias. Edited by Mayeux R, Rosen WG, New York, Raven Press, 1983
16. Berrios GE, Brook P: Delusions and the psychopathology of the elderly with dementia. ACTA Psych Scand 1985; 72:296–301
17. Helms PM: Efficacy of antipsychotics in the treatment of the behavioral complications of dementia. JAGS 1985; 33:206–209
18. Gerner RH: Present status of drug therapy of depression in late life. Affective Disorders (Suppl) 1985; (1)
19. Post F, Shulman K: New views on old age affective disorders, in Recent Advances in Psychogeriatrics. Edited by Arie T, New York, Churchill-Livingstone, 1985
20. Veith RC, Raskind MA, Caldwell JH, Barnes RF, Gumbrecht G, Richie JL: Cardiovascular affects of tricyclic antidepressants in depressed patients with chronic heart disease. N Engl J Medicine 1982; 306:954–959
21. Feighner JP, Herbstein J, Danlougin: Combined MAOI, TCA, and direct stimulant therapy of treatment-resistant depression. J Clin Psychiatry 1985; 46:206–209
22. Ayd FJ: Psychostimulant therapy for depressed medically ill patients. Psychiatric Annals 1985; 15:462–465
23. DePaulo JP: Lithium in the treatment of Affective Disorders, in Clinical Psychopharmacology. Edited by Derogatis LR, Reading MA, Addison-Wesley, 1986
24. Steele C, Lucas MJ, Tune L: Haloperidol vs. thioridazine in the treatment of behavioral symptoms in senile dementia of the alzheimer's type: preliminary findings. J Clin Psychiatry 1986; 47:310–312
25. Post F. Psychotherapy, Electroconvulsive treatments and long-term management of elderly patients, Journal of Affective Disorders, Supplement 1, 1985.
26. Niederehe G, Fruge E: Dementia and family dynamics. J Geriatric Psychiatry 1986; 19:19–53
27. Kalchthaler T, Bascon RA, Quintos V: Falls in the institutionalized elderly, *JAGS* 1978; 26:424–428
28. Berry G, Fisher RH, Lange S: Detrimental incidents, including falls, in an elderly institutional population. *JAGS*, 1981; 29:322–324
29. Squire LR, Butters N: Neuropsychology of Memory. Guilford Press, New York, 1983
30. Feeny R: An Approach to Occupation Therapy for Elderly Psychiatric Inpatients (unpublished report)
31. Watts FN, Bennett D: Theory and Practice of Psychiatric Rehabilitation. Chichester, John Wiley and Sons, 1983
32. Spivak M: Institutional Settings. New York, Human Sciences Press, 1984

20
The Medically Ill Patient

Michael Edelstein
Peter Hartmann

The medical management of psychiatric patients has traditionally been fraught with anxiety on the part of all clinicians concerned.[1] Psychiatric staff tend to become anxious and to overreact to minor medical issues in their patients, while somatically oriented physicians and nurses are unduly frightened by sometimes bizarre thoughts, feelings, and behaviors of psychiatric patients and their violent or self-destructive behaviors. There are additional problems for somatic physicians who provide general medical care in psychiatric hospitals. Often there are only a few of them working in any one institution so that they may experience a sense of professional isolation. When specialty consultation is necessary, it is often difficult to attract qualified practitioners who are willing to come to the psychiatric facility. Of course, patients can be transported to the specialists at their offices or in a general medical hospital; however, this takes time and requires extra staff for transportation. In some cases, the patient's condition or behavior makes it difficult to transport the patient elsewhere; consequently, consultation may not be obtained. Thus, the general medical physician may be forced de facto to manage problems which ordinarily would be referred to subspecialists. In public hospitals, psychiatric patients may have poor hygiene, be uncooperative, be poor historians,[2] or present in an unconventional fashion, perhaps under police guard or handcuffed. These factors can lead to more superficial examinations and a general reluctance of somatic physicians to provide thorough and comprehensive physical care.

A delusional female patient with a florid psychosis stopped her psychotropic medication and insisted she was pregnant. This concern was mixed with delusional material concerning copulation with the devil. Several weeks later, an astute resident drew a serum beta HCG pregnancy test and discovered that she was indeed pregnant. This discovery prompted a rapid reevaluation of therapy, discontinuation of neuroleptics and lithium, and institution of ECT treatment. Fortunately, there was no teratogenicity evident upon birth of the baby.

A depressed patient was admitted with a history of moderate hypertension and noncompliance with antihypertensive medication. Upon admission, the patient's blood pressure was 160 over 90. Under the direction of an anxious night nursing supervisor, the patient was kept awake all night with every two-hour blood pressure measurements. These served only to increase the patient's panic and reinforce his delusional concern that he would shortly die.

Beyond the notion that unfamiliar things are scary, there is often an unspoken, yet very powerful philosophical dichotomy in the way in which psychiatric and somatic physicians solve clinical problems and work in the patient's behalf (Table 1). Diagnosis and treatment by somatic physicians are reductionistic, action oriented, and exclusionary. Diagnosis is a process of beginning with a universe of potential diagnostic entities and establishing a database through history, physical examination, and laboratory work. Deductive reasoning is applied to this database to determine the one or perhaps two causes of a patient's current difficulty. As a rule, intuition and feelings about the patient are not considered relevant.

A 32-year-old nurse was admitted for depression and recurrent fevers. She had been intensively worked up at a local general hospital of excellent reputation by two board-certified internists. No one had seriously considered the diagnosis of fictitious fever, the correct diagnosis, because the patient appeared to her caregivers as "not psychiatric, sincere, a mother, and a highly functional and contributing member of her professional discipline." In fact, the patient had been feigning fever by various guises, such as drinking hot liquids prior to having her temperature taken, rubbing the thermometer vigorously between her fingers when unobserved, and rapidly substituting a thermometer which had previously been dipped in hot water for the one being used to check temperature when the nurse's head was turned. When her temperature was taken with an Ivac electrical thermometer under close supervision of nursing staff, it was invariably normal or nearly so.

Table 1
Clinical Attitudes in Psychiatry vs General Medicine

Psychiatry	General Medicine
Intuitive	Analytic
Inclusive	Reductionistic
High tolerance for ambiguity	Low tolerance for ambiguity
Acceptance of multiple biopsychosocial etiologies	Parsimonious diagnosis
More democratic	More authoritarian
Introspective	Action oriented
More process oriented	More outcome oriented

Thus, correct diagnosis led to abandonment of further, more heroic, unnecessary studies and correct management of depression and borderline personality disorder.

An 18-year-old white female with Type 1 diabetes mellitus since age seven and anorexia nervosa was admitted to the hospital with a history of having maintained weight loss by skipping insulin doses and inducing a ketoacidosis with weight loss. Upon admission to the hospital, the blood sugar was 400, but her electrolytes were within normal limits. She was carefully evaluated by the hospital family physician-psychiatrist and placed on appropriate doses of insulin. Over the next several days, she inexplicably developed ketoacidosis which responded to more insulin. She did well for about one week and then again developed rapidly rising blood sugars, which could not be controlled with seemingly reasonable insulin management. The patient was seen in consultation by an endocrinologist who suggested giving more insulin.

The patient was repeatedly asked by staff whether she was manipulating her insulin, and she vehemently denied acting-out and burst into tears. It was later discovered that the patient had convinced a male nurse during evening shift to allow her to take her insulin unobserved in the upper thigh for modesty's sake. This insulin of course was never injected. When nursing staff began administering all insulin, the patient's diabetes management remarkably improved. The patient never acknowledged her manipulation despite overwhelming evidence of abuse of insulin.

Self-induced medical problems are seen in a variety of situations. The consultation-liaison psychiatrist may find them in the general medical hospital, or they may be seen in a psychiatric hospital when the patient presents with a physical complaint. Fictitious fevers and self-induced ketoacidosis have been cited in the examples above, but there are many other forms self-induced medical problems can take. Patients have deliberately caused infection by injecting feces under the skin. They may pick at their skin creating sores or prevent other skin lesions from healing. They may pull out their hair (trichotillomania) and create a clinical picture which may be confused with other forms of alopecia, such as lupus or alopecia areata or secondary syphilis. Some patients insert objects into body orifices, potentially causing trauma, infection, and/or foul discharge. Ingestion of various nonedible substances or toxins can cause a wide range of physical problems. Sometimes these behaviors result from covert suicide attempts. Thus, the general medical physician must maintain a reasonably high index of suspicion that a physical complaint might be a result of self-induced injury.

Authority in somatic medicine is hierarchical — the cardiologist has more authority than the coronary care nurse — both parties realize this, and the physician's word is final. Decision-making is not by collective consensus. By contrast, much thinking and decision-making in psychiatry involve extrapolation from a behavior to the multiple biopsychosocial determinants of the behavior. Sensitivity and intuitive wisdom are very important; professional credentials perhaps less so. A sign-out supported by the patient's resident and ward chief may be successfully opposed by an experienced mental health worker who perhaps has been working with this population much longer than either physician and has grown wise with experience. "Book learning" and the ability to quote recent journal articles carry little weight. A particular patient may be suspicious and mistrustful of the professional staff but confide thoughts and concerns in the cleaning lady or the hospital barber, and the input of these nonprofessional hospital staff may be sought out and given appropriately serious consideration in clinical decision-making.

Thus, the workings of a psychiatric staff and a somatic medical staff are very different, and one often does not understand or respect the workings of the other. The psychiatric treatment team may see the medical people as brusque, abrupt, and unfeeling, where conversely medical treatment teams may see the psychiatric staff as diffuse, vague, leaderless, and lacking in definition. It is thus very important for physicians, nurses, and other professionals caring for psychiatric patients with medical needs to establish relationships and linkages between the psychiatric and somatic staffs and to meet from time to time as a team to discuss both individual patient care issues and philosophy of work, so that good relationships and mutual respect can be developed.

The overall management of medically ill psychiatric patients might ideally be directed by a physician credentialed in both psychiatry and one of the primary care specialties, such as family practice or internal medicine. An individual with this training would have special competence in applying physical and biological treatments with due sensitivity and attention to relevant psychological and psychodynamic implications, such as the dynamic meaning, for example, of invasive procedures, such as sigmoidoscopy. Conversely, many specialists in psychiatry might not immediately recognize that tachycardia and sweating in a middle-aged male might not mean signal anxiety but an autonomic response to a massive GI bleed, hypoglycaemia, or impending myocardial infarction.

> A 28-year-old, overweight, married white female was referred by her ob-gyn doctor to our institution because of severe, incapacitating anxiety. She felt tense, had trouble sleeping, and would burst into tears for no apparent reason. She trembled so much that her boss sent her home from her job in an optician's store. Upon admission, she had an elevated pulse which was attributed to anxiety. However, when her lab studies were completed, she was found to have an elevated T_3, T_4, and T_7. When reexamined by the hospital family physician, it was discovered that she had an enlarged, smooth thyroid. Once her hyperthyroidism was managed appropriately with radioactive iodine, her "anxiety" symptoms cleared entirely.

While a dual-trained physician would be most ideally suited to supervise the overall management of medically ill psychiatric patients, there are clearly only a limited number of such individuals available, and they are most often found in academic settings. It might thus be necessary to employ a fulltime or part-time general medical physician to provide this service. A person should be selected who has a genuine interest in the somatic care of psychiatric patients and a willingness to learn effective approaches to this sometimes difficult population. Relevant personality characteristics include a capacity to tolerate ambiguity and a willingness to work as a member of a treatment team. It is especially important that such a physician not feel threatened when his conclusions are questioned by nonmedical staff and be able to effectively communicate the thinking behind medical decisions to these nonmedical but very important members of the treatment team.

In those hospitals with a combined medical-psychiatric unit, the medical director may well be a psychiatrist with an above-average interest in somatic illness. Young and Harsch have reported on a successful unit at the Medical College of Wisconsin which is staffed by a fulltime psychiatrist, medical director, a part-time internist, and a resident in internal medicine.[3] Such a facility could provide the individual psychotherapy and milieu therapy required by these patients. Emergency consultations would be available just across the hall from a variety of medical and surgical specialties and subspecialties, and medical coverage on nights and weekends would be readily available. Such a facility might also be a valuable educational resource for psychiatric and primary care residents and psychosomatic fellows, and provide a valuable resource for research. A well-functioning medical-psychiatric unit would favorably influence the comprehensive care provided to patients on the general medical and surgical floors, as residents and others rotating through the service would develop skill and sensitivity in interviewing and in evaluating patients from a broad-based perspective.[4,5]

WHO SHOULD TREAT WHAT AND WHERE

Where should psychiatric inpatients with medical problems be managed? This decision is often based more on pragmatic considerations than on ideals. Many private psychiatric hospitals are located near and have informal relationships with local general hospitals. Over time, the staffs of these institutions develop an informal working relationship, and patients are transferred from one institution to another with relative ease. A problem with such an arrangement is continuity of care. The patient may be upset by the transfer, which often occurs in the middle of the night by ambulance. Psychotherapy and milieu treatment are interrupted, and the staff at the medical facility lack familiarity and comfort with psychiatric medications and the behavioral management of psychiatrically unstable patients.

The issue of acting-out on the part of the psychiatric staff in transferring patients to medical facilities merits special attention. In the authors' experience, patients who develop comparatively minor physical complaints, i.e., temperatures of 102, nonspecific abdominal or chest pains, can be "shipped out" under cover of night to general hospitals by a medically inexperienced junior psychiatric resident bowing to the anxieties and concerns of the evening or night nursing staff. The latter are often medically inexperienced and frightened that their nursing supervisors will hold them personally accountable for any medical harm that might come to a patient. This behavior is especially rampant after a death in the institution, or when the patient's unit is particularly disturbed.

>On the day before her planned discharge, a 19-year-old single black female patient with borderline personality disorder began complaining of crampy abdominal pain. She was sent down to the department of

medicine. Physical examination showed only healed lacerations on her arms from self-cutting, and mild direct tenderness over the left lower quadrant of her abdomen. Rectal exam showed firm stool in the rectum without blood. A flat plate of the abdomen showed large quantities of stool in the left colon. Further questioning revealed that the patient had not moved her bowels for over a week. A laxative was recommended. That evening, the patient complained of worsening of her cramps, and the psychiatric house officer was called. He could find nothing on further physical examination. However, bowing to the pressure from the nursing supervisor, he had the patient sent to the emergency room of the local general hospital. Two hours later, the patient was returned with the diagnosis of constipation. The following day, the director of the emergency room called the medical director of the psychiatric hospital to insist that future referrals to the emergency room be screened by the hospital internist.

On a subsequent day, a depressed patient in his late seventies developed a fever of 103 degrees and a productive cough. That evening, the psychiatric house officer was called to see the patient because his condition was worsening. On examination, he was found to have dyspnea and rales localized to his right lower lung field. Dullness to percussion was noted. As it happened, the house officer had been a residency-trained family physician for ten years prior to his psychiatric residency. He was able to make a confident clinical diagnosis of pneumonia. Yet when he called the emergency room of the local general hospital to arrange for the patient to be evaluated for admission to their hospital, he was pressured to hold the patient, since the psychiatric hospital's internist had not been called to verify that the transfer was "appropriate." Thus, the patient's transfer could have been needlessly delayed. As it happened, the emergency room doctor who made that demand had been the same one who had evaluated the constipated patient in the prior case example.

Patients who are actively psychotic or behaviorally unstable pose special difficulty in both mechanical transfer and management at the receiving general hospital. General medicine nursing staff often do not have the experience to work optimally with these patients, and there is a pervasive notion that if psychiatric patients "shape up and cut the nonsense out, they will simply be okay." Fear gives rise to misdirected hostility toward the patient.

Conversely, medical management at a psychiatric facility can also be difficult. At night, the physician on duty is usually a junior psychiatric resident, who is busy with admissions and has neither time nor expertise to cope with medically complex patients. There is a dearth of stat laboratory and x-ray services available, and ancillary services, such as respiratory therapy, are rarely at hand. Procedures which are routine in a general medical hospital become fraught with anxiety, dynamic interpretation, and milieu concern.

A severely anorectic patient had been refusing food and water for a number of days and was becoming hypotensive. The immediate medical solution was to administer several bottles of intravenous fluids. Implementation of this simple procedure, however, was preceded by several heated team meetings during which a number of issues were raised, especially by the nursing staff. Several staff who were very powerful in team decision-making voiced a concern that giving this unwilling patient IVs would replicate symbolically a rape experience which she had allegedly undergone at the hands of a family member in early adolescence. Another staff member voiced concern that the patient unbeknownst to staff would pull out her peripheral IV line and somehow bleed to death on the unit. Another nursing staff member said, "Oh, my God! What if the IV infiltrates in the middle of the night? What will we do?" There was much dialogue on the effects of this patient's receiving special care and how this special attention might adversely affect the functioning of the milieu and the care of other borderline patients who may vie for attention and act out by delicate self-mutilation and other destructive behaviors.

Many psychiatric patients need ongoing medical evaluation and management, as opposed to acute care of an intercurrent physical illness. Some examples are illustrated in Table 2.

The question frequently arises regarding the advisability of the treating psychiatrist performing the medical history and physical examination on patients admitted to the psychiatric unit. Certainly, the psychiatric physician who is distant from physical medicine or who is uncomfortable performing an admission history and physical examination should defer to his medical

Table 2
Conditions Requiring Ongoing Medical Management

Advanced age with physical illness
Chronic pain
Eating disorders
Electroconvulsive therapy
Drug detoxification
Chronic physical illnesses (e.g., diabetes or arthritis, heart failure)

colleagues. Save for psychiatric residents who are close to their general medical training, approximately one-third of psychiatrists self-report that they no longer feel comfortable performing physical examinations.[6] Unless psychiatrists are willing to reacquire skill in medical history-taking and physical diagnosis, psychiatric hospitals will have to rely on general medical consultants to provide this service. It is important that the treating psychiatrist not rely too much on the medical evaluations performed elsewhere prior to admission.[7] Bunce et al.[1] reported that female patients with chronic psychiatric illness referred to their acute care unit arrived with a correct medical diagnosis only 54% of the time and that an average of 2.7 unexpected physical illnesses per patient were found (see Table 3).

The author's personal experience at our institution supports this finding. In evaluating patients who have been "medically cleared" by referring physicians and hospital emergency rooms, the authors have had to deal with impending drug withdrawal, seizures, unsuspected overdose of psychotropic medications, severe electrolyte disturbance, heart block, profound anemias (with hemoglobins of five and seven), and an undiagnosed carcinoma of the pancreas.

Psychiatric patients may be especially difficult to evaluate physically. For example, chronically psychotic patients may not complain of symptoms even when suffering such serious physical illnesses as incarcerated hernias, burns, fractures, or perforated peptic ulcers.[8] Conversely, some psychiatric patients have somatic delusions and bizarre bodily sensations for which there is no detectable organic focus. If a patient is known to behave in this manner, should he or she then complain of a symptom for which there is an ongoing medical illness, the medical illness is much more likely to be missed. As noted earlier, psychiatric patients may not cooperate with physical exami-

Table 3
Frequency of Medical Illness by Cause

CAUSE	% OF PATIENTS	RANGE OF INCIDENCE PER PATIENT
Infections	55	0–5
Degenerative Condition	50	0–8
Multiple Causes	35	0–4
Nutritional	34	0–3
Trauma	18	0–2
Drug Effect	17	0–2
Neoplastic	3	0–1
Congenital Condition	2	0–1

Reprinted from Bunce DM et al: Medical illness in psychiatric patients: Barriers to diagnosis and treatment. So Med J 75 (8): 943, Aug 1982.

nations or may be perceived by some examiners as unpleasant to work with, so that the history and physical are more likely to be cursory. Perhaps these are some of the reasons why the life span of psychiatric patients is shorter than that of their nonpsychiatrically impaired peers in the community.[9]

While many psychoanalysts and psychotherapists believe that it is counterproductive for them to physically examine their patients, the psychotherapy of most psychiatric inpatients rests on improving reality-testing and attending to the here and now. In that framework, the role of therapist as primary physician with appropriate medical backup can be only helpful. Summers et al.[10] studied the effects of psychiatrists performing physical examinations on their own patients and found no evidence of negative transference or countertransference. Except for emergency situations, however, examination of the genital area, pelvis, and rectum are best done by another physician. These areas of the body are affect-laden, and their competent examination may require considerable expertise. Invasion of body orifices has symbolic significance for some patients and is perhaps best avoided by the primary therapist.

PHYSICAL SYMPTOMS AND ILLNESSES

A number of physical symptoms without organic cause present with unusual frequency in psychiatric patients and are in part a function of sex and age (see Table 4). For example, psychogenic abdominal pain is common in adolescent patients.

Infectious diseases, especially venereal disease, tuberculosis, and increasingly AIDS, present diagnostic challenges, and their management in the psychiatric hospital usually creates much anxiety in patients and staff.

> A 24-year-old white male with paranoid schizophrenia noticed several sores on his penis. He brought these sores to the attention of his psychiatrist, who referred him to the hospital internist for evaluation. The internist was uncertain of the cause of the sores but thought they were due to scabies. Quell lotion was prescribed. The service chief on the patient's unit was concerned about proceeding with the protocol for handling scabies in the hospital, because the diagnosis was uncertain. Preventive measures to protect other patients might create anxiety, he feared. The patient was sent to a dermatologist who said he did not have scabies but might have herpes. A culture was taken, and a herpes titer obtained. When the patient returned to the unit, he announced to the peers that he thought he had herpes. The news of his (probable) diagnosis spread rapidly. As it happened, the greatest impact was on the housekeeping personnel, who refused to continue

Table 4
Common Physical Complaints by Age Group in Healthy Psychiatric Inpatients

ADOLESCENTS	YOUNG ADULTS
Stuffy nose	Stuffy nose
Sore throat, headaches	Sore throat, headaches
Abdominal pain	Chest pain
Vaginal discharge	Pelvic Pain
Painful joints	Vomiting, diarrhea, constipation
Genital Lesions	Impending seizure and faints
Palpitations	
MIDDLE-AGED ADULTS	**ELDERLY ADULTS**
Chest pains	Chest pains
Musculoskeletal pain	Heart fluttering
Dizziness	Coughing blood
Shortness of breath	Blood in stool
Constipation	Dizziness
	Shortness of breath
	Pain in weight-bearing joints
	Constipation
	Generalized weakness
	Difficulty ambulating

cleaning the bathroom that the patient used. A hospital internist arranged to meet with the housekeeping staff and assured them that they were in no danger. However, they would not believe the internist because he worked for the hospital. Over a period of several weeks, the matter seemed to be forgotten, and everything on the unit slowly returned to normal.

Formal inservice presentations to staff which provide actual material about infectious diseases are very important. Staff should have frequent opportunities to discuss thoughts and concerns with the treating physician. These discussions are especially useful when patients are ill with such affect-laden diseases as hepatitis B, AIDS, venereal disease, or tuberculosis. Staff are also reassured by the frequent presence of a somatically trained physician who is ever ready to assume responsibility for the medical care of these patients. The medical physician might occasionally attend a community meeting on the unit housing an individual with an infectious disease to discuss the nature of the infection and rationale behind any isolation procedures found necessary. Several brief presentations are more effective than a long drawn-out lecture, and time should be allowed for questions.

A 42-year-old gay male was admitted for management of acute mania, which began while the patient was in a general hospital for the treatment of pneumonia. During his first group therapy session, the patient announced to the other patients that he had AIDS. Many became frightened and expressed anger at the hospital for exposing them to a patient with this disease. The hospital internist agreed to come to a hall meeting to discuss AIDS with the patients and to allay their fears. He made it a point to shake hands with the AIDS patient and put his hand on the patient's shoulder. This act provided powerful nonverbal reassurance that it was safe to "be around" this patient.

There is often interstaff conflict about when serology for AIDS should be drawn. Clearly, in an asymptomatic patient with neither AIDS nor AIDS-related complex, a documented positive HTLV-III can seriously compromise employability, insurability, and ongoing psychological adjustment. Our recommendation is that these serologies not be drawn routinely in asymptomatic patients in a high-risk group for AIDS unless the patient requests such a study and gives informed consent—documented and signed—clearly explaining the pragmatic life consequences of a positive result. "Safe sex" practices should be taught to all individuals, regardless of their sexual orientation.

While research has demonstrated that the incidence of physical illness among psychiatric patients is significantly higher than among the population at large,[11,12] most psychiatric patients between the ages of 20 through 40 are in reasonably good physical health. As patients approach middle age, evaluation and management become more complex. Patients over 50 are often on a variety of medications and have a variety of illnesses, such as diabetes, hypertension, congestive heart failure, glaucoma, and the like. These illnesses and their management usually complicate both the biological and psychological treatment of the patient's psychiatric disorder and often prolong hospitalization.[13]

The nursing staff can easily become oversolicitous of patients with diabetes, hypertension, and such and end up spending an unreasonable amount of time and energy monitoring patients, with frequent blood pressure checks and urinary glucose determinations. Patients' participation in therapeutic activities may be unnecessarily curtailed. Some patients "act out" around the medical illness in the hospital. Borderline patients with diabetes, for example, will violate their dietary restrictions, and diabetics with eating disorders—a notoriously difficult group of patients to manage—will binge and purge in spite of their diabetes, creating both havoc in the milieu and confusion in their biological management.[14]

A 32-year-old dietitian with type 1 diabetes and a 15-year-history of anorexia nervosa with bingeing, purging, and laxative abuse was admitted for definitive management. Upon admission, her blood sugar was 45 and she was tremulous. She was started on an 1800 calorie ADA diet and carefully followed. After two days, a capillary glucose determination was 600 and serum was positive for acetone. Appropriate amounts of regular human insulin were administered, and by the following day the patient's blood sugar was 200 with normal electrolytes. That evening, however, the patient surreptitiously ingested 30 Correctol laxatives, briefly eloped from the unit, and proceeded to jog around the hospital campus. A staff member incidentally passing by observed her having a hypoglycemic seizure, and she was transferred to the general medical hospital. At that facility, blood glucose was 25, and the patient received glucose IV fluids and was transferred back to the psychiatric institution. The following day, the patient surreptitiously vomited up her breakfast, hid it in a pillowcase, and was found by staff jogging in place in her room. When confronted by staff, she remarked offhandedly, "Don't you know that mental patients can't learn from experience?"

The management of geriatric patients with both psychiatric and medical problems requires special medical expertise. For example, as a result of changes in the level of sensitivity, metabolism, and excretion of drugs in the elderly, lower doses of most medications are indicated in this population. Even aspirin may have a very prolonged half life when high doses are given. Several antihypertensives also may have a longer half life so that the dosing interval must be changed. These agents include propanolol, methyldopa, and quinidine. Lower doses of many psychotropics are required in the elderly because of potentially higher blood levels. Examples include diazepam, amitriptyline, lithium, and chlorpromazine.[15] A good basic rule: The fewer the drugs and the lower the dosage, the better. Many elderly patients suffer from slower gastric motility. They may eat less due to poor dentition or depression or have less bulk in the diet; thus, constipation often becomes a problem. Psychotropic medications, including all antidepressants and antipsychotics, further complicate this problem by slowing gastric motility. Consequently, impactions are a frequent problem in this age group. Starting patients on a bulk agent or perhaps chronulac (sephulac) 15–30 cc at hs can provide excellent prophylaxis and treatment for this problem. Geriatric patients are also more prone to deconditioning (decreased muscle tone and strength, and hypotension) as a consequence of excessive bed rest and are more prone to bed sores, pulmonary emboli, and multiple additional consequences of prolonged immobility. An emphasis on mobility and a milieu program stressing physical movement can pay great dividends.

PATIENT EVALUATION

Since physical illness can easily go undetected in patients suffering from mental disorders,[16,17] how can we improve the chances of making a correct medical diagnosis? Each inpatient should have a full medical history and physical examination within the first 24 hours of admission. Should the patient prove too uncooperative during this time, a screening examination should be done immediately, followed by a comprehensive examination as soon as possible. The clinician must avoid performing a hasty and incomplete assessment on an uncooperative patient and then never returning and completing the examination when the patient is more tractable.

Psychiatric inpatients often provide inaccurate medical histories. Frequently, family members can provide much important information; allowing them to leave the hospital before talking with them can be a time-consuming error.

The physical examination should attend to all organ systems. In psychiatric inpatients, special attention must be provided to the neurological examination and to a careful search for endocrinopathies. Abnormal vital signs must be considered evidence of physical illness until proven otherwise. While an elevated pulse may be secondary to anxiety, it might also represent such entities as anemia or hyperthyroidism. A pulse rate above 120 should not be dismissed as anxiety. An elevated temperature should be investigated thoroughly, as it may represent infection, especially in delusional schizophrenics who do not report bodily sensations accurately. An elevated temperature may also represent early malignant neuroleptic syndrome. An elevated temperature is especially ominous in the geriatric age group, as these patients do not always mount a febrile response to infectious illness. In the elderly population, elevated temperature may also represent the presence of a malignancy or such important and correctable conditions as polymyalgiarheumatica. In some patients, fever is factitious, and obtaining an accurate body temperature may require special maneuvers. Thus, the patient's temperature should be taken with an electronic thermometer which remains at the nurses station to prevent tampering, and when there is reason for suspicion, temperatures should be obtained from multiple body sites, such as the rectum and the axila, as well as the mouth at the same time.

Nausea, vomiting, and diarrhea are frequent complaints among psychiatric patients. Self-reported symptoms may be deceptive, as the patient may be feigning the complaint for secondary gain. It is important that the vomitus, diarrhea, rectal bleeding, etc., be observed by staff prior to institution of an extensive medical evaluation.

Laxative abuse is not uncommon in the psychiatric population and is seen very frequently among young women with eating disorders.[18] It also may be seen sporadically among patients with schizophrenia and character disorders. Patients with eating disorders induce vomiting and diarrhea in an attempt to reduce the absorption of calories and avoid gaining weight. Patients will purloin laxatives on sign-outs or have a confederate bring them in on visiting days. Periodic room searches can be very helpful in preventing surreptitious self-medicating. It is critical to understand that patients with eating disorders, especially those afflicted for a number of years, have developed the art of hiding their disordered eating behavior to a high degree. Additionally, these patients exhibit a very dense denial and even when confronted "red handed" with inducing vomiting or abusing laxatives will often deny the reality of what is going on or respond to their confronter with righteous indignation. It is the experience of the authors that Correctol is especially prone to abuse, as it is less likely to cause severe cramping and is marketed as a laxative for women. Subtle signs of an eating disorder on physical examination include scars on the knuckles from repeated contact with teeth during self-induced vomiting, erosion of the enamel of the teeth secondary to recurrent bathing of teeth in stomach juices, painless swelling of the salivary glands giving rise to a chipmunk appearance, hypothermia, and sinus bradycardia. Laboratory evidence of anorexia include hyponatremia, hypokalemia, low bicarbonate, sinus bradycardia on EKG with rates as low as 30, hypoproteinaemia, and a BUN elevated out of proportion with the creatinine. The medical management of severely anorectic patients is complex and should include a general medical physician from the start. For example, too-rapid refeeding can result in acute congestive heart failure, as the shrunken hypotonic heart struggles to meet the increased metabolic demands caused by refeeding.

> A 24-year-old, single, white female nurse was admitted to the eating disorders unit of a private psychiatric hospital. Her admitting physical examination revealed that she was 10% below her ideal body weight despite her loud protestations that she was too fat. Admission laboratory studies had been unremarkable save for a mild hypochromic anemia and a low serum potassium. A medical consultant wondered if her low potassium might be due to her diarrhea, a symptom about which she had complained intermittently for several weeks. Studies to determine the cause of the diarrhea were proving unrewarding, but a room search performed by the nursing staff revealed several hundred Correc-

tol laxatives concealed in several sanitary napkins. The patient had been secretly abusing laxatives, both to treat a history of "constipation since childhood" and to reduce her absorption of calories from her food. It is noteworthy that the patient denied using laxatives when a careful admission history had been done one week before the room search, and when confronted by staff with the laxatives stated that they were not hers but must have belonged to her roommate.

In addition to the medical history and physical examination, psychiatric inpatients should have basic laboratory screening. A reasonable initial laboratory workup should include an SMA-18 and a urine analysis and a TSH. An elevated TSH is the most sensitive marker for early hypothyroidism in which T_3, free T_4 may be within the normal range. Rarely, one will see a depressed patient with very early hypothyroidism, as indicated by an elevated TSH and normal peripheral thyroid functions in which the depression resolves when the occult hypothyroidism is appropriately treated. In patients taking lithium, an elevated TSH is often the first sign of lithium-induced hypothyroidism.

Venereal disease is again growing in incidence, and an admission serology for syphilis is still advisable. It is important to remember that there are biological false positive VDRL's in the face of various inflammatory and infectious conditions, and FTA should be drawn to establish that the positive VDRL is indeed a marker for syphilis. Macrocytosis on an admission CBC may signify pernicious anemia but is in a psychiatric population frequently an early biological marker of folate deficiency due to alcoholism. A serum folate level and a serum B_{12} level should be drawn when macrocytosis is noted. While pernicious anemia with so-called "megaloblastic madness" can occur in the absence of anemia,[19] such cases are exceedingly unusual, and a busy clinician might see perhaps one in a lifetime. Chest x-rays should be ordered for specific indications and are not done routinely. An admission electrocardiogram for all adult patients is probably reasonable, as most psychotropic agents may potentially alter the EKG, and a baseline tracing for comparison can be invaluable.

Patients remaining in the hospital for over a year should on or about the anniversary date of their admission undergo a repeat physical evaluation and repeat screening laboratory work. It is useful to take vital signs and patient weights weekly even if patients are not medicated. Changes in vital signs or weight is often a first sign of such diverse problems as depression, congestive heart failure, and occult malignancy. Flow charts to display this longitudinal information are a good way to detect significant trends.

SPECIAL COMPLICATING ISSUES

Some psychiatric patients with medical illness refuse medication. This refusal can be life-threatening when the patient is either psychiatrically or medically out of control, as is the case of diabetes or mania. States differ in the legal specifics of management of this problem. A hospital should educate its medical and nursing staff in the particulars of local and state laws and ordinances so that confusion and ambiguity can be avoided. There should be a designated administrator available on call at all times outside of regular business hours to handle unforeseen medico-legal problems. Ideally, the legal firm representing the hospital should provide the number of an attorney designated to be available by phone call during nights, weekends, and holidays, because situations arise in which immediate legal advice can be critical both to the patient and to the institution. In today's increasingly ambiguous and litigious climate, competent legal advice in timely fashion can be critical.

> An insulin-dependent diabetic with bipolar illness was admitted on certificate with a random blood sugar of 700 and a bicarbonate of 12. She refused further studies to clarify her metabolic status and refused insulin. She was floridly psychotic and stated that God told her she was in perfect health. The patient worked as a paralegal and indicated that the first staff member to touch her would be sued. The resident on call wishing to neither compromise the patient's life nor be charged with assault and battery for drawing blood and injecting medications without the patient's consent did not know how to proceed. Fortunately, the institution had just implemented an on-call system, such that the resident was able to talk immediately with a senior administrator. The senior administrator spoke with a representative of the hospital's legal firm who stated that under applicable law in that state, the patient's status constituted a medical emergency and that care was to be rendered. The attorney also indicated to the resident the appropriate content and form of necessary chart documentation should there be subsequent talk of legal action by the patient. From a risk management point of view, the timely availability of this legal counsel was priceless.

REFERENCES

1. Bunce DF, Jones LR, Badger LW, et al: Medical illness in psychiatric patients: Barriers to diagnosis and treatment. Southern Medical Journal 1982; 75:941–944
2. Sternberg DE: Testing for physical illness in psychiatric patients. J Clin Psychiatry 1986; (Suppl) 47:3–9

3. Young LD, Harsch HH: Inpatient unit for combined physical and psychiatric disorders. Psychosomatics 1986; 27:53-60
4. Stoudemire A, Fogel BS: Organization and development of combined medical-psychiatric units: Part 1. Psychosomatics 1986; 27:341-345
5. Fogel BS, Stoudemire A, Houpt JL: Contrasting models for conjoint medical and psychiatric inpatient treatment: Psych/med vs med/psych. Am J Psychiatry 1985; 142:1085-1089
6. McIntyre JS, Romano J: Is there a stethoscope in the house (and how is it used)? Arch Gen Psychiatry 1977; 34:1147-1151
7. Hall RCW, Beresford TB, Gardner ER, et al: The medical care of psychiatric patients. Hosp Community Psychiatry 1982; 33:25-34
8. Talbott JA, Linn L: Reactions of schizophrenics to life-threatening disease. Psychiatric Q 1978; 50:218-227
9. Koranyi EK: Morbidity in rate of undiagnosed psychiatric illness in the psychiatric clinic population. Arch Gen Psychiatry 1979; 36:414-419
10. Summers WK, Munoz RA, Read MR: The psychiatric physical examination—part II: findings in 75 unselected psychiatric patients. J Clinical Psychiatry 1981; 42:99-102
11. Weingarten CH, Rosoff LG, Eisen SV, et al: Medical care in a geriatric psychiatry unit: impact on psychiatric outcome. J Am Geriatrics Society 1982; 30:738-743
12. Karasu TB, Waltzman SA, Lindenmayer JP, et al: The medical care of patients with psychiatric illnesses. Hosp Community Psychiatry 1980; 31:463-472
13. Allodi F, Cohen M: Physical illness and length of psychiatric hospitalization. J Canadian Psychiatric Association 1978; 23:101
14. Rosmark B, Berne C, Holmgren S, et al: Eating disorders in patients with insulin-dependent diabetes mellitus. J Clinical Psychiatry 1986; 47:547-550
15. Ouslander JG: Drug therapy in the elderly. Arch Internal Medicine 1981; 95:711
16. Hall RCW, Gardner ER, Popkin MK, et al: Unrecognized physical illness prompting psychiatric admissions: a prospective study. Am J Psychiatry 1981; 138:629
17. Maguire GP, Granville-Grossman KL: Physical illness in psychiatric patients. Br J Psychiatry 1968; 115:1365
18. Cummings JH: Progress report, laxative abuse. Gut 1974; 15:758-766
19. Reynold EH: The neurology of vitamin B deficiency. Lancet 1976; 2:832-833

21
The Inpatient Care of the Chronic Mentally Ill

John A. Talbott
Ira D. Glick

Inpatient treatment of the chronic mentally ill has undergone many changes in the last few decades. To better understand where we are now, we will begin with a recapitulation of the history of treatment and care of the chronically ill; then we will: selectively review the literature regarding this treatment; present a summary of length of stay studies; discuss the current reasons for admission of chronic patients to inpatient services; review those elements of inpatient treatment that particularly pertain to this population; summarize their long-term treatment; discuss the need for "asylum," as a concept not a building; characterize the discharge planning necessary for their "community survival"; and finally, forecast some future trends in the treatment and care of this population.

HISTORICAL BACKGROUND

Since this country's earliest beginnings, the care and treatment of the chronic mentally ill have undergone radical changes in both locus and method of delivery. In essence we have moved from custodial care in long-term public settings to active treatment and rehabilitation in a multiplicity of settings.

This chapter is adapted from "The Inpatient Care of the Chronically Mentally Ill" by John A. Talbott and Ira D. Glick, published in *Schizophrenia Bulletin*, 12(1), 1986, pp. 129–40.

In colonial times, the severely and chronically mentally ill were for the most part neglected and there were abundant horror stories of persons being locked up in small outhouse-like buildings or "dumped" over town lines into neighboring communities.[1] In time, the mentally ill were housed along with others found deviant by that day's society—the poor, rogues, vagabonds, petty criminals and the like—in poorhouses, almshouses or workhouses. Certainly there was no treatment offered, and care, if it can be called that, was rudimentary.

These locally run "houses" soon became overcrowded and their conditions scandalous. Reformers called for their abolition, and one of the most zealous, Dorothea Dix, suggested that either federal or state governments take over responsibility for the mentally ill.[2] When she failed to convince the United States Congress to act, she embarked on a campaign to convince each state to establish state-operated facilities. In this endeavor she was amazingly successful, and by 1860, 28 of 33 states had at least one public mental hospital.

But given the "silting up" of chronic schizophrenics, absent effective treatment, as well as the influx of new immigrants from Europe, these state hospitals soon became as scandalous as the county institutions they were designed to replace. By the turn of the 20th century, a variety of new institutions began to be established to care for and treat the chronically ill. These included psychopathic hospitals, private mental hospitals, Veterans Administration and Public Health Service hospitals, psychiatric units in general hospitals, and outpatient clinics.[3]

During the first half of the 20th century, all of the aforementioned developments continued: public hospital censuses grew and their conditions became more scandalous;[4] the number of private, largely not-for-profit alternatives to public institutions increased; and while alternatives to inpatient hospital treatment began to appear (e.g. outpatient clinics), hospitals remained the prevailing locus for care and treatment of those suffering from chronic mental illness.

In 1955, all this changed abruptly,[5] for this was the year that the census in public mental hospitals nationwide began to decline for the first time in over one hundred years. The forces that brought about this dramatic shift were several:

1. the community mental health philosophy that it was better, cheaper and more humane to treat and care for the chronic mentally ill in community settings nearer their homes, families, jobs and neighborhoods, than in far distant "warehouses";
2. the technological innovations in the delivery of mental health services in both social (e.g., open doors, therapeutic communities) and

most importantly, pharmacological (e.g., phenothiazine medication) areas;
3. the pressure of civil libertarian forces both within psychiatry and without; and
4. the economic advantages to state governments to shift the responsibility of funding the chronically ill from 100% state tax levy monies to largely federal auspices, with some local contributions, through the provision of Medicaid, Medicare and SSI.[6]

The resultant shift in the locus of treatment and care of chronic patients was characterized both by transinstitutionalization (from state hospitals to nursing homes) and depopulation (of state hospitals to no planned alternative), and these changes, on top of the blockage of new admissions, forced thousands of patients into a variety of substandard community residencies or onto the streets.

The net result of this historic shift in locus of care and treatment of the chronically ill was twofold: *First*, the mental hospital's role was altered from that of the sole place for treatment and care to but one element in the care spectrum (and that, often as a last resort), and *second*, the entire system moved from providing predominately custodial care in asylums to providing active treatment and rehabilitation in the community.

Paralleling this shift in the locus of delivery has been a striking change in our understanding of the treatment of chronic mental illness, which will be summarized in the following section.

A SELECTIVE REVIEW OF THE LITERATURE

While there is an extensive literature on the treatment of chronic mental illness, especially schizophrenia, most of it concentrates on the treatment of acute conditions. In addition, there are few controlled studies. Recently, however, several reviews have appeared which are more applicable to the longer-term treatment of the chronically ill.[7] For example, May[8] concluded that psychotherapy was *not* essential to the inpatient treatment of chronic schizophrenics, but *was* for their outpatient care; that group psychotherapy was *more* effective than individual treatment; and that drugs *alone* were not sufficient to prevent relapses in outpatients.

In addition, Gunderson and Mosher[9] suggested that a highly structured, highly organized, highly expectant milieu that stressed adaptive skills while suppressing symptoms and maladaptive behavior was helpful in the hospital treatment of chronic schizophrenia. Finally, Paul and Lentz[10] demonstrated that patients suffering from chronic schizophrenia who took part in a well-conceived resocialization-relearning program with a behavioral treatment orientation (e.g., token economy) were able to stay in the community much longer than those who received either milieu therapy or traditional state hospital care. Those treated in the behavioral program, which stressed the skills of everyday living essential to community survival, were rehospitalized during the next year less than 10% of the time, compared to 30% of those in the milieu program and 50% of those treated by "traditional" methods.

There now are also a series of studies comparing alternatives to hospitalization with inpatient treatment of chronic schizophrenia. In brief, whether this treatment consists of home care, family treatment, day hospital care, or community-based community support, there is a consistent conclusion[11,12] that alternative care is as effective, if not *more* so, in reducing patients' symptomatology, rehospitalization, interpersonal difficulties, and vocational disablement. While the cost of high quality community care is still quite high, it is a bit less expensive than hospital care plus traditional follow-up,[12] because of the savings in staffing and housing costs. To summarize this literature, although there are strong beliefs, there are no data to support the use of hospitalization instead of outpatient alternatives for most of these patients. Despite this, hospitalization remains a popular treatment in managing the chronic patient—in part, because so many clinicians now practicing were trained in an era when the hospital was seen as the safest, and therefore the most logical, treatment for extremely impaired patients. Further, hospitalizing the patient appears to be a way of stabilizing and calming everyone in the patient's social network. However, before hospitalizing a patient or prolonging hospitalization beyond a brief stay, the clinician must make a careful differential therapeutic decision, considering: the cost; the clinical consequences, i.e., the more an individual is hospitalized, the greater the future use of and dependency on the hospital to solve a crisis; the potential harm to the patient's self-esteem as well as role functioning; and the conditioning effect of hospitalization.[14]

LENGTH OF STAY STUDIES

Length of stay studies have consistently demonstrated no advantage for those chronic schizophrenics (defined as those who have experienced three or more hospitalizations) treated for long (30-90 days) rather than short (under 30 days) periods of hospitalization. In fact, in terms of symptomatology, rehospitalization, and quality of life, short stays seem advantageous.

Several controlled studies of outcome of short versus long hospitalization now exist—one undertaken by Herz, Endicott, and Spitzer,[15,16] a second by Mattes and his associates,[17,18] and the third by Glick and Hargreaves.[19] All of these studies have been reviewed by Riessman, Rabkin, and Struening.[20]

The study by Herz and associates[15,16] excluded patients who were a danger to themselves or others as well as patients without families. Their diagnostically mixed samples of patients were randomly assigned to standard inpatient care (60 days), brief hospitalization (11 days) plus day care upon discharge, or brief hospitalization only. After one year, they found that those assigned to brief hospitalization plus day care showed the least psychopathology, while those who had received standard care showed the most. Significant differences among groups in their levels of symptoms had disappeared after the second year. Patients from the two brief hospitalization groups were more likely to be working at each follow-up, while more members of the standard care group were judged as failing to perform any occupational role, including student or housekeeper, as well as wage earner.

Mattes et al.[17,18] also studied a diagnostically mixed sample of patients. Their patients were assigned to either short-term wards with a 90-day stay or to long-term wards with a mean stay of six months. They found that short-term patients were more improved than the long-stay patients at discharge; however, three years after discharge there were few between-group differences. Long-term patients were rated by relatives as having less pathology, but since they received more individual psychotherapy and this resulted in lower ratings, this was discounted. Another interesting finding was that, among patients who were rehospitalized, long-term patients tended to be rehospitalized more often and for longer periods.

Glick and Hargreaves[19] randomly assigned patients to either short-term inpatient care (21–28 days) or long-term hospitalization (3–4 months). The sample was stratified by diagnosis into patients suffering from schizophrenic disorders, affective disorders, and other non-schizophrenic diagnoses. After one year, with no post-hospital care being provided, the schizophrenics treated for a longer time were doing significantly better than the short-term patients on two global measures. However, discrete symptom scales failed to differentiate the groups, and there was no difference in rehospitalization data. The long-term group received significantly more psychotherapy than controls after discharge, as well as medication at significantly higher dosage levels. The authors concluded that their "work with patients and families during the longer hospitalization period effectively encouraged acceptance of the need for continued psychotherapy and medication." After two years, the clinical global scale again favored the long-term group, but the relationship was weaker than at one year. On further analysis, the investigators found that long-term hospitalization produced a better outcome only in those schizophrenic patients whose prehospital functioning had been relatively good. For those who had relatively poor prehospital functioning, longer hospitalization appeared to be detrimental to outcome. In contrast to the findings with schizophrenics, one and two-year follow-ups of the non-schizophrenic long and short-term groups revealed no significant differences in global ratings, severity of symptom measures, or social and work adjustment.

"All three studies when taken together, have generally failed to show important differences in the effects of 'brief' versus 'standard' hospitalization."[20] Patients treated by either strategy show a rapid reduction in symptomatology, although the speed with which this occurs may be greater during brief hospitalization. Adult roles in the community have been demonstrated to have resumed more quickly by short-term patients in several studies, perhaps because continuity in identity is maintained. Nevertheless, these initial disadvantages of long-term patients are made up as soon as they are discharged. Riessman, Rabkin, and Struening[20] concluded their review of the literature with the opinion that it is now incumbent upon the clinician to justify the use of a hospital stay of more than 60 days. We feel that such a blanket conclusion is premature, especially with respect to the kinds of patients not well represented in the available research; moreover, this recommendation depends upon the adequacy of nonhospital services. We do agree, however, that the evidence suggests that most psychiatric patients who require hospital treatment can be effectively treated in relatively short-term settings, so long as day treatment and supportive residential placement are readily available. With adequate outpatient resources, hospitalization can be avoided altogether for many patients who would formerly have been hospitalized.[21,22]

REASONS FOR ADMITTING CHRONIC MENTAL PATIENTS TO INPATIENT CARE

There are nine reasons why hospitalization is indicated for the chronic mentally ill.

First, chronic patients sometimes require *reevaluation* of their diagnosis, functioning, or treatment plan. Admission to a facility with access to medical technology, careful observation by nursing staff, and 24-hour psychiatric supervision may be indicated when the diagnosis is in question; e.g., organicity or affective illness needs to be ruled in or out. In addition, the patient's functioning in the community may indicate that he is not at the appropriate level of care (e.g., he should be in a more or less structured or supervised setting) or that he is not receiving the appropriate mix of treatment and care services. Finally, the chronically ill require periodic review and reevaluation of their treatment plans, and sometimes the inpatient setting is the most logical place in which to perform this task because it is more comprehensive and structured and equipped with experts.

Second, chronic patients may not be on an optimal *psychopharmacological regimen* and may need readmission to re-equilibrate their medication.

Either too much medication (indicated by the occurrence of undesirable side-effects or the inability to perform the social coping functions necessary to community survival) or too little (indicated by reemergence of psychotic symptoms, inability to function optimally, or behavior that is upsetting or disorganized) may indicate the need for readmission. Since the milieu affects the "optimal medication level," it must, however, be taken into account in assessing this level.

Third, certain chronic mental patients require readmission to effect *changes* in their *treatment plans*. For example, one may want to wash out an ineffective medication and begin a new one, and the hospital structure is invaluable in preventing (or managing) regression during the transition period. Or the person may need to move from one community support element to another and require the structure of a secure setting for this shift.

Fourth, some patients require hospitalization because they *cannot be managed* optimally on an outpatient basis. For example, they may be unreliable in taking oral medications and require the initiation of an intramuscular medication regimen. Or they may become overtly psychotic, homicidal or suicidal, presenting a danger to themselves or others.

Fifth, the chronically ill may require *treatment that is not available* or easy to provide in community settings. While the administration of electroconvulsive therapy is unusual in chronic schizophrenia, there are definite indications for such treatment in other psychiatric disorders, and in these cases inpatient admission may be required. In addition, structure may be required during certain periods, for instance, following the death of a close family member or spouse, when other treatment (e.g., increased medication) would not be helpful.

Sixth, some chronic patients required admission during *transference crises* in their outpatient treatment. At these times, readmission is essential to disentangle the patient from unnecessary complicating ties to the therapist. Conversely, admission may also be helpful when countertransference problems arise. At these times, the hospital serves as consultant to both the patient and therapist.

Seventh, some chronic patients are unprepared or *ill prepared to survive* in the community and require hospitalization to enable them to learn the skills of everyday living that ensure such survival in our complicated contemporary society. Such skills training should usually be circumscribed (e.g., instruction about transportation systems, self-care, etc.) so that the target for discharge can be clearly achieved. While some experts feel that all such training should be *in vivo*, it is our opinion that a case can be made for some patients' receiving such training in the hospital.

Eighth, *detoxification* from alcohol and drugs may necessitate hospitalization to guard against the possibility of adverse reactions, e.g., seizures, coma, death. While this is a little used indication, with the increasing prevalence of polydrug abuse in the new or young chronic mentally ill population, it may become more common.

Finally, inpatient care can be critical to families and community support systems who cannot care for the chronic patient 365 days a year. Such *respite care* although costly in the short run, has been found to be extremely useful to families of the mentally retarded. However, it is currently an underutilized, underoffered and underreimbursed service for the mentally ill. Since too few residential facilities offer such respite care, hospitals *faute de mieux* carry on this function.

In all these instances of hospital inpatient admission, it should be explicitly clear (optimally *prior to* hospitalization) *what the reasons* for rehospitalization are, *what goals* the admission is intended to achieve, and *what plans* are envisioned if the target goals are not reached. Admissions which constitute fishing expeditions or hoped-for magical solutions for "tough cases" are irresponsible and bound to fail.

We also wish to stress that there are specific *contraindications* to admission for this population. These include:[19]

- repeating a treatment that has already failed;
- using the hospital because nothing else works;
- attempting to make major characterological changes;
- attempting to try a new medication, absent any positive indications for its success;
- trying to convince the patient to change living situations;
- treating the patient's unwillingness to follow treatment plans; and
- sheltering malingerers or patients facing legal charges.

THE TREATMENT OF CHRONIC PATIENTS IN THE HOSPITAL

Evaluation/Assessment

Before discussing specific treatment modalities, it is necessary to discuss the evaluation and assessment of chronic illness. Concurrence on a specific diagnosis is essential to the establishment of an effective treatment program. Since withdrawal, depression, lack of spontaneity, etc., are common to chronic schizophrenia, chronic affective disorders, chronic institutionalization, and organic mental conditions, this is one series of differential diagnoses that must be considered from the start, since the required interventions flow from the diagnosis: e.g., socialization for those suffering from institutionalization; appropriate medication for those suffering from affective disorders; and elimination of organic factors, if present, for those suffering from organicity.[23]

In addition, many chronic mentally ill persons have received diagnoses, years before, in public institutions, and regardless of either current thinking about nomenclature or changes in presentation (e.g., affective symptoms), the diagnoses are reapplied thoughtlessly year after year. Also, an Axis II or III diagnosis may be more "treatable" than the Axis I one, and thus provide the critical wedge in a seemingly unbudgeable psychotic condition.

Not only psychiatric assessment, but psychological evaluation, as well as functional assessment, should be conducted. Included should be an assessment of everyday functioning, social functioning, and vocational functioning, and an assessment of the variety of networks used or needed by the patient; a personality or psychodynamic profile is insufficient.

Another critical factor frequently forgotten with the chronically ill is evaluation and *reevaluation* of what treatment and care have or have not worked in the past. This should include an appraisal of what medication the patient and his family members have responded to, since we know members of the same family often are responsive to the same medication.

Medication

There is no question that a primary inpatient treatment modality for the chronic patient is psychopharmacologic. Antipsychotic medication should be considered in most chronic patients exhibiting symptoms of psychosis. It should be noted that, while medication is of great value in symptom suppression in the hospital, it may impede community adaptation on discharge, and thus must be reduced at some point after discharge.[24] Equally important, if the patient has no active symptoms and only residual symptomatology, discontinuance (or low doses) should be seriously considered.

However, since we know from the previously mentioned studies that the two ingredients that prevent or forestall exacerbation of illness and readmission to hospital are medication and some form of talking therapy, i.e., counseling or psychotherapy, medication is critical to the ongoing treatment of this population. Adequate doses, i.e., those that achieve the optimal balance between symptom suppression and side-effects, should be the treatment goal with all chronic patients.

Psychotherapy

As mentioned previously, it appears that individual psychotherapy is not additive to medication among this sample of inpatients but is critical in preventing rehospitalization among outpatients. It is also clear that in outpatients, group therapy is more effective than individual therapy.[8] There are, however, no data about its superiority with inpatients. When utilized, it needs to be targeted to specific goals (e.g., socialization, reduction of anxiety); it should never become a rote, automatic part of a hospital treatment cocktail.

Because of both patient desires and professional prejudices (including the wish not to withhold any treatment that may be beneficial), individual psychotherapy remains common in the inpatient treatment of chronic schizophrenia. Like group therapy, it should be goal-directed, task-oriented, and combine supportive and clarifying elements.[23,25] Milieu treatment is also helpful for the chronic patient, but only if highly structured, well designed, and adequately monitored. There is currently substantial doubt if a short-term inpatient unit can provide the sort of milieu therapy available in longer stay settings.

Family treatment/psychoeducation

Until relatively recently, the families of the chronically ill were seen primarily as noxious agents and important contributors to their relatives' illnesses. After almost 30 years of deinstitutionalization, we are beginning to see their potential contribution as therapeutic allies and are shifting from a psychoanalytic or interpersonal treatment model to a systems or psychoeducational one that stresses information about chronic illness, help in handling the behavior of the patient, and peer-support among families of chronic patients.[26-29] Most current psychoeducational approaches are based upon the recognition that the identified patient with schizophrenia and the family are exquisitely sensitive to each other. This sensitivity, when expressed in a form of high expressed emotion (high criticism, hostility, and emotional overinvolvement) can lead to poor outcome.[30] These newer techniques mobilize strengths of the family and educate family members on what they don't know about the illness rather than what they do know or fantasize.

There are four studies reporting positive results of family psychoeducation techniques in the management of chronic patients. All show positive results, although their details vary. Anderson[26] gives her treatment in a clinic, while Falloon[29] does the interviews at home. Anderson does not include the patient, while Falloon[29] does. What they have in common is an emphasis on crisis management and instruction in problem-solving skills.

What this body of work suggests is that there needs to be a major change in the delivery of inpatient treatment services, with a new form of intervention with families of the chronically ill as a necessary, but not sufficient, component of the treatment package. The modern treatment of chronic mental illness in the hospital involves intensive involvement with families, both to ensure their optimal contribution to the treatment of their relatives and to reduce the stress of their experience dealing with them. This is equally true of those without interested or accessible families, in which case, social networks as they exist, must be utilized.

Finally, it should be mentioned that the emergence of the National Alliance for the Mentally Ill (NAMI) offers mental health providers an enthusiastic organizational ally. Time is well spent speaking to local chapters and offering whatever assistance or information is requested by both groups and individuals.[31] The same usefulness, mutual need, and/or cooperation apply to expatient groups.

Skills of Everyday Living

Whereas at the beginning of the depopulation movement patients were discharged from public mental hospitals without adequate training in how to survive in modern society, today it is recognized that it is critical to know whether or not patients can truly survive outside a sheltering institution before discharging them. Therefore, an adequate inpatient hospitalization both evaluates and trains patients in the skills of everyday living. These include:

- self-care (hygiene, grooming, dressing, etc),
- transportation,
- banking,
- shopping,
- purchasing and preparing food,
- washing and cleaning clothes.

While instruction in these skills can be carried out in a hospital, both direct supervision of the patient's ability to actually perform the activities and actual observation of patients while negotiating community systems are essential. In addition, it should never be taken for granted that the chronic patient, once discharged, will continue to perform these activities without difficulty, and some form of follow-up, continuing assessment, and ongoing interest is critical.

Vocational Rehabilitation

While provision of a full vocational rehabilitation program is not possible within the time available with a short-term hospitalization, both vocational evaluation and prevocational guidance are. After an adequate assessment of the level of functioning of the chronic patient is carried out, assessment of his ability to work in sheltered or competitive employment should be made. Sometimes merely brushing up specific skills (e.g., typing) and/or assistance in generic work areas (interviewing, résumé preparation, appearance) will facilitate transition to either sheltered or competitive work situations.

Socialization

Critical to the community retention of chronic patients is their ability to communicate, get along with others, and develop networks of support. Again, while short-term hospitalization does not allow for full development of socialization skills, it does provide the opportunity to target specific deficits and areas that need improvement and to begin remediation of those areas. Referral to ongoing socialization programs can then follow.

DISCHARGE PLANNING

Planning for discharge from inpatient status is probably the most important process in the inpatient hospitalization of persons suffering from chronic illness. It involves planning the management of the patient's illness over a lifetime rather than for the next 21 or 30 days of hospitalization. This shift in thinking has been hard to come by in psychiatry, and hospital staffs still persist in thinking of the hospital as central to treatment and care, rather than as simply one small portion of it.

Needless to say, such planning should begin at admission, not near or at discharge. Discharge planning with the chronically ill must primarily be based upon an understanding of what functions need to be performed to enable the patient to return to community-based care. As patients move through graded levels of settings and services, one must bear in mind all the services that are required by them. In the following sections we will summarize some of the areas that need to be considered when conducting such planning.

Psychiatric Care

One of the most critical aspects of discharge planning is the psychiatric care of chronic patients post-hospitalization. Since we know that the two ingredients of care that forestall or prevent exacerbation of illness and rehospitalization are continued medication and psychotherapy or counseling, and further that these are carried out less than 50% and 25% fo the time, respectively, provision of each is critical.[32] In addition, provision for crisis intervention and crisis stabilization must be built into any plan or patients will merely spin around in the revolving door or bounce from community to hospital settings and back.[33]

Medical Care

Persons suffering from chronic mental illness have three times the mortality and morbidity from chronic mental illnesses as their age peers.[34] Therefore, provision must be made for continuing medical care. This must involve ease of access to medical care as well as sensitization of mental health personnel to medical issues, because the chronically ill have a seemingly high tolerance for pain and a low level of complaint.[35] The former is difficult to achieve because general physicians often see psychiatric patients as having only mental illnesses, neglecting concurrent medical illnesses.

Housing

A wide range of housing opportunities is needed by the chronic patient population, although such a spectrum is rare in any American community. The guiding principle of placement should be to find the setting that is optimally therapeutic—rather than least restrictive—as it has been shown that the two are not identical.[36] Here, as with all other parts of discharge planning, patient cooperation and collaboration are key. One must always balance the needs of the patient against the services provided by each setting, choosing the best match. In addition, as with all other aspects of community care, the concept of allowing patients the opportunity to progress while not challenging them unrealistically must be born in mind.

Socialization and Social Rehabilitation

Provision must also be made for some form of socialization or social rehabilitation for most chronic patients. Whether this is in a structured (e.g., day hospital) or unstructured (e.g., lounge program) program depends to a large degree on patients' functional levels and personal desires. An ideal way of conceptualizing the social needs of the chronic patient is offered by Cutler and Tatum,[37] who propose five different kinds of social networks, each of which should be considered in planning the post-hospitalization life of chronic patients.

Vocational Rehabilitation and Work

Some constructive activity must be planned for most persons leaving the hospital. This includes vocational rehabilitation, sheltered workshops (both transitional and terminal), and competitive employment (often part-time, which chronic patients can handle more easily than full-time, at least at the start). Constructive activity constitutes such a large part of our contemporary self-image that lack of provision of this aspect of planning can be the most critical in terms of self-esteem and eventual recovery.

Income

If competitive employment does not produce sufficient income for economic self-support, provision must be made for continuing economic support either through home relief, SSI or SSDI. Currently, governmental policy discourages graded assumption of employment, but hopefully public policy will eventually reverse this antitherapeutic practice.

Continuity of Care

In moving from the single institutional umbrella under which all services were provided (e.g., the public mental hospital) to community-based care, we have forced patients into the position of "scrounging" for services. Continuity of care has many dimensions, but in this discussion we are concerned primarily with vertical continuity (pulling together all services needed at one time) and longitudinal continuity (pulling together all services needed over time). To ensure the provision of both types of continuity of care, some person and agency must be designated as the glue that holds services together and enables the patient to have access to them. This concept of the resource or case manager is critical to continuing community survival of chronic patients.[25,28,38,40] It is important to emphasize that the personal relationship between the patient and case manager or case management team is critical.

Community Programs

Optimally, all the sorts of services required by the discharged chronic patient will be offered as part of one community program. Examples of such programs are those offered by psychosocial rehabilitation centers, such as Fountain House and its over one hundred similar models;[39] the Madison, Wisconsin, Training in Community Living Program;[40] and the Southwest Denver Program.[41] The recent NIMH initiative to establish Community Support Programs (CSP's) throughout the country represents another model that, while inadequately funded to date, offers additional promise of providing the glue with which needed services can be stuck together. The growing number of psychosocial rehabilitation programs across the country is an important and critical development in the move toward genuine "community care" of the chronically ill.

LONG-TERM INPATIENT TREATMENT OF CHRONIC MENTAL ILLNESS

While there is little evidence that long-term (i.e., over 30 days) inpatient treatment of the chronic patients is superior to shorter-term treatment, there are special instances where such may be considered.[42] Following are the indications for long-term treatment, the positive aspects of such care, and the detrimental aspects.

Indications

The primary indication for long-term inpatient hospitalization of chronic patients is diagnostic, e.g., to determine what in the patient's personality or family interactions plays a strong role in his current presentation. For example, despite the fact that a patient may exhibit all the signs and symptoms of chronic mental illness, the predominant issue in his life may be a "characterological" one, e.g., passive-aggressive behavior or paranoid ideation. In these cases, it may be beneficial to utilize the structure and milieu of a long-term setting to ameliorate the patient's condition.

Another indication is *behavioral*, that is, when the patient's behavior cannot be controlled or modified in outpatient settings. For example, chronic antisocial or incompetent behavior that either endangers the patient or others may require long-term treatment, usually utilizing a highly structured behavioral modification or social learning program.

Need for *treatment* of a sort not available in outpatient settings is another indication. Here, treatment, whether psychotherapeutic, somatic, or behavioral, is sought within the structure of and making use of the supervision available in inpatient settings. Sometimes, when long-term psychotherapeutic hospitalization has not been attempted in a patient suffering from chronic illness, trying this modality of treatment is warranted.

Rehabilitation of or social learning in severely impaired chronic patients is another indication for long-term hospitalization. For instance, persons who have been institutionalized for many years *or* have severe ego deficits *or* who cannot function at even a minimal level because of their mental disability may require a long-term structured experience like that described by Paul and Lentz[10] in order to progress to another facility or setting (even a halfway house or group home).

Finally, some persons are hospitalized for long periods because they *cannot be treated* nor their symptoms controlled *as outpatients*. Hospitalization is appropriate for those persons with resistant or unremitting symptoms, usually psychotic. Here, however, one must ask whether the hospital is being used for treatment (i.e., for structure which helps medication and psychotherapy effectively control symptoms—a warranted use of this expensive resource) or merely custody (i.e., because the person cannot survive outside

The Inpatient Care of the Chronic Mentally Ill 367

a structured supervision setting — in which case it may not be warranted and care could equally well be provided in a locked facility in the community, an adult home, or foster care.)

The Pros of Long-Term Hospitalization

Long-term hospitalization does offer several advantages over treatment in alternative settings. These include:

- structure
- a therapeutic milieu
- 24-hour-a-day supervision
- use of special medications or combinations of medications
- 24-hour-a-day behavioral modification or social learning
- provision of all services under one roof (housing, therapy, vocational and social rehabilitation, etc.)

The Cons of Long-Term Hospitalization

There are serious reservations about the longer-term inpatient treatment of chronic patients. These include:

- induction into a role of "institutionalized" patient
- overreliance on the hospital to solve social (e.g., housing) problems
- suppression of the development of coping skills
- cost

In conclusion, whereas a few decades ago, long-term inpatient treatment was the preferred, if not the only, treatment for chronic mental illness, current thinking holds that such treatment should be reserved for a very few persons in whom the indications and goals are very specific. For the majority of chronic patients, the rule should be short-term inpatient treatment; for the acutely ill, a trial of long-term inpatient treatment is thoroughly warranted.[19]

THE NEED FOR ASYLUM

As indicated in our first section on the historical development of services for chronic patients in this country, radical shifts have taken place in the three hundred years of American history. Until the 1950s, hospitals were the locus of treatment and care; subsequently and especially during the late 1960s, some individuals maintained that there was no need for *any* hospitals for the mentally ill; only recently has it been realized that there is a need for asylum for some small percentage of our chronic patient population.

By asylum, we do not mean to imply a building or institution, but rather a function. Certainly, in California it has been demonstrated that both Board and Care Homes and what are called "L-facilities" have performed this function of asylum, custody, or supervised sheltered care. Such asylum functions need not be operated by the state. In fact, there is good evidence that, while they should be funded by the state because of their tertiary role in the mental health system, they are probably best operated by local governmental units and located in the community. While the percentage or number of such needed beds is unknown, largely because no system has ever been funded sufficiently and equipped with the entire range of alternative settings, several estimates are available.[41] Wing estimates the number of 15-24 per 100,000, with an additional 300 per 100,000 for the elderly infirm; Beeson and Ford at 18 per 100,000; and the California Model at 40 per 100,000.[43] Consensus, then, among the estimates is in the 15-40 per 100,000 range.

THE FUTURE

Certainly the future of inpatient hospital treatment for chronic patients depends in large part on two factors—reimbursement and scientific research. With the beginning understanding of differential therapeutics,[44] it is becoming increasingly obvious that the practices of both professionals and third parties will be governed more and more by answers to the question: "What treatment works for which patients in what settings?" The current fad of lumping medical diagnoses into large groupings (DRG) is inapplicable to an area such as chronic mental illness, and more sophisticated methods of delineating different subgroups of such patients must be continued.

In addition, it is also clear, regarding the care and treatment of chronic illness, that, while we are miles ahead of where we were a few decades ago, we still have no cure in sight for the basic disease or diseases. As has often been pointed out, scientific advances take place in leaps and bounds and quite spottily, and just as no one would have predicted the current state of understanding and treating many formerly devastating cancerous conditions, no one can predict which mental illnesses will come under control next or when.

However, waiting around for the millenium is an inadequate response to the current problem. Given what we do know about the contemporary care and treatment of chronic mental illness, we are not doing what we could,[6,44] for example: ensuring continuity of care, using short-term hospitalization, combining psychosocial and psychopharmacological interventions, seeing a hospital episode as just one piece of the patient's lifetime vulnerability to illness, and forging a true mental health system. While we await the "cure" for those suffering from chronic illnesses, we have plenty of work simply bringing about their "care."

REFERENCES

1. Dain N: From colonial America to bicentennial America: two centuries of vicissitudes in the institutional care of mental patients. Bull NY Acad Med 1976; 52:1179-1196
2. Rothman DJ: The Discovery of Asylum: Social Order and Disorder in the New Republic. Boston, Little Brown, 1971
3. Talbott JA: Twentieth century developments in American community psychiatry. Psychiatric: Q 1983; 54:207-219
4. Deutsch A: The Mentally Ill in America: A History of Their Care and Treatment from Colonial Times (2nd ed). New York, Columbia University Press, 1949
5. Kramer M: Psychiatric Services and the Changing Institutional Scene. Rockville MD, NIMH, 1975
6. Talbott JA: Toward a Public Policy on the Chronically Mentally Ill. Washington, DC, American Psychiatric Association, 1979
7. Davis JM: Overview: Maintenance therapy in psychiatry: I. schizophrenia. Am J Psychiatry 1975; 132:1237-1245
8. May PRA: Schizophrenia: overview of treatment methods, in Comprehensive Textbook of Psychiatry/II. Edited by Freedman AM, Kaplan HI, Sadock BJ. Baltimore, Williams & Wilkins, 1975
9. Gunderson JG, Mosher LR: Psychotherapy of Schizophrenia. New York, Jason Aronson, 1975
10. Paul GL, Lentz RJ: Psychosocial Treatment of Chronic Mental Patients: Milieu versus Social-Learning Programs. Cambridge, MA, Harvard University Press, 1977
11. Braun P, Kochansky G, Shapiro B, et al: Overview: deinstitutionalization of psychiatric patients: a critical review of outcome American studies. Am J Psychiatry 1981; 138:736-749
12. Kiesler CA: Mental hospitals and alternative care. Noninstitutionalization as potential public policy for mental patients. Am Psychol 1982; 37:349-360
13. Wiesbord BA, Test MA, Stein L: An alternative to mental hospital treatment. III Economic benefit-cost analysis. Arch Gen Psychiatry 1980; 37:400-405
14. Glick ID, Klar H, Braff D: When should chronic patients be hospitalized? Hosp Community Psychiatry 1984; 35:934-936
15. Herz MI, Endicott J, Spitzer RL: Brief vs. standard hospitalization: the families. Am J Psychiatry 1977; 133:502-507
16. Herz MI, Endicott J, Spitzer RL: Brief hospitalization. A two-year follow-up. Am J Psychiatry 1977; 134:502-507
17. Mattes JA, Rosen B, Klein DF: Comparison of the clinical effectiveness of "short" vs. "long" stay psychiatric hospitalization: II. Results of a 3-year posthospital follow-up. J Nerv Ment Dis 1977; 165:395-402
18. Mattes JA, Rosen B, Klein DF, Millan D: Comparison of the clinical effectiveness of "short" versus "long" stay psychiatric hospitalization: III. Further results of a 3-year posthospital follow-up. J Nerv Ment Dis 1977; 165:395-402
19. Glick ID, Hargreaves WA: Psychiatric Hospital Treatment of the 1980's. Lexington, MA, Lexington Books, 1979
20. Riessman CK, Rabkin JG, Struening EL: Brief versus standard psychiatric hospitalization: a critical review of the literature. Community Ment Health J 1977; 2:1-10
21. Riessman CK, Rabkin JG: Hospital vs. home care programs for psychiatric patients: summary of published findings, unpublished, 1977

22. Riebel S, Herz MI: Limitations of brief hospital treatment. Am J Psychiatry 1976; 133:518-521
23. Talbott JA: Therapy of the Chronic Mentally Ill, in Current Psychiatric Therapies. Edited by Masserman JH. New York, Grune & Stratton, 1981
24. Segal SP, Aviram U: The Mentally Ill in Community-Based Sheltered Care. New York, John Wiley, 1981
25. Lamb HRH: Community Survival for Long-Term Patients. San Francisco, CA, Jossey-Bass, 1976
26. Anderson CM: The psychoeducational family treatment of schizophrenia. New Dir Ment Health Serv 1981; 12:79-94
27. Anderson CM, Hogarty GE, Reiss DJ: Family treatment of adult schizophrenia patients: a psycho-educational approach. Schizophr Bull 1980; 6:490-505
28. Boyd JL, McGill CW, Faloon IRH: Family participation in the community rehabilitation of schizophrenics. Hosp Community Psychiatry 1981; 32:629-632
29. Falloon IRH, Boyd JL, McGill CW, Strang JS, Moss HB: Family management training in the community care of schizophrenia. New Dir Ment Health Serv 1981; 12:61-77
30. Goldstein MJ: Short and long-term effects of combining drug and family therapy. New Dir Ment Health Serv 1981; 12:5-26
31. Hatfield AB: Families as advocates for the mentally ill: a growing movement. Hosp Community Psychiatry 1981; 32:641-642
32. Minkoff KL: A map of the chronic mental patient, in The Chronic Mental Patient: Problems, Solutions and Recommendations of a Public Policy. Edited by Talbott JA. American Psychiatric Association, Washington, DC, 1978
33. Talbott JA: Stopping the Revolving Door—a study of readmissions to a state hospital. Psychiatric Q 1974; 159-168
34. Amdur MA: Death in aftercare. Compr Psychiatry 1981; 33:619-626
35. Talbott JA, Linn L: Reactions of chronic schizophrenics to life-threatening disease. Psychiatric Q 1978; 50:218-227
36. Bachrach LL: Is the least restrictive environment always the best? Sociological and semantic implications. Hosp Community Psychiatry 1980; 31:7-102
37. Cutler LD, Tatum E: Networks and the Chronic Patient, in Effective Aftercare for the '80's. Edited by Cutler DL, New Dir Ment Health Serv 1983; 19:13-22
38. Lourie NV: Care management, in The Chronic Mental Patient: Problems, Solutions and Recommendations of a Public Policy. Edited by Talbott JA. Washington, DC, American Psychiatric Association, 1978
39. Glasscote R: What programs work and what programs don't work to meet the needs of the chronic mental patients, in The Chronic Mental Patient: Problems, Solutions and Recommendations for a Public Policy. Edited by Talbott JA. Washington, DC, American Psychiatric Association, 1978
40. Stein LI, Text MA: Use of special living arrangements: a model for decision-making. Hosp Community Psychiatry 1977; 28:608-610
41. Stein LI, Test MA: Alternatives to Mental Hospital Treatment. New York, Plenum, 1975
42. GAP Report: The Chronic Mental Patient in the Community. New York, Group for the Advancement of Psychiatry, 1978
43. Elpers J, Crowell A: How many beds? An overview of resource planning. Hosp Community Psychiatry 1982; 33:755-761
44. Frances A, Clarkin J: Differential Therapeutics. New York, Brunner-Mazel, 1984

IV
Discharge

22
Discharge Planning

Charles P. Peters
Faith B. Dickerson

The discharge of a patient from the hospital is a complex psychosocial event. Though discharge means physical separation from the institution, the patient must still be somehow made to feel therapeutically attached to the milieu which he is about to leave behind. The milieu has been both nurturant and catalytic of change; to expect that the patient will easily duplicate this "holding environment" outside of the hospital is erroneous, even in the best of outpatient therapeutic situations. Further, the patient has interacted with a host of hospital professionals and formed numerous therapeutic alliances with doctors and nurses, adjunctive therapists, and even other patients. A discharge treatment plan, no matter how comprehensive, will inevitably seem barren to a patient who leaves the richness of the hospital.

A crucial part of discharge is the continuation of some form of psychotherapy that has existed within the hospital. This therapy bridges the gulf between hospital and the outside world and hopefully ensures introspectiveness. With the rare expectation of a very high-functioning patient, most individuals will require the professional services of at least one outside therapist.

Psychotherapy can mean many different things, however. The patient with a personality disorder may require a more intensive outpatient treatment than the patient who is hospitalized for adjustment of his antidepressant medication. Some patients require insight-oriented treatment, while others can utilize the supportive services of a therapist. The "brokerage" of patient and therapist is often a delicate and time-consuming process for inpatient staff. Hospital guidelines may recommend that a patient return to the referring doctor upon discharge, but this may not always be workable. In some instances, the patient has been admitted precisely because outpatient therapy has failed, and the patient is not interested in a new therapist. In other instances, the therapist himself may feel that therapy has not been particularly useful or gratifying, and he may suggest another clinician who can take over the case. Therapists from inside the hospital are sometimes picked by the patient, while on other occasions the patient must find someone in his own geographic locale. Whenever a new therapist is chosen, the patient should meet with him and discuss feelings about therapy with the hospital staff. To be suddenly transferred upon discharge to the care of a stranger intensifies the trauma of separation from the hospital.

If drug treatment is to continue after the hospitalization, the psychiatrist who will be prescribing medications is a crucial part of the discharge plan. It is precarious to leave these arrangements until after the patient has left the hospital. Also unwise is the tactic of making last-minute pharmacologic regimen changes, including reduction or discontinuation of medication. Such changes are erroneously predicated on the continuing lack of stress; stress, upon discharge, is bound to be higher, and patients often need the protection of some medication when they leave the hospital.

A thorough medication history should accompany the patient, together with a good narrative summary of his care. Too often, both come very late, following delays in dictation. The drug history itself should document unsuccessful drug trials, including dosage and duration of exposure and currently effective drugs and their titration history, maximum dosages used during acute illness, and maintenance dosages. Without this material, the outside clinician is apt to "start from scratch" in his attempts to control mood or thought disorders.

Many patients will require outpatient care that extends beyond the need for a psychotherapist and somatic treatment. Not infrequently, discharge planning must address the patient's need for a structured daily program and a place of residence. Where the patient sleeps and where the patient spends the bulk of his daytime hours can have a profound impact on the likelihood of relapse versus continued improvement. Gradations of structured daily activity can also be considered. The most regressed patients may require the intensive supervision of a day treatment center or day hospital. Some patients benefit from the structure of a step-down program that affords some of the benefits of inpatient care. The more functional patient may be successfully placed in a volunteer position or part-time job. Many patients combine all three of these activities with gradually increasing autonomy as post-hospital treatment progresses.

The history of previous level of functioning is an important predictor of post-discharge capability. The patient who repeatedly failed to maintain employment prior to admission should be reintegrated into the work force more slowly than the well-functioning patient with an acute illness. There exists a delicate balance between encouraging higher level activities and setting the patient up for failure upon discharge. It is a skilled hospital treatment team that can carefully assess the patient's clinical needs and prescribe a useful blend of caution and challenge to the newly discharged person.

The patient who is unable to return to the previous residence or who is advised against doing so for clinical reasons requires special assistance in the discharge-planning phase of hospitalization. Relocation should be considered when any of the following clinical criteria are met:

1. The patient has been unable to care for himself in the setting from which he was admitted to the hospital, and no other person is able to assume that responsibility.
2. The home or residential environment from which the patient came presents an unhealthy degree of psychopathology that could precipitate relapse were the patient to return.
3. The patient requires more structure or more intensive treatment than can be provided in the previous residence.
4. The patient is not welcome back to the former residence.

Many patients are functioning at a high enough level to assume independent living after hospitalization. Frequently, hospitalization affords the young adult the opportunity to plan transition from parents' home to an individual apartment or a house shared with peers. When independent living is not indicated, a halfway house or supervised boarding home should be considered. Indications for these faculties include:

1. The patient requires assistance in maintaining personal care in areas of grooming, nutrition, and compliance with treatment that extends beyond that which can be provided by family or friends.
2. Continual clinical assessment is required that exceeds the skills of untrained individuals.
3. The patient would benefit from the structured community of a professionally operated residential facility.
4. The level of psychopathology existing after discharge exceeds that which would be tolerated in a less formal treatment environment.

Once a place of residence is selected that is affordable, the patient should have the opportunity to visit or spend a number of nights at the new home before discharge. Many early problems can be averted if the patient is comfortable with the living situation before being discharged from the hospital.

A sound discharge plan frequently requires attention to other significant individuals in the patient's life. The parents of a young patient may benefit from an opportunity to meet regularly with a mental health professional to discuss their reactions to the illness of their child and to seek guidance in dealing with the disruption to the family unit that the illness has precipitated. Families may benefit from family therapy with or without the patient in the early post-hospital period. Couples therapy or counseling of children of an ill parent may be a useful preventive measure in helping the spouse and children understand and adapt to the implications of mental illness.

One consideration in assessing the patient's readiness for discharge concerns the sources of stress that may have led to the need for hospitalization. For some patients, there may not be any clearly identifiable precipitants. For other patients, there are relationship, vocational, or other life problems which can be directly linked to the onset of illness leading to hospitalization. The possible sources of stress are multiple, from the death of a family member to unemployment to change in outpatient therapist—to any other loss or major life change. In some cases, the stress not only may have contributed to the patient's psychiatric problems but may also be secondary to them. For example, the manic patient who spends excessive money winds up with significant financial as well as psychiatric problems.

Psychosocial stressors are acknowledged in *DSM-III* among Axis IV designations.[1] The importance of this for the clinician is that patients must come to understand and grapple with the dynamics of the stressor as a condition for discharge. For example, a patient may come to realize that using marijuana made him psychotically decompensate, while another patient may come to understand the fact that his wife's abandonment of him gave rise to the rage for which he was admitted to the hospital. Understanding the dynamics gives a "handle" to the patient in terms of prevention; without some appreciation of his own vulnerabilities, the patient is at risk for relapse. Patients, however, differ widely in their ability to deal with stressors; some have good insight into these events while others seem almost disdainful of them and see precipitating events as unrelated to mental illness.

A 22-year-old man with a schizotypal personality was admitted with an acute psychosis following the use of drugs in college. He had smoked marijuana heavily a week prior to admission and on route home had become paranoid and delusional. He was committed to the hospital and experienced a stormy hospital course. Once recovered, he showed little insight regarding his drug use and on a weekend pass home again undertook the use of drugs.

Discharge in the above case was delayed until the patient had better understanding of his self-destructive behavior and tolerated weekends home better.

Discharge planning with the acutely psychotic patient begins at the time that the patient is free of disruptive symptoms. If the hospitalization is a long-term affair, then some resolution of the dynamics giving rise to the illness is possible; in other instances, the most that can be accomplished is a few meetings with family to sensitize them to the issues at hand. Discharge may be compromised by time constraints and financial issues, leading staff to purposely ignore the larger psychosocial issues surrounding the patient's psychosis. Attention to compliance may be more important but achieved with difficulty.

A 24-year-old man, was admitted on an emergency basis after becoming acutely paranoid while working for his father's company in a distant town. Upon admission, he was agitated, psychotic, and grandiose, but settled down quickly with the aid of neuroleptic medication. Once he was less symptomatic, he pressed insistently for discharge. He minimized and externalized his recent difficulties ("I was just under a lot of stress on the job"). He also resisted educational efforts about affective disorder, which was the final diagnosis, and about the need for continued medication. He did reluctantly agree to continue medication but had only a vague plan about returning to work and was subsequently discharged.

This case illustrates the problems inherent in treating the acutely ill patient, difficulties often compounded by the patient's denial and that of his family, who see the process as "medical" and do not wish, or cannot tolerate, psychological exploration.

The criteria for discharging the chronically psychotic patient are somewhat different from those for discharging the acutely ill patient. With chronic patients symptom relief is seen as more limited. Instead, the goal is to provide good aftercare arrangements to prevent relapse and to work with the family regarding future hopes and rehabilitation.[2] Medication compliance is another agenda, though the emphasis is more on maintenance. Discharge of the patient with a chronic psychotic illness is often an imperfect one. Social programs invariably are difficult to arrange for, and the patient himself may sabotage efforts or seek situations that are unrealistic and not predicated on past achievements. *DSM-III* also acknowledges the highest level of psychosocial functioning in Axis V, and this may be used at discharge time to assess a psychosocial milieu conducive to the limits of rehabilitation. Even then, compromise dictates much of what occurs at discharge time.

> A 28-year-old male with ten previous hospitalizations since adolescence was admitted for exacerbation of a chronic schizophrenic disorder compounded by alcohol abuse. After several months in the hospital, the patient was stabilized with a structured inpatient program and weekly depot antipsychotic drug injections. The patient continued to have residual psychotic symptoms and experienced difficulty on sign-outs off grounds. Discharge planning was commenced in the face of limited insurance benefits. Because the patient had failed repeatedly while living with his parents, the social worker pursued halfway house placement. Unfortunately, the patient could either not afford or was not accepted at any of the area halfway houses, so he was discharged to his parents' home with a commitment to medication compliance and day treatment attendance.

This case illustrates the limits of aftercare and also shows how hospital staff, cognizant of the limits of discharge plans, may have to simply relinquish their care of the patient and hope for the best. Optimal aftercare plans are difficult to achieve.

Inpatient programs for the treatment of alcohol and drug problems tend to be more standardized than those for other disorders and discharge plans may be part of the program format. Readiness for discharge is usually based on the patient's acknowledgment of the chemical dependence and a reduction in his denial about the addiction and its adverse effects. Sobriety and a commitment to continued abstinence are also expected before discharge, along with a commitment to regular Alcoholics Anonymous or Narcotics Anonymous meetings.

Despite regular AA or NA attendance, it remains difficult to accurately assess the readiness for discharge, given the patients' use of denial and, at other times, manipulation concerning drug use and cravings. Perhaps more useful than verbalized ideation is behavior during actual sign-outs for weekends. Sometimes, multiple discharges and admissions are required before the patient comes to meaningfully admit the true nature and extent of his illness and to seriously engage in treatment.

Patients with primitive personality disorders present discharge problems. Borderline patients, for example, are rarely free of long-standing pathology and in some respects resemble the chronically psychotic patient. Yet, there are some guidelines for discharge; these include the attenuation of rage and the ability on the part of the patient to reduce self-destructive acts, at least within the hospital. The ability of the patient to tolerate ambiguity and to see the world as grey, rather than black or white, is some indicator of health, as is the ability of the patient to verbalize affect and interact meaningfully with some other patients and staff. Indeed, the staff's subjective feelings about the patient often signal to the therapist the patient's actual internal improvement.

A 19-year-old female with multiple short-term hospitalizations since age 17 was admitted following an overdose attempt precipitated by a romantic rejection. This was the fourth such suicide attempt in two years, and all were related in some way to the demise of a stormy and chaotic interpersonal relationship. At the time of admission, the patient was dysphoric, easily enraged, and prone to self-destructive ideation and behavior. Responses to others were dramatic and polarized, with most people and situations seen as all good or all bad.

Following extended hospital treatment, discharge was considered when the patient evidenced greater impulse control, modification of defenses such as devaluation and negativism, and an ability to engage in therapy. The patient still had self-destructive thoughts but did not act on them. Her interpersonal responses in the hospital indicated a greater tolerance for and appreciation of multiple sides to any one person.

A discharge plan was formulated to include individual psychotherapy regular attendance at a day treatment center and a part-time job. The patient was successfully discharged.

The above case is illustrative of improvement within the hospital and readiness for discharge; however, outpatient treatment continued at a very intensive level, with medication prescribed as well.

Discharge for the patient with recurrent affective disorder is complicated by the unpredictable course of the illness and the use of complex pharmacologic regimens. Assuming adequate remission of the acute affective episode, discharge planning with this patient population must include special attention to pharmacological management. Titration of medication should be accomplished in the hospital for patients with refractory or poorly controlled illnesses. The patient should be carefully instructed in the use and potential risks of antidepressant medications or of lithium or carbamazepine. Only after the patient has shown the ability to comply with medication usage and appreciates the need to responsibly adhere to laboratory monitoring schedules should he or she be considered ready for discharge. While many patients can be started on these medications on an outpatient basis, the patient who has been hospitalized for the treatment of his illness is usually one with markedly impaired judgment due to mania or manic psychosis, or with suicidal intent for which his medication could serve as a lethal instrument.

Aside from considerations unique to particular diagnostic groups, there are general clinical criteria used to assess the patient's readiness for discharge. These criteria are based on the patient's current level of functioning in the hospital and his responsiveness to treatment. A basic concern in discharging a patient is the likelihood of his hurting himself or others. The prediction of dangerousness constitutes the clearest grounds for continuing hospitalization and postponing discharge to the community. Assessment of danger may be based on the patient's actual behavior in the hospital. Thus, the patient who mutilates himself or assaults others needs to have a significant destruction-free period before discharge is commenced. In other instances, the assessment of prospective danger is based on the patient's response to increased autonomy from the hospital staff or verbalized statements about the future. While dangerousness is notoriously difficult to predict, it exerts a powerful effect in the assessment of discharge readiness.

Other considerations based on the patient's functioning within the hospital include the patient's capacity to follow a daily routine and care for self, to participate in expressive and task-oriented activities, to engage in a relationship with the psychotherapist or treating psychiatrist, to forge interpersonal ties with staff members and other patients, and to successfully manage increasing degrees of autonomy from the close supervision of the nursing staff. While the expectations in each of these areas may vary with the particular patient and diagnostic group, there needs to be some competence demonstrated in each area prior to discharge.

There are several categories of discharge; some, such as those labeled against medical advice (AMA) are universally applied at all hospitals. Others are unique to individual hospitals and include other types of administrative discharges that reflect the problematic nature of the discharge. The AMA discharge generally implies dissatisfaction by the staff with the timing or nature of the patient's discharge (see Chapters 6 and 16).[3] One tactic used to reduce abrupt departure of the hospital by the patient is a three-day notice. Here, the patient makes a contract with the hospital to submit a handwritten notice of intent to leave. Once so submitted, the hospital begins to attempt to persuade the patient to remain, thus forestalling a potential AMA discharge. Patients put in three-day notices for many reasons, including dissatisfaction with staff or other patients, conflicts arising out of therapy or ward meetings, or outside pressures with spouse or family. Three-day notices take up a considerable amount of the hospital staff's time and come to be richly symbolic of many dynamic issues concerning the patient's interaction with staff.

A 30-year-old male was hospitalized for suicidal ideation within a borderline personality disorder. About a month after admission and slight improvement, the patient put in a three-day notice to leave the hospital. He expressed intense anger that he was not permitted by the treatment team to return to work full-time and threatened to hurt himself if he could not go back to his job immediately. The patient's family, also the target of his anger, did not support continued hospitalization. The patient was viewed by staff as manipulative and not truly a danger to himself, so he was discharged against medical advice.

An AMA discharge is at times a safety valve for the hospital but more often represents a therapeutic failure. Education focused on reducing AMA discharges pays off in lessening the draining effects such maneuvers have on hospital staff.[4] After all, the staff have put large amounts of energy into the patient's care, only to have him leave precipitously. Of course, this very process of "caring" may be what propels the patient out of the hospital. Patients who are paranoid or intolerant of intimacy or highly anxious are at risk for leaving the hospital. Adolescents may recreate the need to flee "the family."

There are a couple other kinds of situations in which the patient is discharged prior to the point of sufficient improvement for discharge to the community. In some cases, a patient may leave to be transferred to another hospital setting. Transfer may be made to a more specialized inpatient program which better matches the patient's needs or to a medical facility if so indicated. The patient may also be moved between the private and public sectors as dictated by insurance availability or the expiration of funds.

In yet another set of circumstances, the patient may be asked to leave the hospital regardless of discharge readiness or available aftercare plans. Administrative discharge or discharge at staff request is an unusual event and occurs only when the patient has significantly violated hospital rules or caused harm to others in the hospital setting. Assault with bodily harm of other patients or staff, fire-setting, and drug/alcohol abuse within the hospital milieu are the kinds of destructive behaviors that may lead to such a discharge. There are few hard and fast rules about the criteria for administrative discharge, and decisions are usually made on a case-by-case basis and influenced by assessment of such variables as the harmfulness to other patients and the malicious intent involved.

A 25-year-old male was admitted for paranoid symptoms within a chronic schizophrenic disorder. He had no history of physically aggressive behavior. On the unit the patient was seclusive and verbally hostile towards the staff. One day, after a minor confrontation with staff, he punched a nurse several times in the head. Although she was not seriously injured, the incident was highly traumatic for her and the other staff and patients on the unit. Once in seclusion, the patient was paranoid and nonremorseful. After considerable anguish by the treatment team, it was decided that the patient could not stay on the unit because strong negative feelings about him precluded therapeutic interactions.

As the patient approaches the final stages of hospitalization, certain clinical phenomena are frequently observed. These include the predischarge exacerbation of symptoms. It is not uncommon for the symptoms that necessitated hospitalization to reemerge as discharge approaches. While not symptomatic with the same intensity, the previously depressed patient may begin having milder signs of sleep disturbance and difficulty concentrating; the borderline patient may feel more anxious and empty; the substance-abusing patient may report dreams of drug use or drug-craving episodes. The clinician must keep in mind that this is an expected occurrence and does not always indicate premature discharge. Often the patient will show greater ability to master these signs and symptoms than he did prior to admission. The patient must be advised of the possible occurrence of this type of worsening to prevent demoralization if it does occur. Likewise, the treating team should appreciate this phenomenon and avoid anxiety over a suddenly less optimistic clinical picture.

Regarding the issue of separation and how it is approached by patients and staff, a number of points can be made. However brief the hospitalization, most patients develop a strong attachment to the hospital and staff. This attachment may be dealt with by denying any feelings of loss at the time of discharge or by experiencing profound anxiety at the prospect of navigating without the support of the hospital and staff. Ideally, the inpatient unit provides an ongoing forum for discussing the events and emotions leading up to discharge. A predischarge group made up of patients preparing for discharge and patients recently discharged helps to provide support to smooth the way to post-hospital living. Patients ready for discharge can test their fears and expectations with those who have made the transition, while those recently discharged benefit from the link back to the stability of the hospital.

Staff are also encouraged to discuss their feelings about separating from patients to whom they have become attached. The recurring and often relentless separation from patients in whom the staff has become invested is a draining emotional experience. In some situations, patients may be encouraged to visit staff after discharge as a continuation of a healthy treatment alliance. In other settings, such contact may be frowned upon as fostering excessive dependency. Whatever contact does occur, it is apt to be informal and casual and not the result of scheduling. Thus, a discharged adolescent may visit another patient on the ward or may return to see a staff member with whom he had felt close. Visits of this type are somewhat encouraged, but the staff must tread the narrow line between being sympathetic and setting limits on some patients who inappropriately use the hospital as a refuge. While there are post-discharge groups which can help patients with the continuing problems of adjustment in society, the post-discharge contact with the hospital is a part of discharge planning.[5]

REFERENCES

1. Diagnostic and Statistical Manual, Third Edition. American Psychiatric Association, Washington, DC, 1980
2. Caton CL, Goldstein JM, Serrano O, Render R: The impact of discharge planning on chronic schizophrenic patients. Hosp Community Psychiatry 1984; 35:255–262
3. Smith HH: Discharge against medical advice (AMA) from an acute care private psychiatric hospital. J Clin Psychology 1982; 38:550–554
4. Targum SD, Capodanno AE, Hoffman HA, Foudraine C: An intervention to reduce the rate of hospital discharges against medical advice. Am J Psychiatry 1982; 139:657–659
5. Austad CS, Shapiro RS: Treatment implications of the postdischarge contact. Hosp Community Psychiatry 1986; 37:839–840

23
Following Hospitalization: Residential Aftercare

Richard D. Budson

Modern care of the psychiatric patient today often requires comprehensive aftercare services following hospitalization. Essential among these services is sheltered housing or community residential care serving many different kinds of patients. The technical knowhow is available to provide services not only for different diagnostic groups, but also for different levels of disability, as well as for selected age groups. Thus, programs may be specifically designed for patients with chronic psychotic disorders, borderline character disorders, neuropsychiatric disorders, or problems with alcohol and substance abuse, to name only a few. So, too, are there programs specifically for long-term patients, and programs for those recovering from first acute breakdowns, as there are special programs for adolescents and the elderly. These different types of patients, then, can be placed in any one of a variety of community residential programs which have been specifically conceived, planned, and implemented to serve them. Thus, a spectrum of services is potentially available in a range of community residential programs.

The establishment of these programs can often be a difficult and frustrating task. There are complex administrative challenges, which may well vary from place to place. Two issues predominate—legal and financial. The legal issues include zoning and building code regulations, which are usually determined at the local community level. Local resistance to the starting of a new program can sometimes be expressed through overly restrictive determinations of building inspectors, as well as through the denial of requests for special permits from local zoning appeals boards. Licensing and determination of need requirements are usually decided by state agencies, which may or may not be supportive and helpful, depending on state policy, which in turn is responsive to the political climate at the time.

Contributing to the complexity of finding operational monies for these programs is the fact that, in general, the financing of mental health care is in a state of flux and rapid change. The sources of income for these programs have been variable, their extent has been very uneven, and there have been significant differences between the private and public sectors. Until recently, only in the public sector has there been support and subsidization of these programs. This support has come in two primary ways — through state subsidies directly to the programs themselves, and through federal subsidies to clients in the form of federal Supplemental Security Income. Financing in the private sector has been primarily limited to patients paying out-of-pocket. One exception to this is that some rare private insurance companies have included community residential care in their benefit packages, often because it was included in a partial hospitalization benefit mandated by state legislation.

New on the scene, and potentially very significant in terms of community residential care, is the development of health maintenance organizations (HMOs), which are funded on a capitation basis. Through this mechanism a health service provider contracts to provide necessary services for an annual, fixed amount of funds per subscriber. In this situation, it is incumbent upon the provider to keep costs low. Since a community residential program is often able to care for an inpatient who cannot otherwise be discharged, at only one-quarter to one-fifth the cost of inpatient hospitalization, a strong incentive exists for such health care providers to develop community residential services. Consequently, we may be on the threshold of a rapid development of privately operated community residential programs serving HMOs nationwide.

Once in operation, complicated and unique administrative situations can arise, such as legal quandaries regarding the rights of a program to exclude a disruptive resident. In this instance, there has to be a determination if housing law, invoking tenants' rights and regulations regarding eviction, is to be relevant. On the other hand, the program may be considered to be not primarily housing but rather a mental health service which has a right, as well as a clinical responsibility, to exclude disruptive and uncooperative residents or patients. Several court decisions are beginning to establish that the latter is the case. New programs need to incorporate into their administrative structure the execution of a contract with each new patient, establishing the fact that the patient is desiring a mental health service and that there are mutual obligations and responsibilities by both parties in this arrangement—service to be rendered by the program and adherence to programmatic policies by the client.

It should be observed that some of these legal and financial issues are problems because community residential programs for the mentally ill are relatively new on the mental health scene. Only in the last 20 years have they been developed in the United States. Thus, their legal identity and financial place in the health care delivery system are in the midst of an evolutionary process. Building codes in many states are just being drafted for these facilities, zoning bylaws do not usually take them into account, and the health care industry is just beginning to realize their potential as a cost-effective way to deliver quality service.

At the same time, these facilities do not represent an entirely new departure when viewed from a long-term clinical perspective. In fact, the roots of their clinical philosophy can be found in the origins of moral treatment as it was established in the 18th century in Europe. In particular, one can find in Samuel Tuke's 1813 *Description of the Retreat* (at York)[1] many of the principles also described in this author's work, *The Psychiatric Halfway House—A Handbook of Theory and Practice*, published in 1978.[2] The commonality which bridges almost two centuries is the conviction that family values brought to bear in a homelike environment are helpful to the rehabilitation of mental patients. As described by Samuel Tuke in 1813, the Retreat espoused these values in common with our current thinking: staff eating and living in the same quarters with patients; a focus on enhancing the self-esteem of the patients; a sense of the importance of productive work to mental health; a family-like set of values and known consequences to aberrant antisocial behavior; and a presumption that the patient, as any developing person in a family, wished to be well thought of. In the 18th century, moral treatment at the Retreat replaced conditions at the local lunatic asylum where, "It was believed . . . that the general treatment of insane persons was, too frequently, calculated to depress and degrade, rather than to awaken the slumbering reason, or correct its wild hallucinations."[1] In recent years, I have similarly described the community residence as replacing long-term hospital care which, to the patient's detriment, sustained an environment based on a universal medical model, where all activity was viewed in terms of the patient's pathology instead of focused upon building his or her strengths.

DIFFERENT TYPES OF COMMUNITY RESIDENCES

Seven different types of post-hospital housing are currently in use throughout the country. These include:

1. transitional halfway houses;
2. long-term group residences;
3. cooperative apartments (satellite housing, landlord supervised apartments, post-halfway house accommodations);
4. lodge programs;
5. total rural environments (work camps);
6. foster care (family care);
7. board-and-care homes.

Private psychiatric hospitals mostly use transitional halfway houses, long-term group residences, and cooperative apartments (options 1-3), although they may occasionally use total rural environments, foster care, and nursing homes (5-7). Public hospitals are more likely to use all of these programs with the exception of the rural programs.

The National Institute of Mental Health has defined the transitional halfway house[8] as a "residential facility in operation seven days a week with round the clock supervision (often a staff member living on the premises) and providing room, board, and assistance in the activities of daily living." Nonprofit corporations usually operate these facilities in large old houses, with 10-20 residents, who generally participate daily in a planned program outside the dwelling. Whereas some facilities are increasingly acting as an alternative to hospitalization, the "halfway house" has conventionally been used as just that — a transitional facility from hospital to the community. Quality programs usually provide individual counseling, house meetings, and recreational activities, with emphasis on mutual support and understanding among house residents. The transitional halfway house is likely to have a relatively young population whose problems are of recent onset, and whose potential for reentry into the community and total independent living is quite high.[3-11]

Although the long-term group residence resembles the transitional halfway house in many particulars, its residents are usually sufficiently lacking in living skills, or sufficiently symptomatic, to require a higher on-site staff/resident ratio. In addition, the duration of residence in these facilities may exceed one year, in contrast to the transitional facility, which may be only six to eight months. This facility, however, is designed to care for those difficult patients who otherwise would be detained in a psychiatric inpatient setting.

Cooperative apartments are distinctive in that they have no on-site staff and are usually comprised of groups of four per unit. There is a regular staff visit from the sponsoring mental health agency to oversee the living arrangement as well as the required outside daily program. Cooperative apartments are often developed as outward community extensions of staffed residential programs. These programs may be designed not only to broaden the scope of these core community care programs, but also to avoid various constraints — to minimize startup costs, lower operating costs, avoid community opposition, and circumvent restrictive building codes. These programs are among the least expensive for the patient.[12-15]

It has been found that patients known to each other in the hospital can more easily move into the community as a group. Fairweather developed such a model, the group establishing economic independence by organizing itself to operate a self-sustaining business. The hospital staff prepares the group for both the living and business aspects of the community program prior to leaving the wards. "Patients function together as a cooperative, communal society, running the household and working together to earn money."[17]

Total rural environments are non-hospital residential facilities which offer total supervised living, including daily on-premises farming chores. An operational farm provides ongoing, reality-based responsibilities focused on the fulfillment of rehabilitative goals. Such facilities are particularly suitable for those clients who, although not needing a hospital, cannot reliably or safely manage in a more independent community setting. Gould Farm in western Massachusetts and Spring Lake Ranch in Vermont have been pioneers in this area.[20,21]

Foster or family care, one of the oldest community placements, entails the location of ex-patients in private homes. The Veterans Administration has relied more heavily upon foster care than the state systems. Up to four residents may be placed in one foster home. The patient is supervised by the family caretaker, who is in turn supervised by a visiting social worker from the referring institution. One continuing concern about foster home care is that it provides primarily a custodial function. A significant study on foster homes in Canada by Murphy et al.[22] showed that there was no, or only minimal, improvement in social functioning or community participation.[23,24]

Board-and-care homes have been the recipient of many discharged mental patients from the public hospitals. They are generally proprietary rooming houses which provide a wide range of care, depending upon the interest and motivation of the proprietor. Some of these facilities provide little more than room and board in dingy surroundings, with no semblance of a rehabilitative program whatsoever. Other programs have well kept, pleasant surroundings and maintain close alliance and consultation with referring mental health agencies. Special efforts have been made to improve these facilities, which are so important to the public sector in several large metropolitan cities.[25-28]

The reader should keep in mind that well planned and financed services primarily use the three first mentioned types of facilities: the transitional halfway house, the long-term group residence and the cooperative apartment. These will be described in greater detail later in the chapter. The following description of clinical issues relates primarily to these three types of facilities.

PATIENT TYPES TREATED IN COMMUNITY RESIDENCES

These facilities can care for patients with various diagnoses. The community residence carries out certain therapeutic tasks and addresses certain particular issues for each diagnostic group. The level of disability, irrespective of the diagnosis, is usually the primary determinant of the type of community residence to which the patient would be referred. In other instances, there are diagnostic specific facilities, such as for neuropsychiatric patients, eating disorders, etc. The universal goal of the community residence is relapse prevention, along with a simultaneous strengthening of the patient's capacity to function in a healthy and adaptive manner.

Schizophrenics are a major group cared for in post-hospital community residential care programs. Placement may follow an initial acute psychotic episode or, for a long-term chronic patient, one of many hospitalizations. Within this diagnosis, two groups can be differentiated — those patients who can tolerate a social push program (which they may need to prevent desocialization) and those patients who must have a low intensity program (because they relapse in the face of any high intensity program). This differentiation of schizophrenic patients reflects the work of Vaughn and Leff[29] and Wing,[30] who showed that patients returning to families with high expressed emotion (high EE), characterized by lack of acceptance of the illness, criticalness, and demands for higher performance, relapsed at a much higher rate than patients who returned to low EE homes where there were few demands made upon the patients and in general a greater acceptance of their limitations. At the same time, it is known that some patients deteriorate in the face of too little stimulation. Thus, program design and operation, as well as sophisticated patient referral, require careful assessment so as to differentiate which patients should go to which program.

A common feature of all programs for schizophrenic patients is careful monitoring of antipsychotic medication, since many patients either deny their illness or have paranoid thoughts about their medication being poison — both of which impel the patient to stop the medicine. There should also be thoughtful alertness to adverse reactions to family visits or interactions, which can precipitate relapse in many patients. In addition, during the evaluation, a careful history is always taken to determine two clinical facts:

first, the previous precipitants to relapse (these often are typical and predictable), and second, the previously noted early signs of impending relapse. Knowing the latter can give the clinicians and even fellow patients early warning that trouble is brewing, thereby facilitating early intervention.

Manic-depressive patients who have had numerous relapses are prime candidates for post-hospital community residential care. These are often patients who have so enjoyed the euphoria of their illness that they are prone to stop taking their lithium to reexperience that pathologic mental state. The results are usually disastrous. The residential community works together in being alert to the early signs of relapse—such as a manic-depressive patient suddenly becoming very humorous and making everyone laugh. This is usually a sign of impending mania. Monitoring of the taking of lithium is a sine qua non. Further, the careful delineation of a very structured daily routine is important so as to contain a potentially expansive mental state. It is often felt that it is best to keep these patients on the slightly depressed side of things to prevent relapse into mania.

Patients with unipolar depression are often referred to community residential care when the history is that of repeated serious suicide attempts. One of the most important clinical tasks in this case is for the clinician in the program to form—usually before the patient enters the program—an antisuicide alliance with the patient. This requires an informed and close working relationship with the patient. The patient makes a contract with the clinician that, when the patient feels suicidal, he or she will inform the clinician, rather than taking action. Additionally, part of the evaluation of the patient includes a careful history of likely precipitants of suicidal feelings. Antidepressant medication is routine, the taking of which sometimes needs to be monitored. Diet has to be carefully watched when the patient is on MAO inhibitors to ensure the absence of tyramine-containing foods, which can provoke a hypertensive crisis.

The community residence and, in particular, the high expectation halfway house have become therapeutically powerful in the treatment of the borderline personality disorder. Here the community can become a safe, secure, and stable holding environment for a patient who has often had a stormy course of repeated hospitalizations in response to impulsive, self-destructive acts. The staff is alert to splitting maneuvers and the entire community works to gradually help the patient experience others as real people who are neither idealized nor devalued. This is also an environment which sets limits and offers real interpersonal feedback to obnoxious, demanding, and narcissistic behavior.

Patients recovering from alcohol and other substance abuse disorders also can use community residential care. There are various levels of care for such programs. All have very strong traditions of peer group cohesion, support, and structure. Strict abstinence is usually required. Regular AA meetings can be fruitfully integrated into the residential program. Often Antabuse is used, as well as unscheduled urine checks for other substance abusers.

The clinician must be alert to the patient who has antisocial features and who, in particular, lies. There is no room for a person who cannot be trusted in a residence which operates as a small family-modeled community. All of the community members must be dependable for the program to operate successfully. Time and again, we have had the clinical experience of the referring clinical team not being aware of or fully recognizing this element in a patient's background, to the ultimate detriment of the recipient program — not to mention the patient.

Two additional diagnostic groups deserve some mention. We are currently planning at the McLean Hospital to build a community residence for patients with neuropsychiatric disorders. There is a special need for programs for these patients, who often have secondary neurological deficit from disease (meningitis, brain tumor, etc.) or accident (automobile, motorcycle, skiing, etc.) superimposed upon a personality disorder. Such a program would combine psychiatric counseling to manage the underlying personality disorder and treatment of the psychological consequences of the inflicted secondary deficit. The latter would usually entail mourning the loss of function and the injury to the ego ideal, followed by enlisting the ego's energy in accepting the newly experienced limitations, as well as in making a maximal effort at physical rehabilitation. The program would be physically set up to provide these services.

Women with eating disorders may also need a special residential program. For several reasons these patients, currently being managed in more generic community residences, might be better managed in their own programs. First, when in a generic program, the eating habits of bulimics may be so extreme that other residents experience the bulimics as an intrusion into their space. This is due to the objectionable odor of vomitus in the bathrooms, as well as to finding much of the residence's food supply missing on particular mornings. Second, the problems of the eating disorder patients are so unique, with such a panoply of physical complications, that group support in dealing with this mutual problem is potentially helpful. Anorectic/bulimic patients need weight monitoring, close supervision, and an opportunity to develop warm social relationships, often with a support group of other motivated women, to help bring their disorder under control.

CLINICAL CONDITIONS WARRANTING REFERRAL

Under what conditions should community residential care be considered? First, there are clinical considerations specific to the illness suggesting that successful outcome requires community residential care. These include the illness's severity, its duration, the history of relapse, and the history of previous attempts at discharge to other sites.

An example in regard to severity would be an unrelenting schizophrenic illness. For instance, a patient is still delusional despite pharmacologic and other psychotherapeutic efforts during hospitalization. Such a patient will need to be discharged from the hospital, as there is nothing more than can be done there. However, it may be impossible for a family to provide sufficient supervision at home. A group residence would be the ideal solution. The same argument would hold true for severe manic depressive illness, unipolar depression, or any of the personality disorders.

Clearly, whatever the diagnosis, when a patient has a history of repeated relapse following discharge from the hospital to either the home or other types of independent living, alternative plans for placement into a community residence ought to be considered. Usually a little investigation reveals either a particularly noxious family situation or inadequate structure and supervision at home or in more independent living situations. The isolation of living alone is particularly deadly for most patients with psychiatric illnesses. A community residential placement often goes a long way in preventing breakdown from this kind of isolation.

Other aspects of the patient's life situation, less related to the precise nature of the illness, are often deciding factors leading to community residential referral. These factors include the life phase of the patient (adolescent, adult, or elderly) and the particular family situation (whether the adult is single or divorced or whether there is an intact family home).

For example, an adolescent from a home which itself is so pathological that it is a primary precipitant of disturbed behavior (which may represent a cry for help) may be placed in an adolescent group home especially to afford him or her the opportunity for a more healthy development. A young adult who is recovering from a psychotic episode may need to work at developing the capacity to care for himself away from the family home, as he is at the stage of development where fostering autonomy from the family home is essential. The elderly patient may be widowed, isolated, with a severe depression. This would suggest the possibility of a community residential stay in the post-recovery period; from there longer term planning could be accomplished. Those people who have acute psychiatric illnesses in the face of a recent divorce may have no intact home to which to return. Here again a residential interim stay may give the patient and the treatment team time to plan a better living situation.

We now have the situation, often involving HMOs, where funding for inpatient care is restricted and an alternative must be found to sending the patient home when that is clinically impossible. New, more intensive care group residences may well serve this population.

UNIQUE CLINICAL FEATURES OF COMMUNITY RESIDENTIAL CARE

What is it that community residential care *uniquely* provides for the patient? Community residential care provides a living environment which closely approximates an actual independent living situation in a manner which is likely to allow the replication of the patient's characteristic behavioral patterns. These patterns are subject to early therapeutic intervention because they are observed by a trained staff. Some of these patterns are particularly pathologic and ultimately would result in relapse without intervention. Some have the seeds of strength, which can be developed into rehabilitative gains. Staff members learn, during the evaluation before admission, of previous *precipitants* to relapse. They then help the patient to *avoid* known noxious situations when possible and to carefully *prepare* for such situations when they are unavoidable.

In addition, during the evaluation the early *signs* of impending decompensation are elicited, so that staff members are alert to that eventuality. Examples of this would include a patient suddenly beginning to incessantly smoke and drink large amounts of coffee or a patient who had previously been meticulous, neat, and punctual becoming messy and missing or being late for his or her obligations.

Those of us with experience in this type of care would argue that these subtle changes would most likely either be missed if the patient were only seen in outpatient visits or be discovered so late in the decompensatory course that hospitalization could not be prevented. In the residential care facility the rectifying therapeutic intervention can be made, therefore, much earlier than would otherwise be possible. If the intervention is made before the patient has become so psychotic that he or she is unable to truly collaborate in the endeavor of relapse prevention, this is a new *learning* experience. The patient gains mastery of the situation and the ego is given a chance to deal more effectively with more disruptive, primitive parts of the psyche. All of this represents a powerful therapeutic event which could not otherwise have occurred.

In addition, the community residence has an ideology which is different from that of the hospital, which I have described in detail elsewhere.[2] Residential care, in contrast to the hospital, is conceived of as small, family-modeled, integrated within the community, and an open society. This means, for one thing, that the community of patients is involved in decision-making in the facility — from choosing wallpaper and fabrics in decorating the house, to selecting food preferences, to choosing weekend activities, to having a role in deciding details of house policies. This kind of participation in the life of the house gives the patient an opportunity to prepare for independent living. This is in contrast to hospital practices, which usually keep the patient very remote from decision-making regarding the hospital ward which is the patient's milieu. The residential staff, too, is small, stable, and committed to this philosophy. As in any home, they act as role models for the residents of the facility.

Ideally the milieu fosters a continual process of self-discovery and mastery of the ability to care for oneself. This usually means learning about one's vulnerabilities and strengths, and learning how to balance them to preserve health. This may mean grieving the lost ego ideal and coming to terms with realistic goals. The milieu also believes in the concept of altruism, which in this context means caring about one's fellow house residents. This caring fosters the development of true social relationships, which, in turn, promote the forming of an extended psychosocial kinship system.[3] This social network of patients can help foster mutual caring among friends; we believe this has a profound effect in helping patients to stay well. Patients also note adverse changes in their friends and act upon these observations by either intervening themselves or calling for help.

The community residence stay is long enough for rehabilitative work to occur. It provides the time for working at the newly developed self, time for working through new relationships with the family, time for gaining support while developing new work skills and life skills both within the residence and in the community.

Finally, there is another unique dynamic which sometimes is seen in community residential care. Within the context of the community social setting, the patient often unconsciously repeats characteristic, stereotypic behaviors reflecting family patterns which has distorted his or her life relationships in a very detrimental manner. Commonly these are reactions to both the staff of the community residence, who are experienced as parental figures, and the residents, who are experienced as siblings. Sibling rivalries and jealousies, or raging, distrustful, paranoid attitudes towards parents, or playing one parent against another (often in characteristic sexual patterns), with one idealized and one demeaned—all of these are played out with house managers and residents. On the spot, the staff has a golden opportunity to interpret these reactions—and to illuminate the nature of the distortions. House meetings with fellow residents can be instrumental in clarifying distorted views of a frightened, distrustful, or angry resident.

THE THREE PRIMARY TYPES OF COMMUNITY RESIDENCES

Transitional Halfway House

The high expectation transitional halfway house cares for some of the healthiest patients when judged by their capacity to function in the community. Thus, it requires the resident to have a 30-hour-a-week daily program outside of the house. This requirement is met by competitive or volunteer employment, a school program (usually college, but possibly high school), or participation in a psychiatric day center. That all of the residents comply with this requirement creates an ethos of pride in the milieu. The residents' self-satisfaction in their ability to function in the community creates a spirit of group cohesion which impels new members of the community to sustain this standard of health.

The healthy part of the residents notwithstanding, it is clear that a therapeutic program is needed, for the reader must not forget that these residents may have any one of the diagnoses considered above. The crucial difference here is that the schizophrenia or the manic-depressive illness, the depression or the personality disorder, is not so disabling as to prevent the patient from benefiting from a high expectation program. At the same time, this kind of program is able to provide structure for the manic-depressive, support for the schizophrenic, limit-setting for the borderline personality disorder, and an alliance against suicide with the severely depressed.

Since these patients are all out of the facility during the day at their respective activities, the therapeutic life of the house takes place during the evening hours. We have had a motto, in fact, summarizing the essence of the program: "Day time is for work; evening is for support." The clinical program includes dinner, family-style, each evening. In this informal group setting, a great deal of emotional sharing and support occur as the efforts, successes, and failures of the day are naturally exchanged over the meal.

Another evening program is a weekly house meeting. This is a time for everyone to get together and review issues common to all. In addition, individual problems, where appropriate, may be reviewed so as to enlist group support for a resident going through particularly difficult times. In addition, each resident is seen by a primary clinician once a week in an "administrative interview." The individual interview should include a number of standard areas of inquiry for a population of discharged mentally ill patients: how the patient is feeling; how things are going with other clients in the residence; how things are going with the client's daily activity (job, day program, etc.); how the client is physically, including medication side-effects; how things are with the client's family; how preparations are going for any impending change in the client's life, such as in work, housing, family, or health; how things are going financially; how things are going with any other mental health system member. In effect, the clinician checks the pressure points for stress that could ultimately lead to relapse.

The clinician in the community residence, even the entire clinical team of the residence, may work collaboratively with an outside therapist of a patient to enhance the psychotherapy in several ways. First, clinical data obtained from direct observation in the living situation can be made available to the psychotherapist to fill in his picture of how a patient is seen by others and correct distortions in the patient's self-portrayal. Second, the community residence provides a therapeutic environment which either prevents crises or manages crises if they arise, so that therapy can focus on psychodynamic issues instead of being caught up in the direct management of crises.

The staff of the high expectation community residence is often a live-in person or couple who makes the facility his or her primary domicile. This allows for true role model figures in the facility. It is the degree of health of the clients which permits such a live-in situation without undue burnout or hardship. At the same time, it should be noted that patients can come to the halfway house who are too sick to enter an apartment program with only visiting staff. For many patients the reassurance, availability, and structure offered by live-in staff make all the difference between community survival and return to the hospital. Additional staff members include an executive director of the program who is a clinician and other clinicians or counselors as required by the size of the program. There needs to be a psychiatrist affiliated with the program to handle pharmacologic issues, but other clinicians may be social workers, psychologists, or psychiatric nurses.

The halfway house is located usually off the hospital grounds and is best in an urban situation close to public transportation and near first-level job opportunities, such as fast food restaurants, shops, and stores, etc. The program is often considered to be a transitional facility, rather than a long-term one. The program is best located in a large house with many bedrooms. Size varies according to available housing. Our experience has been very favorable with a program of up to 20 residents in a halfway house. This number allows for development of enough pooled ego strength in the population to foster a strong group process motivated toward positive rehabilitative goals. Other halfway house programs vary in size from 12 to 20 residents.

The Cooperative Apartment

The cooperative apartment provides the most independent residential care situation for the mentally ill. This is because its aim is to provide as much independent living as possible, while at the same time providing support, supervision, and structure, which can make all the difference between successful community tenure and relapse. In this instance the staffing is only one social worker or other clinician supervising each two-family unit. At McLean Hospital we have used two-family homes. The program includes a weekly psychiatric interview as outlined above and two weekly group meetings — one for each separate apartment and one with both apartments meeting together. A 30-hour-per-week program is required outside of the house, exactly as at the halfway house. In this program, however, the residents have to take responsibility for themselves in shopping, cooking, handling utilities, neighbor relations — all of those issues which are entailed in independent living.

The Long-term Group Residence

The long-term group residence is actually a functioning quarterway house. It is designed to care for the most severely impaired patients. Here care is provided for ambulatory schizophrenic patients who have not had a good therapeutic result in spite of all pharmacologic and psychotherapeutic efforts. These patients require round the clock supervision and programming. Some are able to be rehabilitated and eventually move on to a more independent level of residence. Others, even though they may improve in their adaptation in this setting, may need to stay indefinitely. Nevertheless, for these latter patients, there is no question but that prevention of hospitalization is a major accomplishment of this program.

The staffing of this type of program is usually around the clock shifts of counselors, usually two at a time on duty, with a single person awake at night. During the day multi-disciplinary professional staff facilitate the various rehabilitative components required in the program. Included are a psychiatrist, a psychiatric nurse, a social worker, a rehabilitation counselor, and a psychologist. Program components include life skills as well as prevocational skill training. Life skills include all of those involved in daily living — dressing, eating, cleaning, management of money, and those skills needed in the community, such as use of transportation, shopping, banking, and utilization of such community resources as sheltered workshops, libraries, community centers, recreation, and entertainment. Using both work time and leisure time is a focus in community residential care. Our most successful group residence has been a program for 12 residents, living in a large renovated dwelling on the grounds of the psychiatric hospital. Alternatively, large homes near a psychiatric hospital could be used. It is useful to be near a hospital partly because the residents often feel more secure. In addition, they often continue to use various hospital facilities, including psychopharmacologic and rehabilitative services.

A WORD ABOUT COSTS

Our experience has been that costs for these three programs run in multiples of the cost for the cooperative apartment program. The cooperative apartment program costs in 1986 about $25–30 per day; the halfway house program costs about $50–60 per day; and the group residence costs about

$100–120 per day. All of these costs are reflections primarily of the staffing intensity and the size. The cost of the number of full-time-equivalents of staffing plus other significant costs (including rent or amortization of the building, food, utilities, taxes, secretarial and accounting services) divided by the number of residents determines the cost per resident.

CLINICAL CARE IN THE COMMUNITY RESIDENCE

Evaluation at Admission

When the admission of a prospective resident is to be discussed, the clinical team that referred the applicant should be present, along with some representatives of the auxiliary services. Thus, in addition to the community residence staff and the consultant, the applicant's therapist, representatives of the inpatient backup facility, the applicant's social worker, vocational counselor, and representatives of hospitals where the applicant has previously been treated should meet together. Discussion should air any disagreements among the staff involved in prior treatment, as well as differences that may crop up during the meeting between these prior caregivers and residence staff. Critical issues to be reviewed include: history of the prospective resident; the dynamics that contributed to the acute illness; the family's relationship to the applicant; the community residence's approach to the family; the role of continuing psychotherapy; the status of medication; services required to ensure that medication is maintained and monitored; the applicant's physical health; his or her proposed outside daily program and transportation to that program; the history of peer relationships and interpersonal difficulties; arrangement for potential inpatient backup, if necessary; the applicant's special talents, interests, and strengths; and planning for the applicant's transition from the inpatient unit into the community residence.

Experience has shown that, if at all possible, there should be no more than one significant change in the applicant's life at any time in four key areas: residential circumstances, job or other daily program, therapy, and medication. Since changes in these areas create stress, careful support and preparation are necessary in dealing with them. We have tried to have a two-week interval between changes. Otherwise the clinician is often hard pressed to understand the cause of an impending decompensation, rendering it all the more difficult to therapeutically intervene.

The community residence clinical staff, together with the applicant's clinical team, decides whether the applicant is suitable for the program. The conditions that often disqualify an applicant for admission include: poorly controlled destructive impulses toward the self, others, or property; ongoing substance abuse; and sexual promiscuity. The characterological trait of lying habitually also usually disqualifies a candidate.

The Clinical Program

Moving in is the first activity of the new resident. Where possible, moving in gradually is preferable to a sudden move, especially if the patient has become attached to the inpatient milieu he or she is leaving. This allows for adjusting to the new environment and saying goodbye to the old.

We have found that double bedrooms are preferable to singles. It is advantageous for the new resident to live with a roommate. This facilitates socialization and creates a "buddy" system, making the residence a safer place. Roommates, over time, increasingly tend to look after each other's well-being. A resident will come to the house managers if he feels that the roommate is in some secret difficulty. This can range from suicidal feelings, through drug problems and surreptitious avoidance of the daily program, to despondency over a lost lover or friend. Double occupancy, then, provides checks and balances with regard to the house's clinical program and its behavioral codes, helping prevent illicit drinking, sex, drugs, or antisocial behavior.

In the initial clinical phase the primary clinician makes a very strong effort to get to know the resident well and to form a strong therapeutic alliance. Everything else flows from that alliance. In addition, a problem list is developed which identifies the patient's deficiencies and the specific ameliorative therapeutic efforts to be implemented. Depending upon the level of the program, there are life skill development schedules drawn up or outside activity schedules identified. Chores to be done by house residents are reviewed. Administrative interviews are held, and family-style dinners are shared. Subtly, through all of the daily routines, the patient, in contact with fellow residents and with staff, gradually becomes more confident of an emerging self which has grieved over a lost ego ideal and has adjusted to a new notion of what is within realistic reach.

The house meeting can be seen as a paradigm for the entire program. All programs have house meetings. These house meetings can be important therapeutic events in four ways. First, each patient, in spite of his or her shyness or isolation, may learn how to speak about meaningful issues with an entire group. Second, through the feedback the patient gets, it is discovered that he or she is not so strange or his or her problem so unique. He or she is not alone. Third, through the help of housemates, the resident learns both to master the problems themselves and to improve his capacity to relate them effectively. Finally, by listening and relating to others, the resident learns that those who may have seemed unapproachable or hostile were really troubled about matters in which he or she was not involved. Thus, each person's sharing diminishes isolation, enhances self-understanding, and promotes accessibility. Each of these gains for the individual carries a reciprocal gain for the whole group. Openness on both the individual and the group levels facilitates a mutuality, a closeness, a common helping and support, that carries into the milieu, beyond the limits of the house meeting. This effect, too, is reciprocal: Group solidarity and increasing pride in the milieu contribute to a feeling of strength and capacity in the group to do further meaningful work.

Crisis Management

When a resident experiences acrisis, the precipitating event must be identified and explored, along with the reason for the resident's particular vulnerability to the event. Hopefully, through insight into how a present event triggers a past painful experience the resident will master the situation. Alternatively, the resident may have to confront one of the persons allegedly causing the disturbance. If staff intervention does not help the situation, sometimes a small amount of antianxiety or antipsychotic medication, as appropriate, can help. Sometimes a crisis can be alleviated by enlisting the support of a resident's family and significant others in a joint meeting to identify the nature and solutions to the crisis.

If the resident, in spite of these efforts, remains agitated or severely depressed, with suicidal potential requiring continuous attention from staff, inpatient backup for short-term hospitalization may often shorten the duration of the disturbance. Whenever possible, such action should be taken with the cooperation of the resident and with the explicit understanding that the bed at the community residence will remain available for immediate return upon the resolution of the crisis.

Leaving the Community Residence

Ideally, the resident should depart to a living situation within the context of a social network. This network should be drawn from a postresidence program with several features. Ex-residents should move into a living arrangement with known others; they should not live alone. They should have a daily program of familiar activities. They should maintain a therapeutic relationship with a significant clinician whom they trust and to whom they can turn in time of trouble. Their medication should be stabilized and provisions should be made for medical monitoring where appropriate. There should also be some stabilization of the ex-resident's relationship with the family of origin, so that old pathological patterns will not reemerge without some provision for checking them and preventing relapse. Finally, a continuing relationship with the community residence through an ex-resident program and personal ties to the house is desirable. In sum, the program of the resident who is moving out should be intact and stable.

REFERENCES

1. Tuke S: Description of the Retreat. London, Dawsons of Pall Mall, 1964
2. Budson RD: The Psychiatric Halfway House: A Handbook of Theory and Practice. Pittsburgh, University of Pittsburgh Press, 1978
3. Budson RD, Jolley RE: A crucial factor in community program success: the extended psychosocial kinship system. Schizophrenia Bull 1978; 4:609-621
4. Budson RD: Community residential care for the mentally ill in Massachusetts: halfway house and cooperative apartments, in New Directions in Mental Health Care: Cooperative Apartments. Monograph. Edited by Goldmeier J, Mannino FV, Shore MF, NIMH Study Center, DHEW Pub No (ADM) 78-685. Adelphi, Md: 1978
5. Budson RD: Challenging themes in community residential care systems, in New Directions for Mental Health Services: Issues in Community Residential Care, no. 11. Edited by Budson R, San Francisco, Jossey-Bass, 1981
6. Wechsler H: Halfway houses for former mental patients: a survey. J Social Issues 1960; 16:20-26
7. Landy D, Greenblatt M: Halfway House. US Dept of Health, Education, and Welfare, Vocational Rehabilitation Administration, Washington, DC, 1965
8. National Institute of Mental Health: Reference Data on Halfway Houses for the Mentally Ill and Alcoholics, United States. Washington DC: Superintendent of Documents, US Govt Prtg Office, 1973
9. Rothwell ND, Doniger JM: The Psychiatric Halfway House: A Case Study. Springfield, Ill, Charles Thomas, 1966
10. Raush HL, Raush CL: The Halfway House Movement: A Search for Sanity. New York, Appleton-Century Crofts, 1968
11. Glasscote RM, Gudeman JE, Elpers JR: Halfway Houses for the Mentally Ill. Washington, DC, Joint Information Service of the APA and NAMH, 1971
12. Goldmeir J, Mannino FV, Shore MF (Editors): New Directions in Mental Health Care: Cooperative Apartments. Monograph, NIMH, DHEW Pub No (ADM) 78-685, Adelphi, MD, 1978
13. Sandall H, Hawley T, Gordon GL: The St. Louis homes. Am J Psychiatry 1975; 32:617-622
14. Chien C, Cole JO: Landlord supervised cooperative apartments: a new modality for community based treatment. Am J Psychiatry 1973; 130:156-159
15. Arce AA, Vergare MJ, Adams RS, Lazarus L: A Typology of Community Residential Services, Washington, DC, American Psychiatric Association, 1982
16. Mannino FV, Ott S, Shore MF: Community residential facilities for former mental patients: an annotated bibliography. Psychosoc Rehab J 1977; 1:1-43
17. Fairweather GW, Sanders DH, Maynard H: Community Life for the Mentally Ill: An Alternative to Industrial Care. Chicago, Aldine, 1969
18. McDonald L, Gregory GW: The Fort Logan Lodge: International Community for Chronic Mental Patients NIMH Final Report. Grant No. 1 R01 MH1 5853-02, Rockville, MD, NIMH, 1971
19. Anthony WA: Efficacy of Psychiatric Rehabilitation. Psychol Bull 1972; 78:447-456
20. Huessy HR: Spring Lake Ranch — The pioneer halfway house in Mental Health with Limited Resources, Edited by Huessy HR, New York, Grune & Stratton, 1966
21. Wechsler H: Transitional residences for former mental patients: a survey of halfway houses and rehabilitation facilities. Mental Hyg 1961; 45:65-67
22. Murphy HBM, Engelsmann F, Tcheng-Laroch F: The influence of foster home care on psychiatric patients. Arch Gen Psychiatry 1976; 33:179-183
23. Goldmeir J: Community residential facilities for former mental patients: a review. Psychosoc Rehab J 1977; 1:1-45
24. Linn MW: Can Foster Care Survive? in New Directions for Mental Health Services: Issues in Community Residential Care, no. 11. Edited by Budson R, San Francisco, Jossey-Bass, 1981
25. Lamb HR: Maximizing the potential of board and care homes, in New Directions for

Mental Health Services: Issues in Community Residential Care. no. 11. Edited by Budson R, San Francisco: Jossey-Bass, 1981
26. Lamb HR: Board and care home wanderers. Arch Gen Psychiatry 1980; 37:135–137
27. Shadoan RA: Making board and care homes more therapeutic, in Community Survival for Long Term Patients. Edited by Lamb HR, et al, San Francisco, Jossey-Bass, 1976
28. Tunaka B, Shaefer I: The community boarding house as a traditional residence during aftercare. Curr Psychiatr Ther 1965; 2:235–239
29. Vaughn CE, Leff JP: Patterns of emotional response in relatives of schizophrenic patients. Schiz Bull 1981; 7:43–44
30. Wing JK: The Social Context of Schizophrenia. Am J Psychiatry 1978; 135:1333–1339

Index

accreditation, hospital, 9, 13, 32, 34, 66–67, 253, 255
activity therapies, 170, 179–207, 216, 217, 222, 233, 237
   assessment in, 182–88
   benefits of hospitalization and, 181–82
   case histories of, 184–88, 201–5
   children and adolescents and, 301, 317
   creative art therapies in, 196–97
   economic trends and, 205–6
   future of, 205–6
   geriatric treatment and, 206, 330–31
   group therapy in, 192–95
   history of, 179–81
   insurance and, 181–82, 205
   knowledge base of, 205
   modalities of, 196–204
   occupational therapy in, 197–98, 330–31
   population trends and, 206
   recreation therapy in, 198–99
   staff role in, 190–92
   therapeutic value of, 189–90
   treatment assumptions in, 188–89
   treatment planning in, 182–88
   vocational planning in, 199–201
   work therapy in, 199–201
Adler, Wolfe N., 109–28
admissions process, 88–95
   AMA discharges and, 89
   certificates of need in, 92
   children and adolescents in, 303–5
   families in, 89–90
   forensic hospitals and, 60
   forensic issues in, 93
   general hospitals and, 43, 45, 46
   informed consent in, 93
   institutional transfers in, 93–94
   insurance in, 91, 92–93
   patient acceptance criteria in, 91–92
   patients' anxieties about, 88, 89, 90
   patients' economic status and, 92–93
   patients' rights in, 93
   private hospitals and, 14, 17
   public hospitals and, 29
   reasons for admission in, 14, 88, 181
   smoothness of, 89
   three-day notices in, 90, 272, 380–81
   see also emergency rooms, psychiatric; involuntary commitment
adolescents, *see* children and adolescents, treatment of
affective disorders, 14, 18–19, 272, 359
   diagnostic process and, 102–3
   discharge planning and, 379–80
   geriatric treatment of, 322–24, 328
   psychopharmacology in, 165, 169, 171, 172, 174–75, 176, 379–80
   residential aftercare and, 390
   suicide and, 292, 293–94, 380
aftercare, *see* discharge planning; residential aftercare
age grouping, inpatient, 9, 17, 43, 260, 300–301, 308, 384
Aichhorn, A., 302
AIDS (acquired immune deficiency syndrome), 344–45
Alcoholics Anonymous, 133, 378, 390–91
alcoholism, 9, 30, 106, 177, 259, 272, 378, 390–91
ALI (American Law Institute), 54
Alzheimer's disease, 324, 326
Alzheimer's Disease and Related Disorders Association, 331
AMA (against medical advice) discharges, 16, 89, 272, 278–79, 380–81
American Academy of Psychiatry and the Law, 68
American Bar Association, 50, 273

American Bar Association (*continued*)
  Commission on the Mentally Disabled of, 55
American Board of Psychiatry and Neurology, 128
American Journal of Insanity, 4
American Journal of Psychiatry, 4
American Law Institute (ALI), 54
American Nurses' Association, 211, 212, 298
American Psychiatric Association (APA), 4, 27, 255, 259, 268, 269, 285
  CHAMPUS Peer Review Program of, 253, 256, 259
  National Advisory Committee of, 256
  Task Force on Psychiatric Aspects of Restraint and Seclusion, 298
American Psychological Association, 256
Anderson, C. M., 361
anorexia nervosa, *see* eating disorders
antisocial personality disorder, 9, 14, 46, 391
anxiety disorders, 146, 155–56, 164–65
Appleton, W. S., 173
assertiveness training, 146–47
attitude therapy, 209–10
Auburn State Lunatic Asylum for Insane Convicts, 50
Auger, N., 17
autism, 162, 163

Bachrach, L. L., 35
Bach-Y-Rita, G., 295
Bandura, Albert, 138
Barter, James T., 22–38
Bassuk, E., 88
Baxstrom v. Herold, 50
Beck, Aaron, 138, 143
Beck Depression Inventory, 140, 141
Bedlam, 48, 51
Beeson, 368
behavior therapy, 137–38, 285
Behavior Therapy and Beyond (Lazarus), 138
Bellevue Hospital, 300
Belmont Hospital (England), 111
Bettelheim, B., 302
Bleuler, Eugen, 228
Bloomingdale Asylum (New York Hospital), 4
Blue Cross, 181–82, 253–54, 255, 256, 259, 260–65, 269
  Federal Employees Program (FEP) of, 255, 258
Blue Shield, 259
board-and-care homes, 368, 375, 388
Bond, T. C., 17
borderline personality disorder, 9, 19, 177, 272, 345–46
  activity therapies and, 181, 201–3

cognitive behavior therapy and, 148, 158–61
discharge planning and, 378–79
general hospitals and, 46
milieu therapy and, 117, 126
psychotherapy of, 131–32
residential aftercare and, 390
Boronow, John J., 228–50
Bradley Hospital, 300
Bridgewater State Hospital, 50
Brigham, Amariah, 4
Brody, M., 15–16
Brooks, Ann Marie T., 208–27
Bucher, B., 163
Budson, Richard D., 384–402
bulimia, *see* eating disorders
Bunce, D. F., 342
Burlingame, C. Charles, 5
burnout, staff, 86–87, 94, 308
Burns, David, 161
Butler Hospital, 4

California, 26, 27, 292, 368
Canada, 388
capitation, 7, 28, 269, 385
Carpenter, W. T., Jr., 173, 231
catastrophic insurance, 20
CHAMPUS, 253, 256, 258, 259
character disorders, 6, 17, 19, 46
Charcot, Jean-Martin, 228
Chestnut Lodge, 5, 8, 15, 18
children and adolescents, treatment of, 17, 79, 102–3, 259, 260, 300–321, 343, 392
  activity therapies in, 301, 317
  admission criteria in, 303–4
  admissions process in, 303–5
  age grouping in, 17, 43, 308
  aggression management in, 307, 317–18
  assessment/evaluation in, 309–11, 318–19
  behavior problems in, 319–20
  cognitive behavior therapy in, 162–63
  diagnostic grouping in, 308–9
  diagnostic process and, 102–3
  discharge planning in, 320–21, 381
  families in, 301, 310–11, 314–15
  general hospitals and, 43, 46
  length of stay in, 17, 301–2
  level system in, 315–16
  locked vs. open system in, 307–8
  milieu therapy in, 127, 301, 302, 312–13
  nurses in, 212, 312
  overview of, 301–2
  physical environment in, 17, 216, 306–8
  post-discharge aftercare in, 320–21
  preadmission interview in, 304–5
  private hospitals and, 9, 17, 19
  process of, 311–20

Index   405

psychopharmacology in, 172, 176-77, 316
psychotherapy in, 301, 313-15
psychotic children and, 162-63
reevaluation in, 318-19
regression at discharge in, 321
residential centers in, 302, 303
school in, 301, 316, 320-21
sex grouping in, 308
staffing in, 302-3
team approach in, 311-12
chronic mentally ill, inpatient care of, 6, 8, 18-19, 45, 80, 206, 352-70
   assessment/evaluation in, 357, 359-60
   behavioral problems and, 358, 366
   cognitive behavior therapy in, 147, 355-56
   contraindicated admissions in, 359
   detoxification in, 358-59
   discharge planning in, 363-65, 377-78
   families and, 361-62
   future of, 368-69
   history of, 352-54
   length of stay studies of, 355-57
   literature on, 354-55
   long-term, 366-67
   need for asylum in, 35, 367-68
   psychoeducation and, 361-62
   psychopharmacology in, 357-58, 360
   psychotherapy in, 360-61
   public hospitals and, 30, 35
   reasons for admission in, 357-59
   research on, 26, 229, 241
   respite care in, 359
   social rehabilitation of, 358, 362, 363, 364, 366
   transference crises in, 358
   treatment availability in, 358, 366
   treatment in, 359-63
   treatment planning in, 358
   unremitting symptoms in, 366-67
   vocational rehabilitation in, 362-63, 364-65
Clifton T. Perkins Hospital Center, 49, 51, 55, 59-60, 63, 65
cognitive behavior therapy, inpatient, 136-68, 285, 295, 355-56
   anxiety disorders and, 146, 155-56, 164-65
   assertiveness training in, 146-47
   assessment in, 139-45
   behavior therapy and, 137-38, 285
   borderline personality disorder and, 148, 158-61
   chronic mentally ill and, 147, 355-56
   clinical application of, 149-63
   cognitive therapy and, 138
   contingency contracting in, 148
   contingency management in, 147-48
   definition of, 137-39

eating disorders and, 146, 156-58
environmental control in, 137
flooding in, 137, 146
imitation learning therapy in, 147
initial target behaviors in, 145
mental health professionals and, 163-64
microcomputers in, 141-43, 162
modeling therapy in, 147
obsessive-compulsive disorders and, 146, 155-56
operant conditioning in, 147, 154
organic mental disorders and, 161-62
origin of, 138-39
patient and staff acceptance of, 166-68
prolonged exposure in, 137, 146
psychodynamic therapies and, 165, 166, 168
psychopharmacology and, 164-65
psychotic children and, 162-63
reinforcer identification in, 143-44
response prevention in, 137, 146
schizophrenia and, 149-55
self-assessment and monitoring in, 144-45
social skills training in, 147
symptom substitution and, 165-66
systematic desensitization in, 145-46
techniques of, 145-48
therapeutic effects of assessment in, 144
therapeutic self-instruction in, 148
token economy in, 128, 136, 137, 143, 147, 148, 152, 237, 354
community hospitals, 39, 44-45
community mental health movement, 6, 22, 23, 24, 29, 33, 34, 353
community residences, *see* residential aftercare
Community Support Programs (CSPs), 365
competency to stand trial, 48, 52-53, 60, 62
confidentiality, 16, 18, 61, 75, 252, 266-67, 285-88, 354
   forensic issues and, 271, 280, 285-88
   insurance and, 267, 286
   medical records and, 257, 266, 267, 285-86
   research units and, 242, 247
Conn, L. M., 294
contingency contracting, 148
contingency management, 147-48
cooperative apartments, in aftercare, 387-88, 389, 396-97
cost containment, 7, 17, 136, 205-6, 224, 251-56, 259, 265, 266, 268, 269
county hospitals, *see* public hospitals
court-ordered patients, 280-81
   see also forensic hospitals
creative art therapies, 196-97
criminal responsibility, 48, 52, 53, 62
Cutler, L. D., 364

dangerousness, patient, 14, 63, 64, 88, 91, 93, 272, 273, 275, 279, 380
Dannemora State Hospital, 50
Dawkins, J. E., 226
day hospitals, 16, 18, 19, 128
Defense Department, U.S., 256
deinstitutionalization, 6, 25, 29, 30–31, 45, 67, 73, 80, 93, 136, 181, 206, 258, 269, 354, 361
delirium, 322, 323, 328
dementia, 322, 324–25, 328
Description of the Retreat (Tuke), 386
diagnostic grouping, inpatient, 9, 43, 126–27, 260, 308–9, 384, 389–91
diagnostic process, 99–108, 170, 335
  adolescents and, 102–3
  affective disorders and, 102–3
  diagnostic labeling in, 106–7
  differential diagnosis in, 322–23
  "DRG creep" in, 100
  drug dependency in, 106
  DSM-III in, 99
  families in, 103–4, 347
  geriatric treatment and, 322–23
  medically ill patients and, 105–6, 335–36, 342, 347–49
  reevaluations in, 100–103, 239
  rehospitalizations and, 100–101
  staff observations in, 104–5
Diagnostic Related Groups (DRGs), 7, 29, 100, 136, 267–69
Dickerson, Faith B., 373–83
discharge planning, 45, 269, 373–83
  acute vs. chronic patients in, 377–78
  administrative discharges and, 381–82
  AMA (against medical advice) discharges in, 16, 89, 272, 278–79, 380–81
  children and adolescents and, 320–21, 381
  chronic mentally ill and, 363–65, 377–78
  court-ordered patients in, 280–81
  diagnostic groups in, 378–80
  discharge categories in, 380–82
  elopement and, 279–80
  families in, 376, 377
  forensic hospitals and, 55–56, 64–65
  forensic issues in, 278–81, 283
  geriatric treatment and, 331
  living arrangements in, 374–76
  patient "contract to stay" and, 272
  private hospitals and, 15–16, 19
  psychopharmacology in, 176, 374, 379
  psychosocial stressors in, 376–77
  psychotherapy in, 373–74
  readiness for discharge in, 380
  regression at discharge in, 382
  risk/benefit notes in, 278
  separation difficulties and, 382–83
  structured daily programs in, 374
  Tarasoff considerations in, 288
  three-day notices in, 90, 272, 380–81
  transfers in, 381
Dix, Dorothea, 353
Docherty, John P., 231
DRGs (Diagnostic Related Groups), 7, 29, 100, 136, 267–69
drug-free periods, 173, 238–40, 246
DSM-III, 99, 286, 302, 360, 376, 377–78
DSM-III-R, 124
Dunton, William Rush, 180

eating disorders, 9, 43, 215–16, 260, 345–46, 348–49
  activity therapies and, 184–88
  cognitive behavior therapy and, 146, 156–58
  milieu therapy and, 126
  physical symptoms of, 348
  residential aftercare in, 391
Edelstein, Michael, 334–51
Ekblom, B., 298
elderly, treatment of, *see* geriatric treatment, inpatient
electroconvulsive treatment (ECT), 24, 255, 282, 283, 284, 326
Ellis, Albert, 138, 143, 160
elopement, patient, 279–80
emergency procedures, forensic, 275, 283
emergency rooms, psychiatric, 73–87, 94
  ambulances and, 84
  burnout and, 86–87
  crisis intervention in, 81–82
  dispositions in, 82–83
  evaluations in, 76
  families and, 82
  hospitalizing patients and, 82–83
  interview rooms in, 74
  involuntary commitment and, 83
  medical equipment in, 76
  patient "dumping" in, 77–78
  patient populations of, 77, 78, 79–81
  psychopharmacology in, 76
  referrals to, 77–78, 80
  repeater patients in, 80
  restraints in, 74, 75–76
  seclusion rooms in, 74
  security in, 79
  staffing of, 77–79
  stresses unique to practice in, 85–86
  structural requirements of, 74–76
  team approach in, 78–79
  transportation and, 84
  violence in, 74–75, 77, 83
Endicott, J., 18, 355

Index

enforced treatment, 283-84
expert witnesses, 49, 53, 54
Extein, I., 9-10

Fairweather, G. W., 388
Falloon, I. R. H., 361
families, patient, 16, 23, 82, 167, 218
   admissions process and, 89-90
   children and adolescents and, 301, 310-11, 314-15
   chronic mentally ill and, 361-62
   diagnostic process and, 103-4, 347
   discharge planning and, 376, 377
   forensic issues and, 272, 273, 289
   geriatric treatment and, 322, 323, 327
   psychopharmacology and, 175-76
   research units and, 241, 243
   residential aftercare and, 389, 400
family therapy, 63-64, 301, 314-15, 361-62
Farview State Hospital, 50
Fear Survey Schedule, 140, 141
fee-for-service treatment, 28, 182
Feeling Good (Burns), 161
Feigelson, E., 88
feminism, 210-11
flooding technique, 137, 146
Fogel, B. S., 44
Folstein, Marshal F., 322-33
Ford, 368
Ford v. Wainwright, 67
forensic hospitals, 48-69
   admissions process in, 60
   architecture and milieu of, 56-60
   competency to stand trial and, 48, 52-53, 60, 62
   conditional release in, 55-56
   criminal responsibility and, 48, 52, 53, 62
   custody exchange in, 60-61
   dangerousness and, 63, 64
   death penalty and, 67
   discharge planning in, 55-56, 64-65
   domain of, 48
   emergency evacuation in, 66
   etymology of, 48
   evaluation in, 51-55, 61-62, 66
   expert witnesses and, 49, 53, 54
   future trends in, 66-68
   governance of, 49
   history of, 50-51
   insanity tests and, 54
   internal disturbances control in, 65-66
   malingering in, 52
   malpractice litigation and, 48, 67
   mission of, 51-56, 66
   patients' rights in, 64, 67
   patient transportation and, 65
   programming in, 60-66
   referrals to, 49, 60
   regulation of, 49, 63, 67
   residential aftercare and, 55
   restraints in, 58, 61, 65
   sally ports of, 57-58, 59, 61
   security in, 57-60, 63, 64
   treatment in, 55, 58, 62-64, 66
   typical admissions to, 49
   uniqueness of, 49
   violence and, 64-65, 292
   ward environments in, 59-60
   weapons in, 58, 65
forensic issues, 93, 271-90, 291, 292
   AMA discharges in, 272, 278-79
   attorneys and, 274, 280, 282, 289, 350
   colleague reviews in, 289
   commitment hearings in, 275-77
   confidentiality in, 271, 280, 285-88
   court-ordered patients in, 280-81
   dangerousness in, 272, 273, 275, 279
   discharge planning in, 278-81, 283
   elopement in, 279-80
   emergency procedures in, 275, 283
   enforced treatment in, 283-84
   First Amendment in, 282-83
   incident report in, 288-89
   involuntary commitment in, 272, 273-77, 283, 289
   malpractice prevention in, 271, 288-89
   medically ill patients and, 345, 350
   medical records in, 279, 280, 281, 283, 285-86
   parens patriae concept in, 273, 274
   patient rights in, 271, 281-87
   police power concept in, 273
   privileged communication in, 286-87
   restraints in, 271, 285
   right to refuse treatment in, 17, 64, 271, 282-85, 350
   right to treatment in, 17, 271, 281-82
   risk/benefit notes in, 278
   risk management in, 289
   seclusion in, 271, 285
   staff rights in, 271
   Tarasoff case (duty to warn) in, 79, 287-88
   violence in, 272, 273, 275, 279, 291
   voluntary hospitalization in, 271-72, 283
for-profit hospital chains, 7, 11, 19
foster care, residential, 388
Fountain House, 365
Franklin School, 300
Freed, H., 291
Freud, Sigmund, 56
Friends Hospital, 4
Fromm-Reichmann, Frieda, 5

Gelpi, Jose A., 48-69
general hospitals, psychiatric units of, 10, 14,
    39-47, 267, 268, 287, 353
  acute intervention in, 46-47
  admissions process in, 43, 45, 46
  adolescents in, 43, 46
  age grouping in, 43
  characteristics of, 40-42
  common problems of, 45-47
  community hospitals and, 39, 44-45
  deinstitutionalization and, 45
  discharge planning in, 45
  history of, 39
  insurance and, 40-41, 45
  length of stay in, 44, 45-46
  liaison problems in, 41
  medical-psychiatric units in, 43-44
  nurses in, 41, 44, 45
  patient population of, 40, 43
  shift of care to, 39
  specialized, 42-44
  staff conflicts and, 41-42
  training programs in, 40
geriatric treatment, inpatient, 6, 30-31, 35,
    43, 322-33, 346-47
  activity therapies in, 206, 330-31
  affective disorders in, 322-24, 328
  Alzheimer's disease in, 324, 326
  behavior problems and, 328-30
  combativeness and, 329
  community facilities and, 331
  delirium in, 322, 323, 328
  dementia in, 322, 324-25, 328
  demographic effects in, 322
  differential diagnosis in, 322-23
  discharge planning in, 331
  ECT in, 326
  falls and, 329
  families and, 322, 323, 327
  Geri-chairs in, 329
  management techniques in, 328
  milieu therapy in, 127, 331
  nurses in, 327-28
  private hospitals and, 9, 16
  psychopharmacology in, 169, 175, 177,
    324-26
  psychotherapy in, 326-27
  public hospitals and, 30-31, 35
  setting design in, 331-32
  sleep disturbances and, 329-30
  strokes in, 324
  suicide and, 323-24
  team approach in, 327-28, 331
  wandering and, 329, 331, 332
Geri-chairs, 329
Gerson, S., 88

Gibson, Colleen, 322
Gibson, Diane, 179-207
Gibson, Robert W., 251-70
Glick, Ira D., 18, 192, 352-70
Gold, M. S., 9-10
Gould, E., 192
Gould Farm, 388
Gralnick, A., 8
Greenblatt, M., 34
Grob, G. N., 4
group residences, *see* residential aftercare
group therapies, 15, 29, 45, 63, 119, 120,
    126, 161, 192-95, 255, 313-14, 360
Guide to Rational Living (Ellis and Harper),
    161
Gunderson, J. G., 118, 354
Gutheil, T. G., 298

halfway houses, transitional, 387, 389, 394-96
Hall, R. C. W., 10
Hargreaves, W. A., 355, 356
Harper, R., 161
Harsch, H. H., 338
Hartford Retreat, 4, 5
Hartlage, L. C., 91
Hartmann, Peter, 334-51
health maintenance organizations (HMOs),
    19, 269, 385, 392
Hegyvary, S., 223
Hemphill, B. J., 205
Herz, M. I., 18, 355-56
Hoge, S. K., 298
Holmes, W., 89
hospitals, mental, 1-79
  accreditation of, 9, 13, 32, 34, 66-67, 253,
    255
  age grouping in, 9, 17, 43, 260, 300-301, 308
  cost containment and, 7, 17, 205-6, 224,
    251-56, 259, 265, 266, 268, 269
  court-ordered patients in, 280-81
  diagnostic grouping in, 9, 43, 126-27, 260,
    308-9
  DRGs and, 267-68
  influence of insurance on, 215, 255-56,
    258-65, 267-70
  locked vs. open systems in, 216, 307-8, 353
  outcome studies of, 18-20, 252
  patient/staff ratios in, 282
  prospective pricing systems and, 267-69
  regulation of, *see* regulation, governmental
  right to treatment and, 281-82
  risk management in, 289
  safety standards in, 252, 253
  specialized services in, 8-9, 17, 42-44,
    126-27, 260, 300-301, 308-9
  utilization review criteria for, 254

Index

illness education, 120–21, 212, 215, 361–62
imitation learning therapy, 147
incident reports, hospital, 288–89
infectious diseases, 343–45
informed consent, 93, 120, 230, 240–44, 247, 284, 345
insanity tests, 54
Institute of Living, 5, 10, 14, 17
Institutional Review Board (IRB), 230, 240, 243
insulin coma therapy, 24, 255
insurance, health care, 19, 215, 239, 251–70, 300, 385
   activity therapies and, 181–82, 205
   admissions process and, 91, 92–93
   arbitrary limits in, 255–56, 258
   capitation in, 7, 28, 269, 385
   catastrophic, 20
   claims denials in, 255, 257, 259
   claims review in, 255, 258–60
   confidentiality and, 267, 286
   cost containment and, 251–56, 259, 265, 266, 268, 269
   fee-for-service treatment in, 28, 182
   future of, 269–70
   general hospitals and, 40–41, 45
   influence on hospitals of, 215, 255–56, 258–65, 267–70
   length of stay and, 181, 258, 260, 266–67, 269
   managed care in, 258, 265–67
   Maryland experience in, 260–65, 268
   medical records and, 256–58, 261–66
   milieu therapy and, 127, 255
   on-site vs. off-site review and, 265–66
   patient stress and, 266
   peer review in, 13, 254–55, 256, 261, 265
   preadmission requirements of, 266–67
   private hospitals and, 6–8, 13, 18, 19
   prospective pricing systems and, 267–69
   public hospitals and, 28, 29
   quality assurance and, 13, 255–58, 268
   retrospective review and, 261
   specific treatment modalities and, 259
   utilization review in, 251–55, 258, 259, 264, 268
Interpersonal Relations in Nursing (Peplau), 209
in-vivo procedures, 140, 146, 228, 358
involuntary commitment, 17, 34, 46, 52, 83, 91, 93, 244
   forensic issue of, 272, 273–77, 283, 289

Joint Commission on Accreditation of Hospitals (JCAH), 9, 13, 66–67, 253, 255
Joint Commission on Mental Health, 300

Jones, Maxwell, 6, 111
Jung, Carl G., 228

Kayton, L., 291
Kings Park Hospital, 300
Kirkbride, Thomas, 4
Krieger, G., 292

Labor Department, U.S., 200
Langley Porter Hospital, 18
laxative abuse, 348
Lazarus, Arnold F., 138, 141
least restrictive environment, concept of, 136
LeBow, M. D., 15
Leehey, K., 33–34
Leff, J. P., 389
legal insanity, 48, 52, 53, 62
Lentz, R. J., 128, 354
Leopold, Bruce, 99–108
level system, 121–23, 315–16
Levenson, A., 7
Levine, I., 15
L-facilities, 368
Lindsley, O. R., 137
Lion, John R., 99–108, 169–78, 218, 291–99
Lovaas, O., 163

McGee, James, 136–68
McGlashan, T. H., 18
McHugh, Paul, 322*n*
McLean Hospital, 4, 208, 391, 396
McNamara, Mary Eileen, 73–87
Macro Systems, 268
Main, T. F., 6
malingering, 52
malpractice litigation, 34, 48, 67
   prevention of, 271, 288–89
managed care, 258, 265–67
Marshall, Patricia A., 22–38
Maryland, 241, 260–65, 268, 275, 283–84, 298
Maryland Foundation for Health Care, 254
Massachusetts, 281, 282
Mattes, J. A., 355, 356
maximum security institutions, 57–59, 63, 64
Maxmen, J. S., 10, 15
May, P. R. A., 354
Medicaid, 24, 28, 253–54, 268, 354
Medical College of Wisconsin, 338–39
medically ill psychiatric patients, 10, 334–51
   continuity of care problems in, 339–40
   diagnostic evaluation of, 105–6, 335–36, 342, 347–49
   dual-trained physicians and, 338
   forensic issues and, 345, 350
   geriatric, 346–47
   incidence of, 345

medically ill psychiatric patients (*continued*)
  infectious diseases in, 343–45
  intimate examinations of, 343
  laxative abuse by, 348
  medical-psychiatric units and, 43–44, 338–39
  medical vs. psychiatric facilities and, 339–43
  medical vs. psychiatric staffs and, 334–35, 337
  misdiagnosis of, 342
  ongoing medical management of, 341–42
  psychogenic illness in, 343
  self-induced injury in, 335–37, 345–46
  staff discussions of, 344
  suicide attempts in, 337
  therapists as primary physicians to, 343
  transfers of, 339–41
medical-psychiatric units, hospital, 43–44, 338–39
medical records, 13, 18, 252, 256–58
  confidentiality and, 257, 266, 267, 285–86
  forensic issues and, 279, 280, 281, 283, 285–86
  insurance review of, 256–58, 261–66
  quality assurance and, 256–58
  suicide and, 292
  working notes vs., 286
Medicare, 9, 16, 24, 28, 92, 181–82, 253–54, 261, 265, 267, 268–69, 354
medication, *see* psychopharmacology
Menninger, Karl and William, 4–5
Menninger Foundation, 4–5, 16, 209, 216
Mental and Physical Disability Law Reporter, 55
Meyer, 228
Mezzich, J. E., 14
microcomputers, 141–43, 162
milieu therapy, 45, 109–28, 268, 339, 373
  aggression management in, 112
  children and adolescents and, 127, 301, 302, 312–13
  chronic mentally ill and, 355, 361
  cognitive behavior therapy and, 167, 168
  community meetings in, 111, 125–26
  diagnostic grouping in, 126–27
  functions of, 112–21
  future of, 127–28
  geriatric treatment and, 127, 331
  insight in, 119–20
  insulation and asylum in, 112–13
  insurance and, 127, 255
  involvement in, 118, 121
  level system in, 121–23, 315–16
  medical milieu model in, 109–10, 112
  milieu characteristics in, 127
  nurses in, 210, 214–18
  patient-role induction in, 114–15
  private hospitals and, 6, 15
  problem-solving in, 113, 118–19, 126
  psychoeducation in, 120–21, 212, 215
  psychosocial milieu model in, 110–12
  public hospitals and, 24–25, 29
  research units and, 235, 237, 240, 245–48
  social reintegration in, 113–14
  specialized vs. general programs in, 126–27
  structure in, 115–16, 121
  support in, 116–18, 121
  training programs in, 128
  treatment teams in, 123–25
Mini-Mental State Exam, 323
Misiaszek, J., 33–34
M'Naghten insanity test, 54
modeling therapy, 147
Moos, Rudolph, 127
moral treatment, concept of, 3, 9, 18, 24, 179, 386
Mosher, L. R., 19, 354
municipal hospitals, *see* public hospitals
Murphy, H. B. M., 388

Narcotics Anonymous, 378
National Alliance for the Mentally Ill (NAMI), 16, 28, 92, 362
National Association of Private Psychiatric Hospitals (NAPPH), 7, 17, 269, 302
National Association of Psychiatric Hospitals, 268
National Institute of Mental Health (NIMH), 229, 235, 236, 237, 240, 243, 268, 365, 387
  Division of Biometry, 31
National Mental Health Act, 209
neuropsychiatric disorders, 391
New York, 50
New York State Hospital Association Task Force, 252
nurses, psychiatric, 110, 208–27, 264, 265, 312
  attitude therapy in, 209–10
  clinical role of, 218–23
  cognitive behavior therapy and, 163–64
  contemporary perspective on, 210–12
  cost containment and, 224
  definition of, 212
  essential elements of care by, 223
  feminism and, 210–11
  forensic, 68
  future of, 226
  general hospitals and, 41, 44, 45
  geriatric treatment and, 327–28
  history of, 208–10
  milieu management by, 210, 214–18
  nursing practice/staffing models and, 223–24

Index

paraprofessionals and, 224–25
psychopharmacology and, 210, 215
public hospitals and, 32
recruitment of, 211–12
research units and, 234–35, 239, 246
role in 1980s of, 212–13
role stress of, 226
staff development of, 225–26
standards of, 212
suicide and, 219, 292, 293
training of, 209, 210, 211
treatment and, 219–20
treatment teams and, 217, 218
violence and, 218, 298
nursing homes, 6, 30–31, 35, 44, 206, 331, 354, 387

obsessive-compulsive disorders, 146, 155–56
occupational therapy, 197–98, 330–31
Okin, R. L., 35–36
Olin, G. B., 93
Olin, H. S., 93
operant conditioning, 147, 154
Oregon, 65
organic mental disorders, 161–62, 295, 359
O'Sullivan, A. O., 15–16

PADs (protective aggression devices), 174
paraprofessionals, psychiatric, 32, 224–25
parens patriae, 273, 274
patients' rights, 17–18, 34, 67, 93, 136, 252, 267, 281–87, 354
  confidentiality in, *see* confidentiality
  emergency procedures in, 275, 283
  enforced treatment and, 283–84
  restraints in, 271, 285
  right to refuse treatment in, 17, 64, 271, 282–85, 350
  right to treatment in, 17, 271, 281–82
  seclusion in, 271, 285
  Wyatt v. Stickney and, 25, 281, 282
Paul, G. L., 128, 354
Payne Whitney Clinic (New York Hospital), 236
peer review, 13, 254–55, 256, 261, 265
Peer Review Improvement Act, 254
Penna, Manoel, 39–47
Pennsylvania Hospital, 4
Peplau, H., 209
Peters, Charles P., 373–83
Phipps Clinic, 228
phobic disorders, 9, 145–46, 155–56
Pinel, Philippe, 3, 228
police power, of state, 273
Post, Robert M., 231
Pottash, A. C., 9–10

Premack, D., 143, 150
President's Commission on Mental Health, 300
Principles of Behavior Modification (Bandura), 138
private hospitals, 3–21, 40, 92, 93, 260, 269, 353, 387
  ability to pay in, 4, 7, 9
  accreditation of, 9, 13
  administration of, 12
  admissions process in, 14, 17
  boards of trustees of, 11
  chief executive officers of, 11–12
  children and adolescents in, 9, 17, 19
  confidentiality guarantees in, 16, 18
  court-ordered patients in, 280–81
  diagnostic and treatment process in, 14–16
  discharge planning in, 15–16, 19
  distinguishing features of, 8–11
  economic influences on, 7–8
  evaluation in, 14, 15
  families and, 16
  for-profit (investor-owned) chains of, 7, 11, 19
  free-standing status of, 10, 20
  future of, 18–20
  geriatric patients in, 9, 16
  history of, 3–8
  humanism vs. economics in, 8
  insurance and, 6–8, 13, 18, 19
  involuntary commitment in, 17
  length of stay in, 10–11, 15, 18–19
  marketing strategies of, 8
  medical directors of, 12–13
  medically ill patients in, 10
  medical records in, 13, 18
  medical staffs of, 13
  moral treatment concept in, 3, 9, 18
  organizational structure of, 11–13
  outcome studies of, 18–20
  patient population of, 7, 14
  patient prognoses and, 14
  patient/staff relationships in, 17
  primary treatment modalities in, 15
  quality assurance in, 13
  regulation of, 7–8, 9, 18
  reputations of, 8
  research in, 5, 9–10
  right to treatment lawsuits and, 281
  sizes of, 10
  special issues in, 16–18
  specialized services offered by, 8–9
  staffing of, 10
  state hospitals vs., 6, 8, 9
  training programs in, 9–10
  treatment planning in, 14–15

private hospitals (*continued*)
  voluntary (not-for-profit), 7, 20
privileged communication, 286-87
Professional Standards Review Organizations (PSROs), 253-54
prolonged exposure therapy, 137, 146
proprietary hospitals, *see* private hospitals
Prosen, Melvin, 129-35
prospective pricing systems, 267-69
protective aggression devices (PADs), 174
Psychiatric Halfway House—A Handbook of Theory and Practice, The (Budson), 386
psychiatric institutes, 26
psychiatrists, 31-32, 33, 216, 228, 233-34, 281
  cognitive behavior therapy and, 164
  commitment hearings and, 275-77
  expert witnesses and, 49, 53, 54
  forensic, 4, 68, 281, 289
  practice models and, 13, 31, 44, 45, 217
  violent assaults on, 298
psychoanalysis, 5, 15, 167
psychodrama, 197
psychoeducation, 120-21, 212, 215, 361-62
psychologists, 32, 68, 136, 163-64, 216, 233
psychopharmacology, inpatient, 6, 15, 24, 29, 32, 63, 76, 169-78, 255, 282, 285, 354
  affective disorders and, 165, 169, 171, 172, 174-75, 176, 379-80
  affective states and, 171-72
  children and adolescents and, 172, 176-77, 316
  chronic mentally ill and, 357-58, 360
  cognitive behavior therapy and, 164-65
  compliance in, 45, 120, 169-70, 212, 215, 377
  diagnostic clarification and, 170
  discharge planning and, 176, 374, 379
  dosages in, 174
  drug-free periods in, 173
  drug reactions in, 173
  excessive use of, 174
  family pathology and, 175-76
  geriatric treatment and, 169, 175, 177, 324-26
  nurses and, 210, 215
  premature discharges and, 176
  residential aftercare and, 389, 390
  staff conflicts in, 177-78
  substance abuse and, 177
  target symptoms in, 170-71
  training patients in use of, 176-77
  violence and, 173, 298
psychosurgery, 255, 282
psychotherapy, inpatient, 15, 63, 129-35, 165, 166, 168, 339
  aggression management in, 133-34

children and adolescents and, 301, 313-15
chronic mentally ill and, 360-61
confrontation in, 131-32
discharge planning and, 373-74
geriatric treatment and, 326-27
group influences in, 132-33
insight in, 134
public nature of, 129, 132
reactions to hospitalization in, 129-30
supportive therapy in, 132-33
therapist's experience level in, 130-31
transference in, 131, 132
Public Health Service, 353
public hospitals, 22-38, 39, 92, 93, 258, 269, 282, 334, 387
  accreditation of, 32, 34
  acute illness in, 30
  administration of, 26-27, 34
  admissions process in, 29
  alcoholism in, 30
  asylum function of, 25, 35
  characteristics of, 23-26
  chronic mentally ill in, 30, 35
  civil service system in, 27
  clinical care in, 29-32
  community mental health movement and, 22, 23, 33, 34
  cost of care in, 28-29
  custodial role of, 24, 25
  deinstitutionalization and, 29, 30-31
  detention and seclusion function of, 24, 25, 35
  economic benefits of, 26
  functions of, 24-26
  funding of, 24, 27, 28-29
  future of, 24, 34-36
  geriatric treatment in, 30-31, 35
  governance of, 23
  leadership in, 27, 34
  length of stay in, 25, 30
  locations of, 23
  malpractice litigation and, 34
  milieu therapy in, 24-25, 29
  numbers of, 24
  operations of, 26-29
  patient population of, 29-30, 33
  patient types in, 30-31
  pros and cons of working in, 32-34
  referral patterns in, 29
  regulation of, 28-29
  research in, 25, 26
  social undesirables and, 24, 25, 35
  staffing of, 31-32
  substance abuse in, 30
  training programs in, 25-26, 33
  treatment in, 24-25

Index

quality assurance, 13, 255-58, 268
quiet rooms, 160, 317-18

Rabkin, J. G., 355, 357
Rachlin, Stephen, 282
rapid titration dosage technique, 174
Rappeport, Jonas R., 271-90
rational emotive therapy, 138
Ray, Isaac, 4
recreation therapy, 198-99
Redl, F., 302
regression at discharge, 321, 382
regulation, governmental, 9, 13, 251-70
  accountability and, 137, 251
  current approaches to, 253-55
  documentation in, 13, 253, 254
  enforced treatment in, 283-84
  forensic hospitals and, 49, 63, 67
  future of, 269-70
  patients' rights in, see patients' rights
  peer review in, 13, 254-55, 256, 261, 265
  private hospitals and, 7-8, 9, 18
  privileged communication statutes in, 286-87
  prospective pricing systems in, 267-69
  public hospitals and, 28-29
  quality assurance in, 13, 255-58, 268
  residential aftercare and, 384-86
  restraint and seclusion in, 285
  safety standards and, 252, 253
  staff and, 252-53, 268
  suicide and, 292
  treatment mandating by, 266
  utilization review in, 251-55, 258, 259, 264, 268
  work therapy and, 200
Reid, W. H., 218
reinforcer identification, 143-44
research units, inpatient psychiatric, 5, 9-10, 24, 25, 26, 40, 228-50
  architecture of, 236-38
  biological vs. psychodynamic approaches in, 231, 234, 248
  clinical considerations in, 238-40
  drug-free periods in, 238-40, 246
  ethical considerations in, 238-40, 244
  families and, 241, 243
  hospital community perceptions of, 248-49
  informed consent in, 240-44
  institutional support of, 236-37
  involuntary patients in, 244
  milieu in, 235, 237, 240, 245-48
  motivations to conduct research and, 229-33
  nurses in, 234-35, 239, 246
  practical considerations in, 238-40

  prerequisites for, 233-38
  professional staff in, 230-31, 233-35, 237, 246, 248
  skewed samples in, 236
  study controls in, 238-39
  subjects in, 235-36
  suitable studies for, 229
residential aftercare, 16, 19, 29, 55, 128, 206, 368, 375, 284-402
  age grouping in, 384
  board-and-care homes in, 368, 375, 388
  clinical care in, 398-400
  clinical conditions warranting referral to, 391-92
  clinical programs in, 399-400
  cooperative apartments in, 387-88, 389, 396-97
  costs of, 388, 397-98
  crisis management in, 400
  diagnostic grouping in, 384, 389-91
  establishment of, 384
  evaluation in, 389-90, 398-400
  families and, 389, 400
  foster care in, 388
  funding of, 384-86
  goals of, 389
  history of, 386
  leaving from, 400
  legal issues in, 384-86
  L-facilities in, 368
  long-term group residences in, 387, 389, 397
  patient contracts in, 385-86
  psychopharmacology and, 389, 390
  regulation of, 384-86
  relapse and, 389, 390, 392
  residence types in, 386-91, 394-97
  total rural environments in, 388
  transitional halfway houses in, 375, 387, 389, 394-96
  unique features of, 393-94
response prevention therapy, 137, 146
restraints, physical, 46-47, 58, 61, 65, 74, 75-76, 174, 218, 295, 296, 317-18
  patients' rights and, 271, 285
Retreat (England), 386
retrospective review, 261
Richards, Linda, 208
Riessman, C. K., 355, 357
right to refuse treatment, patients', 17, 64, 271, 282-85, 350
right to treatment, patients', 17, 271, 281-82
risk/benefit notes, 278
risk management, hospital, 289
Rogers, Carl, 161
Rogers v. Commissioner, 282
Rorschach Test, 310

Ross, Donald, 129-35
Rovner, Barry W., 322-33
Rudnick, Barry, 88-95

safety standards, hospital, 252, 253
Saidel, Donald H., 300-321
Sarles, Richard M., 300-321
schizophrenia, 5, 6, 18-19, 80, 126, 272
  activity therapies and, 192-93, 203-5
  cognitive behavior therapy and, 149-55
  residential aftercare and, 389
  suicide and, 292
Schizophrenia Bulletin, 352n
Schwartz, D. A., 292
Schwartz, M. S., 8, 110-11
Science, 232
seclusion rooms, 74, 173-74, 216, 218, 237, 298, 317-18
  patients' rights and, 271, 285
security, hospital, 57-60, 63, 64, 79
sequential parenteral dosages, 174
sheet packs, sedative cold wet, 246-47, 248, 317-18
Sheppard and Enoch Pratt Hospital, 4, 5, 180, 237, 248-49, 252
Silver, Stuart B., 48-69
Skinner, B. F., 137, 138
Slaby, Andrew, 73-87
Slagle, Eleanor Clarke, 180
Slovenko, R., 50
snow phenomenon, 173
social breakdown syndrome, 136
social rehabilitation, 113-14, 147, 358, 362, 363, 364, 366
social workers, 32, 41, 68, 164, 216, 233, 331, 388
Soloff, P., 298
Solomon, Ari, 73n
Solomon, H. C., 137
Solomon, P., 89
Soteria House, 19
Southwest Denver Program, 365
special observation, of patients, 122, 222, 292
Spitzer, R. L., 18, 355
Spivak, M., 331
Spring Lake Ranch, 388
Stanton, A. H., 8, 110-11
State Cost Review Commissions for Hospitals, 9
state hospitals, 4, 6, 8, 9, 39, 200, 206, 241, 280, 354, 355
  see also public hospitals
Stein, E. M., 16
Steinglass, P., 89
Strauss, J. S., 231
Struening, E. L., 355, 357

substance abuse, 6, 9, 17, 30, 80, 106, 126, 177, 215-16, 259, 272, 378, 390-91
suicide, 79-80, 91, 288, 289, 291-96, 390
  affective disorders and, 292, 293-94, 380
  forensic issue of, 291, 292
  geriatric treatment and, 323-24
  medically ill patients and, 337
  medical records and, 292
  nurses and, 219, 292, 293
  staff denial of, 292
  staff risk-taking and, 293
  sublethal self-destructive behaviors in, 294-96
Sullivan, Harry Stack, 5
Summers, W. K., 343
Supplemental Security Income (SSI), 354, 385
Supreme Court, U.S., 50, 67
Sweeney, D., 9-10
Symptom Checklist 90, 141
symptom substitution, 165-66
systematic desensitization, 145-46

Talbott, John A., 33, 36, 352-70
Tarasoff, Tatiana, 287
Tarasoff v. Regents, 79, 287-88
tardive dyskinesia (TD), 239, 285
Tatum, E., 364
teaching hospitals, *see* training programs, psychiatric
Thematic Apperception Test (TAT), 308
therapeutic environment, *see* milieu therapy
therapeutic self-instruction, 148
third-party payers, *see* insurance, health care
three-day notices, 90, 272, 380-81
"Titicut Follies" (Wiseman), 50
token economy, 128, 136, 137, 143, 147, 148, 152, 237, 354
total rural environments, 388
Toward Quality in Nursing (U.S. Public Health Service), 210
Training in Community Living Program, 365
training programs, psychiatric, 9-10, 19-20, 24, 25-26, 33, 40, 41, 128, 232, 249, 268
transfers, patient, 30-31, 93-94, 295, 297-98, 339-41, 381
transinstitutionalism, 30-31
transitional halfway houses, 375, 387, 389, 394-96
triage, 77, 85
Tucker, G. J., 15
Tudor, G. A., 209
Tuke, Samuel, 3, 386
Tupin, Joe P., 169-78

unconditional positive regard, 161
University of Maryland Hospital, 40

Utica State Hospital, 50
utilization review, 251–55, 258, 259, 264, 268

Van Rybroek, G. J., 174
Vaughn, C. E., 389
Veno, A., 295
Vera, M. I., 89
Veterans Administration (VA), hospitals of, 6, 46, 353, 388
  see also public hospitals
violence, inpatient, 46, 91, 218, 234, 288, 291, 292, 295–98
  administrative discharges and, 381–82
  assaults on staff in, 272, 298
  emergency rooms and, 74–75, 77, 83
  forensic hospitals and, 64–65, 292
  forensic issue of, 272, 273, 275, 279, 291
  management of, 112, 133–34, 291, 296–98, 317–18
  patient transfers after, 295, 297–98
  psychopharmacology and, 173, 298
  snow phenomenon in, 173
  staff denial of, 291
  see also dangerousness, patient

vocational rehabilitation, 199–201, 362–63, 364–65
voluntary hospitalization, 14, 17, 93, 271–72, 283
Voluntary Hospitals of America (VHA), 19–20, 25–26

Wadeson, H., 173
Ward Atmosphere Scale, 127
Webb, William L., Jr., 3–21
Weinman, J., 143
Wilson, A., 15
Wineman, D., 302
Wing, J. K., 368, 389
Wiseman, Frederick, 50
"With Liberty and Psychosis for All" (Rachlin), 282
Wolpe, Joseph, 137
work therapy, 199–201
Wyatt v. Stickney, 25, 281, 282

Young, L. D., 338